AF899722

Bioarchaeology and Social Theory

Series Editor

Debra L. Martin
Professor of Anthropology
University of Nevada, Las Vegas
Las Vegas, NV, USA

More information about this series at http://www.springer.com/series/11976

Lorna Tilley • Alecia A. Schrenk
Editors

New Developments in the Bioarchaeology of Care

Further Case Studies and Expanded Theory

Springer

Editors
Lorna Tilley
School of Archaeology and Anthropology
Australian National University
Canberra, ACT, Australia

Alecia A. Schrenk
Department of Anthropology
University of Nevada, Las Vegas
Las Vegas, NV, USA

Bioarchaeology and Social Theory
ISBN 978-3-319-39900-3 ISBN 978-3-319-39901-0 (eBook)
DOI 10.1007/978-3-319-39901-0

Library of Congress Control Number: 2016947724

© Springer International Publishing Switzerland 2017
This work is subject to copyright. All rights are reserved by the Publisher, whether the whole or part of the material is concerned, specifically the rights of translation, reprinting, reuse of illustrations, recitation, broadcasting, reproduction on microfilms or in any other physical way, and transmission or information storage and retrieval, electronic adaptation, computer software, or by similar or dissimilar methodology now known or hereafter developed.
The use of general descriptive names, registered names, trademarks, service marks, etc. in this publication does not imply, even in the absence of a specific statement, that such names are exempt from the relevant protective laws and regulations and therefore free for general use.
The publisher, the authors and the editors are safe to assume that the advice and information in this book are believed to be true and accurate at the date of publication. Neither the publisher nor the authors or the editors give a warranty, express or implied, with respect to the material contained herein or for any errors or omissions that may have been made.

Printed on acid-free paper

This Springer imprint is published by Springer Nature
The registered company is Springer International Publishing AG Switzerland

We dedicate this book to Tony Cameron, partner of Lorna Tilley, and David Beane, fiancé of Alecia A. Schrenk.

Foreword

This collection of case studies represents a companion volume to Lorna Tilley's *Theory and Practice in the Bioarchaeology of Care* (2015) published in this same series, *Bioarchaeology and Social Theory*. The one-two punch of these volumes cements the future of this paradigm-shifting approach in bioarchaeology. The continued working of the theoretical underpinning for approaching the notion of caregiving in communities from both the deep past and more historical yesteryears provides a wealth of caveats, approaches, suggestions and confirmations of what can be learned by asking the twin questions: How did severe ailments affect individuals, and were there caretakers involved? This follow-up volume offers a wholly new paradigm for the identification, careful analysis and interpretation on temporally specific case by case, locality by locality, bases. With the publication of this edited volume, I do not think there will be any question that this theoretical framework and methodological approach is here to stay and that it opens up new avenues of study into the lived experience of individuals in the past.

This volume also tests the rigour that was built into Tilly's online index of care instrument that became available in 2014 (http://indexofcare.org/intro.aspx). These studies demonstrate that the standardization of the approach permits a great deal of flexibility and responsiveness to nuance and circumstance. Most of the chapters here expand upon, evaluate and redesign the approaches using a wide range of case studies both from the ancient as well as the historic periods of time and from locations all over the globe. Some case studies demonstrate the utility of using the index of care, while some of the chapters expand beyond the available empirical data into new theoretical and applied areas. Most importantly, several chapters explicitly explore the ethical dimensions involved in doing (and not doing) these kinds of critical inquiries into health, healthcare, human caregiving and the resiliency of individuals with severe morbidity burdens.

For example, readers will be able to emphasize with Worne's study (Chap. 4) involving a detailed exploration of an elderly female who survived several traumatic injuries. She recovered while also dealing with a number of age-related degenerative conditions. The mapping of this woman's life history on to the known clinical literature provides a profoundly nuanced and engaged interpretation of the kind of life she lived and some of the suffering she endured. Roberts' study (Chap. 5) walks the reader through a case involving a middle-aged man with leprosy living in medieval England. Here we see the challenges of reconstructing care even with extensive archival and ethnohistoric information.

From susceptible children (Chap. 10) to the vulnerable elderly (Chap. 11), a range of challenges and possibilities are exposed in attempting to move beyond individuals to subgroups at risk within the larger population. Examining the forces and structural nature of the violence that often targets the most vulnerable, these chapters seek to integrate the broader societal institutions within which injuries and debilitations occur. The care for inmates in historic asylums in New York also demonstrates the kinds of societal structures that can be implicated in producing bodies that are debilitated and injured (Chap. 13). In another case study, we see the violence underlying the lack of care given to injured participants in projects mandated by colonial rule (Chap. 12). New approaches by these authors led them to refinements in how the index of care was operationalized and the other kinds of data that were brought to bare on the topic.

In all cases, rigorous science and empirical data underlies these approaches for delineating individuals with severe ailments and the care they may or may not have gotten. The integrated use of multiple methodologies involving ethnohistoric documents, clinical literature, historical sources and elaborated contextual information enriches each study's potential. This collection of studies straddles the literature in palaeopathology and bioarchaeology but goes well beyond the approaches normally recruited to carry out studies. One of the more provocative messages in this volume is that bioarchaeologists and palaeopathologists have a moral duty to interrogate the past using these kinds of integrated methods and encompassing questions. To not do so greatly limits our ability to recognize past people's full humanity.

Debra L. Martin
University of Nevada, Las Vegas
Las Vegas, NV, USA

Acknowledgments

First and foremost, we want to acknowledge the cooperation and hard work of all the authors in this volume. It was well worth it; every chapter meets the challenge of advancing the reach and vision of bioarchaeological research into health-related care provision in the past. All authors responded to our editorial cajolement (and sometimes harassment) with a promptness and generosity of spirit that allowed us to meet deadlines that outsiders initially judged 'impossible' and enabled us to send this volume to print within nine months of the Society for American Archaeology *Building a Bioarchaeology of Care* symposium (April, 2015) at which it was conceived. Our very sincere thanks to each and every one of you.

Others also deserve our gratitude. In particular, we would like to thank Debra Martin, in her role as the editor of the Springer *Bioarchaeology and Social Theory* series, who has been consistently encouraging and supportive. We were also very fortunate in obtaining assistance from a number of experts from areas of bioarchaeology, archaeology, philosophy and communications who acted as 'anonymous reviewers', adding value to many individual chapters and thereby to the volume as a whole. In particular, two reviewers took on the responsibility of reviewing *all* chapters—a Herculean task in the tight timeframe given and one that is greatly appreciated. Our only regret is that, for obvious reasons, we cannot name the reviewers to express our thanks directly.

Many friends and colleagues provided encouragement and support as we put this book together. In this regard, we would particularly like to thank the following (in alphabetical order): David Beane, Tony Cameron, Virginia Esposito and Robyn Longhurst. We would also like thank Teresa Krauss and Hana Nagdimov, of the Springer editorial staff, for their responsiveness and their patience.

All of the above have contributed to the process of constructing a robust and dynamic bioarchaeology of care.

Lorna Tilley
Alecia A. Schrenk

Contents

Contributors

Ronald Beckett, Ph.D. Bioanthropology Research Institute, Quinnipiac University, Hamden, CT, USA

Graduate Faculty, Rush University Medical Center, Chicago, IL, USA

Jelena Bekvalac, B.A. Hons., M.Sc., F.S.A. Centre for Human Bioarchaeology, Museum of London, London, UK

Jo Buckberry, Ph.D. School of Archaeological Sciences, University of Bradford, Bradford, UK

Jane Buikstra, Ph.D. Center for Bioarchaeological Research, Arizona State University, Tempe, AZ, USA

Gerald Conlogue, M.H.S., R.T(R.)(M.R.)(C.T.) Diagnostic Imaging Program, Quinnipiac University, Hamden, CT, USA

Bioanthropology Research Institute, Quinnipiac University, Hamden, CT, USA

Karina Croucher, Ph.D. School of Archaeological Sciences, University of Bradford, Bradford, UK

David Doat, Ph.D. Department of Ethics and Philosophy, Catholic University of Lille, Lille, France

Centre for the Study of Science and Philosophy, University of Namur, Namur, Belgium

Ramon Gonzalez, M.D. Diagnostic Imaging Program, Quinnipiac University, Hamden, CT, USA

Rebecca Gowland, Ph.D. Department of Archaeology, Durham University, Durham, UK

Ryan P. Harrod, Ph.D. Department of Anthropology, University of Alaska Anchorage, Anchorage, AK, USA

Sarah Jolly, M.A. Department of Anthropology, University of Pittsburgh, Pittsburgh, PA, USA

Brenda Koverman, M.B.A., M.S., O.T.R/.L. Rush University Medical Center, Chicago, IL, USA

Tomasz Kozłowski, Ph.D. Department of Anthropology, Nicolaus Copernicus University in Toruń, Toruń, Poland

Kenneth Kramer, M.D. Connecticut Orthopaedic Specialists, Hamden, CT, USA

Danielle Kurin, Ph.D. Department of Anthropology, University of California, Santa Barbara, Santa Barbara, CA, USA

Keith Manchester, D.Sc. (Hon.), M.B.B.S. School of Archaeological Sciences, University of Bradford, Bradford, UK

Debra L. Martin, Ph.D. Department of Anthropology, University of Nevada, Las Vegas, Las Vegas, NV, USA

Magdalena D. Matczak, Ph.D. Department of Anthropology, Nicolaus Copernicus University in Toruń, Toruń, Poland

David Joseph Mennear, M.Sc. Author of web-blog These Bones of Mine, Consultant Bioarchaeologist, Hartlepool, UK

Marco Milella, Ph.D. Department of Anthropology, University of Zurich, Zurich, Switzerland

Kenneth Nystrom, Ph.D. Department of Anthropology, State University of New York at New Paltz, New Paltz, NY, USA

Marc Oxenham, Ph.D. School of Archaeology and Anthropology, Australian National University, Canberra, ACT, Australia

Dario Piombino-Mascali, Ph.D. Department of Cultural Heritage and Sicilian Identity, Palermo, Italy

Charlotte Roberts, B.A., M.A., Ph.D., S.R.N., F.S.A. Department of Archaeology, Durham University, County Durham, UK

Alecia A. Schrenk, M.A. Department of Anthropology, University of Nevada, Las Vegas, Las Vegas, NV, USA

Melinda Sharkey, M.D. Yale University School of Medicine, New Haven, CT, USA

Rebecca Storm, Ph.D. School of Archaeological Sciences, University of Bradford, Bradford, UK

Lorna Tilley, Ph.D. School of Archaeology and Anthropology, Australian National University, Canberra, ACT, Australia

Lori A. Tremblay Critcher, Ph.D. Department of Anthropology, The Ohio State University, Columbus, OH, USA

Mark Viner, F.C.R., M.Sc., H.D.C.R., M.C.S.F.S., S.R.R. Barts and London School of Medicine and Dentistry, Queen Mary University of London, London, UK

Cranfield University Forensic Institute, Swindon, UK

Julie K. Wesp, Ph.D. University of California Institute for Mexico and the US (UC MEXUS), Riverside, CA, USA

Mexico's Consejo Nacional de Ciencia y Tecnología (CONACYT), Mexico City, Mexico

Alyssa Y. Willett Department of Anthropology, University of Alaska Anchorage, Anchorage, AK, USA

Anna Willis, Ph.D. School of Archaeology and Anthropology, Australian National University, Canberra, ACT, Australia

Andrew S. Wilson, Ph.D. School of Archaeological Sciences, University of Bradford, Bradford, UK

Heather Worne, Ph.D. University of Kentucky, Lexington, KY, USA

About the Editors

Alecia A. Schrenk has an M.A. in bioarchaeology and is currently a Ph.D. student at the University of Nevada, Las Vegas Department of Anthropology. She has co-organized a symposium focusing on the Index of Care and furthering Bioarchaeology of Care methodology at the Society for American Archaeology 2015 Annual Meeting. She has recently published research on an 18–20-year-old female with paraplegia from Bronze Age Tell Abraq, using isotopic analysis to give a perspective on the role that immigration and mobility may have on increased risk of disease and healthcare ("Differential diagnosis of a progressive neuromuscular disorder using bioarchaeological and biogeochemical evidence from a bronze age skeleton in the UAE"). Her research interests include palaeopathology, bioarchaeology of care, the Index of Care, subadult health and mortuary practices.

Lorna Tilley came to archaeology with an honours degree in psychology and work experience in areas of health practice, health status and health outcomes assessment and health policy development. She was awarded a graduate diploma in archaeology from the Australian National University in 2006 and a Ph.D. from the same institution in 2013. She has been sole or primary author of several articles on the bioarchaeology of care approach; the first of these (Tilley & Oxenham, 2011) was awarded *Most Influential Paper (2011–2015)* by the *International Journal of Paleopathology* in April 2015. Her book *Theory and Practice in the Bioarchaeology of Care* (based on her Ph.D. dissertation) was published by Springer in September 2015.

Chapter 1
Introduction: New Developments in the Bioarchaeology of Care

Lorna Tilley and Alecia A. Schrenk

> *Health is among the most important conditions of human life, and a critically significant constituent of human capabilities which we have reason to value.*
>
> *(Sen, 2002, p. 660).*
>
> *[O]ur response to the health needs of others embodies a wealth of information about ourselves and our community ... It follows from this that where healthcare practice can be identified in the archaeological record it has the potential to provide important – and possibly unique – insights into the lives of those under study.*
>
> *(Tilley, 2012, p. 39)*

The experience of serious illness or injury can have far-reaching consequences for both the individual and the community. At a personal level, disease impacts may range from temporary discomfort through to a permanent disability affecting any or all aspects of an individual's life, including perception of self and the nature of relationships with others, the ability to participate in society in a way that is fulfilling and, in the worst case scenario, the capacity to manage basic tasks necessary for day-to-day independent living. At a population level, the effects of disease may be measured in increased rates of morbidity and mortality and reductions in average lifespan, with repercussions for political stability, economic performance, cultural activity, social practice and social relations.

Given the ubiquity of disease throughout human existence, and the potential contribution that knowledge of the way disease operated in the past can make to our understanding of the way it operates in the present, it is easy to understand why the study of pathology is a popular focus for archaeologists and anthropologists. Within this focus on disease in the past, however, palaeopathology has concentrated on

L. Tilley, Ph.D. (✉)
School of Archaeology and Anthropology, Australian National University, Canberra, ACT, Australia
e-mail: lorna.tilley@anu.edu.au

A.A. Schrenk, M.A.
Department of Anthropology, University of Nevada, Las Vegas, Las Vegas, NV, USA

© Springer International Publishing Switzerland 2017

L. Tilley, A.A. Schrenk (eds.), *New Developments in the Bioarchaeology of Care*, Bioarchaeology and Social Theory, DOI 10.1007/978-3-319-39901-0_1

increasingly technical description and diagnosis. It has stopped short of considering one integral behavioural component of the 'health and disease' equation – the provision of care to those suffering the impacts of pathology.

Putting this another way, palaeopathology has overlooked the distinctively *human* response to the presence of disease that is as equally ubiquitous throughout history, and as equally relevant for modern times, as the presence of disease itself. It is a truism that at some stage during our lives almost every one of us will experience the need for health-related care; many of us will require such care on more than one occasion, and some of us will require extensive, long term or recurrent care provision (IHME, 2016; World Health Organization, 2004). Health-related care provision, whether by family, friends, neighbours or within a more formal health-care system, is critical to the way societies operate today, and it is very unlikely to have been different in the past. Yet it is only in the last five years that this subject has started to gain acceptance as a legitimate topic for archaeological research. Previously, some reports had contained occasional observations to the effect that evidence for survival, found in conjunction with evidence for severe pathology, indicated that an individual had likely received care – but this was never the main point of the corresponding study and, ironically, more effort overall may have been dedicated to arguing that neither the experience of disability, nor the provision of care, is accessible through the archaeological record (this observation is discussed in more detail in Chap. 2).

Work in bioarchaeology is now breaking down past paradigms of what is possible, making the identification and interpretation of past caregiving the centre of research effort, and using an evolving approach – the bioarchaeology of care – that is both responsive and rigorous to achieve this. In its broadest sense, the bioarchaeology of care refers to the process of analysing human remains, within, and with continual reference to, the parameters of the corresponding lifeways context, for the purpose of identifying and interpreting the experience of disability and of any associated health-related caregiving. Because the willingness to give care, and the nature of the care given, is a product of the cultural, social, economic and physical environments in which this behaviour occurs, bioarchaeology of care theory argues that analysing the characteristics of caregiving may provide a route into past communities and cultures, group and individual (caregiver and care-recipient) identities, unattainable through other means. The first bioarchaeology of care study was published in 2011 (Tilley & Oxenham, 2011). It was followed in early 2014 by the Index of Care, an online instrument developed to support the bioarchaeology of care methodology (Tilley & Cameron, 2014), and in 2015 by *Theory and Practice in the Bioarchaeology of Care* (Tilley, 2015), a book which details the foundations, development and application of the bioarchaeology of care approach and which is part history, part theoretical argument, and part 'user-manual'.

This present volume, New Developments in the Bioarchaeology of Care: Further Case Studies and Extended Theory, is a major milestone in bioarchaeology of care research. Its genesis lies in a symposium titled Building a Bioarchaeology of Care, which took place during the 2015 annual meeting of the Society for American Archaeology and which united an international and cross-disciplinary cast of scholars (from the USA, Europe and Australia) in applying their experience, perspective, style and expertise to considering health-related care provision in the past. Including the Introduction, there are 19 chapters in this book: fifteen represent expanded versions of symposium presentations, and three (Chaps. 5, 7 and 11) are invited contributions from researchers unable to participate in this session. Chapter 2 provides a summary of the bioarchaeology of care approach up to the time of the symposium, and Chapter 19 draws out the significance for bioarchaeology of care development of the chapters that make up the body of the book. These latter - Chapters 3-18 - reveal the potential scope of a research focus on past care provision. They include case studies of care that date (variously) to prehistoric, precolonial and historic periods; novel applications of the bioarchaeology of care methodology; new directions for bioarchaeology of care theory; cross-disciplinary approaches to bioarchaeology of care analysis; and examination of the philosophical basis for, and ethical imperatives of, research into past care provision. Together, these chapters investigate, evaluate, refine and redesign concepts and practices in this new field of research.

To provide orientation for the reader, the 'core' 16 chapters are organised under three headings: (1) *Case studies: applying and adapting the bioarchaeology of care methodology;* (2) *New directions for bioarchaeology of care research* and (3) *Ethics and accountability in the bioarchaeology of care.* However, to some extent chapter allocation is arbitrary. For example, all '*Case study*' chapters raise (different) issues with implications for aspects of method and/or theory; some of the case studies incorporate the type of '*New directions*' envisioned under the second heading, and others touch on concerns belonging under the third heading. Case studies are grouped together on the basis that they are primarily focused on the experience of a single individual, but it would be a mistake to ignore the broader considerations they raise. Similarly, some of the chapters in the '*New directions*' section use case study material to illustrate their arguments, which, if expanded, might place them under the '*Case studies*' heading, and others hint at issues of ethical concern that might, with some enhancement, see them fall into the '*Ethics and accountability*' category.

This Procrustean dilemma – the problem of slotting individual chapters into neatly bounded repositories – most likely arises because caregiving is one of the most integrated, complex and multifaceted of human behaviours. It is impossible to restrict research to an exclusive focus on one particular question, and even if this *were* possible, the answer would probably make little sense. This dilemma may, in part, also reflect the fact that bioarchaeological research into health-related care provision is such a recent undertaking that it lacks a substantial body of work to which reference can be made and, like explorers entering new territory, the authors in this volume have cast their nets wide.

New Developments in the Bioarchaeology of Care: The Chapters

Chapter 2, by Lorna Tilley, provides background for the chapters that follow. It is the first substantive chapter, but it is primarily intended for readers coming to bioarchaeology of care analysis for the first time. Using examples from earlier research, it recapitulates the bioarchaeology of care approach and the role and content of the Index of Care; discusses the principles, scope and limitations of the bioarchaeology of care methodology; and briefly considers the relevance of research into past caregiving to modern public debate.

Case Studies: Applying and Adapting the Bioarchaeology of Care Methodology

In the first case study, Alecia A. Schrenk and Debra Martin (Chap. 3) apply the Index of Care to the remains of a severely disabled young woman from a Bronze Age site in the United Arab Emirates. Differential diagnosis suggests two equally likely candidates for explaining indicators of pathology – one a congenital and the other an acquired disease. Both conditions could have resulted in broadly similar functional impacts by time of death, but age of onset and initial symptomatology would have been very different, and therefore features of the care provided, and possibly the attitudes towards caregiving, may have varied significantly. Uncertainty in diagnosis is common in palaeopathology, and research into past caregiving will often have to work around this problem. The authors offer one approach for dealing with this quandary.

Both the second and third case studies apply the Index of Care to the remains of a (different) woman displaying serious pelvic injury, in addition to other traumatic and degenerative pathologies, recovered from sites in the late pre-contact period southern US (New Mexico and Tennessee, respectively). Alyssa Willett and Ryan Harrod (Chap. 4) consider the case of a young female who suffered extensive trauma (likely as the result of violence) that permanently limited her mobility and compromised participation in traditional work-related and cultural activities. Concluding that their subject received support along a continuum from emergency care to rehabilitation, they use ethnographic data to discuss care options. Heather Worne (Chap. 5) examines the case of an older woman, who survived multiple, activity-limiting, traumatic injuries which would have necessitated care and whose recovery was likely complicated by age-associated degenerative factors. Worne examines the implications of deliberate versus accidental cause of injury for interpreting care provision in the context of the role and status of older females in the subject's community.

This description makes the two studies appear very similar, but nothing is further from the truth. Because the subjects are different women, from different lifeways, it is inevitable that the experience of each will also be different. While both studies situate their subjects within their corresponding lifeways, and both emphasise the use of clinical information in estimating disability impact, the approaches taken to analysis and the interpretations of the results of this analysis are quite distinct. A bioarchaeology of care approach demands much more than quantitative description, and all researchers will bring their own personal perspectives, interests and goals to their work; these two case studies illustrate the richness that can result from this.

Chapters 6, 7 and 8 move bioarchaeology of care research into the historic period, allowing use of documentary sources to help inform understanding of the context of caregiving. In Chap. 6, Charlotte Roberts applies the Index of Care to the case of a middle-aged man from late Mediaeval England diagnosed with lepromatous leprosy. Roberts is cautious about the extent to which it is possible to assess disability and consequent need for care on the basis of skeletal lesions alone, emphasising the importance of remembering that individuals respond *individually* to the experience of disease and that therefore only the minimum effects of any disease can ever be assumed. This study demonstrates that, although there can be no 'one size fits all' answer in a bioarchaeology of care analysis, discussion of likely disease impact and possible care provided can be both nuanced and convincing.

In Chap. 7, Magdalena Matczak and Tomasz Kozłowski present two subjects from different sites in Mediaeval Poland. Both are adult females, one diagnosed with lepromatous leprosy and the other with gigantism, and both had also sustained and recovered from moderately serious traumatic injury(ies) some time prior to death. The authors develop a detailed osteobiography for each subject. They then use the evidence of each woman's mortuary treatment, combined with consideration of what this may suggest about the social status of the subject and/or perceptions of her disabled state, to reflect upon both the nature of possible care provided and the contemporary understandings of disease.

Gerald Conlogue, Mark Viner, Ronald Beckett, Jelena Bekvalac, Ramon Gonzalez, Melinda Sharkey, Kenneth Kramer and Brenda Koverman (Chap. 8) apply the Index of Care in analysing the remains of a mature adult male that date to late eighteenth to early nineteenth century London and which display evidence of severe spinal deformity and other physical anomalies. This collaboration includes specialists in imaging, medicine, bioarchaeology, forensics and orthopaedics. The team's combination of expertise has produced an historically and socially contextualised analysis of disease and its likely impact on function that is rich in content and meticulous in detail, and which illustrates the power of a multidisciplinary approach in researching past care provision.

In the final chapter of this section Sarah Jolley and Danielle Kurin (Chap. 9) present the likely experience of a young male from the conflict-ridden Late Intermediate Period in Peru, whose remains display multiple healed trepanations as well as evidence for survival following severe postcranial trauma. As part of their case study, the authors provide a comprehensive overview of the physical and behavioural implications of traumatic brain injury, trepanation surgery and post-surgical rehabilitation. They also use their description of the contemporary social and political lifeways as a platform for considering the way that 'care' might be conceptualised (and its motivations understood) within a context of organised violence.

New Directions for Bioarchaeology of Care Research

To date, bioarchaeology of care analyses have relied exclusively on skeletal evidence in identifying likely candidates for receipt of care. Ken Nystrom and Dario Piombino-Mascali (Chap. 10) make a commanding case for extending the bioarchaeology of care approach to mummified remains. The number of pathologies that manifest in bone is limited. Evidence from preserved soft tissue offers the prospect of being able to identify a much wider range of disease conditions likely to have required care and, in some cases, even the opportunity to identify traces of the actual treatment provided – such as evidence for consumption of substances with known medicinal properties, use of therapeutic topical applications, or tattooing in locations associated with disease symptom manifestation. In brief, this chapter provides the groundwork for a promising new area of bioarchaeology of care research.

Chapters 11 and 12 argue the benefits of focusing bioarchaeological research into disability and care on specific sectors of the population – albeit those from opposite ends of the demographic spectrum. Focusing on the experience of children, Marc Oxenham and Anna Willis (Chap. 11) discuss the complex question of distinguishing between 'normal' altricial care and specifically *health*-related care, particularly in infancy and early childhood. The authors ask whether, in the situations of elevated child morbidity and mortality often characterising prehistoric communities, the bioarchaeology of care model could be used to explore provision of care to children at a population level, and they employ data from the Vietnamese Neolithic community of Man Bac and other contemporary east Asian sites to assess the feasibility of doing this.

In a theory-driven chapter, Rebecca Gowland (Chap. 12) identifies another specific population likely to reward a dedicated bioarchaeology of care focus – the elderly, an often neglected group in archaeology, which, when thought about at all, is often thought of as in need of 'special' care by virtue of the frailty we often automatically associate with old age. The author discusses concerns commonly linked to the health, safety, disability and care of the elderly (highlighting the elderly's vulnerability, past and present, to neglect and abuse). She also addresses the issue of power dynamics between care-recipient and caregiver, especially relevant to the experience of the elderly who may end up being looked after by family members over whom they once had authority. Central to her thesis, Gowland argues that, for elderly subjects in particular, a life course perspective is essential for understanding the interplay between impairment and identity.

Julie Wesp engages with one of the most problematic concerns in reconstructing care practice based predominantly on physical evidence from human remains. Where disease impact can be estimated in terms of bodily dysfunction, then identification of broad parameters of the care required can be defended. However, psychological, emotional and spiritual forms of caregiving, invisible in the archaeological record, may be equally essential for the individual concerned. In Chap. 13, the author demonstrates how (bio)archaeology might be able to identify these intangible aspects of care, situating discussion in the period when Christian institutions responsible for providing both medical *and* spiritual care were being established in the early post-contact Americas. Wesp refers to skeletal remains from the first hospital established in Mexico for the treatment of the indigenous population, as well as historical sources, to discuss physical and religious care provision, and the way this may have been perceived and *re*ceived by patients.

Most bioarchaeology of care research to date has concentrated on identifying need for care, the detail of the probable care provided, and the broader social implications of this care. In Chap. 14, Lori Tremblay Critcher describes a modified version of the bioarchaeology of care model that she developed with the aim of assessing, at both individual and population levels, the *efficacy* of the care received by the inmates of historic period institutions providing long term treatment and shelter. She applies the adapted methodology to data collected previously at the Rome State Custodial Asylum (New York), where she analysed the remains of patients making up part of the asylum population in the early decades of the twentieth century. The author discusses the results of the first test of her new approach, reporting on its strengths and weaknesses and identifying areas for future refinement.

Chapter 15 presents an ambitious proposal – the development of a potentially predictive, biocultural model for helping to explain the evolutionary origins and the operation of health-related care behaviours. Employing modern hunter-gatherer social systems as a proxy for early modern human forms of social organisation, Marco Milella uses published data on modern hunter-gatherer group environment, demography, mobility and epidemiology to test relationships between these variables and infant and juvenile mortality rates. He suggests that lower mortality in some circumstances may be an indicator of caring or nurturing practice.

In Chap. 16, Andrew Wilson, Keith Manchester, Jo Buckberry, Rebecca Storm and Karina Croucher describe *Digitised Diseases*, an open access online resource providing three-dimensional images of chronic disease manifestations in bone, with brief text explanations alongside these. A major goal of *Digitised Diseases* is to help achieve a wider understanding of public health in the past through supporting research into the clinical and social implications of the lived experience of disease. One of the particular strengths of this application is its ability to help researchers visualise the effects of disease on bone, which in turn helps in identifying the possible range of a particular pathology's impact on functional capability – making it a valuable practical tool in bioarchaeology of care research.

Ethics and Accountability in the Bioarchaeology of Care

This last section of the book comprises two chapters that ask the reader to think about the intellectual and ethical responsibilities which accompany any research effort touching on aspects of human experience.

In Chap. 17, the philosopher David Doat renders transparent the assumptions, values and beliefs that underlie past objections to the archaeological inference of care, then subjects the bioarchaeology of care methodology to the same systematic scrutiny to test the resilience of the principles on which it is based. The author argues that (bio)archaeologists have a moral *duty* to provide an account of the past that offers a more balanced representation of our ancestors, pointing out that those with disabilities are often written out of the (pre)historic record, and certain 'softer' behaviours, such as caregiving, are overlooked. At the same time, he asserts that it is archaeologists' moral *responsibility* to ensure this account is as accurate as possible.

In Chap. 18, David Mennear, author of a popular bioarchaeological blog, urges bioarchaeology of care researchers to recognise that clear, inclusive, two-way, public communication of research findings is an ethical responsibility. Noting widespread community interest in archaeological research, Mennear points out that information about past experience of disease, disability and care has a particular relevance for many people, and argues that every effort should be made to share acquired knowledge on this subject matter in the public domain. The author offers practical advice on using effective and easily accessed social media, as well traditional media and education outreach strategies, to address the widest possible audience.

Conclusion

In the final chapter, Jane Buikstra (Chap. 19) situates the bioarchaeology of care approach generally, and the contents of this book in particular, within the wider practice of bioarchaeology. There is no-one better placed to do this: it was Buikstra who, 40 years ago, first defined the discipline of bioarchaeology (Buikstra, 1977), and she has since been a leading figure in this new discipline's exponential growth in research output and influence (Rakita, 2014). The author discusses the history and impact of the bioarchaeology of care model and briefly reviews all chapters, concluding that, collectively, these contribute substantially to advancing the bioarchaeology of care methodology.

Common Themes, Shared Concerns, and New Horizons

New Developments in the Bioarchaeology of Care: Further Case Studies and Extended Theory presents the reader with original and wide-ranging content. Chapters are innovative in approach and argument, and they consolidate, add to, and expand upon, existing achievements in bioarchaeology of care research. Many of the authors challenge traditional perceptions of what is possible and what is permissible in archaeological research, either by their choice of subject matter or the way they choose to address it, and this opens the door for exploring an even greater diversity of issues in relation to the giving and receipt of care in the past.

Several themes appear repeatedly across chapters, although sometimes these themes are implicit rather than explicit. A handful of examples are identified below.

The first of these examples is the theme of 'motivation for caregiving'. How do we explain, however imprecisely, *why* people in the past provided health-related care? In many of the cases that are archaeologically visible the support required was costly in terms of effort and emotion, and in at least some of these cases there may have been little prospect for (complete) recovery. All chapters in this book address some aspect of the 'motivation for care' enigma, from the first case study by Schrenk and Martin (Chap. 3), who observe that elements of the motivation for Lesley's care would very likely have differed depending upon whether she experienced a congenital or an acquired disease, to the chapter by Mennear (Chap. 18), which notes an avid public interest in understanding how the willingness to provide care in the past sits with modern practice. Wesp (Chap. 13) discusses the balance between the twin motivations of 'saving the soul' and 'curing the body' that defined the care provided to the indigenous people of Mexico under early Spanish colonial rule; in looking at ways to assess the efficacy of past institutional care Tremblay Critcher (Chap. 14) incorporates the formal goals of an institution (these are arguably a formal expression of 'motivation') in design of evaluation criteria; Oxenham and Willis (Chap. 12) focus on cultural practices – and perforce the social motivations behind these – for the health-related care of infants and children; and in developing a biocultural model for explaining care, Milella (Chap. 15) offers an evolutionary explanation for factors 'motivating' selection of caregiving behaviours. From a different perspective, the accumulation of knowledge and the hands-on skills development reflected in trepanation surgery (Jolly and Kurin, Chap. 9), as well as in traditions of therapeutic tattooing and pharmaceutical remedies (Nystrom and Piombino-Mascali, Chap. 10), also speak to societies' 'motivations' in investing in health-related care for (certain members of) the community.

A second common theme revolves around the 'need for rigour in research' into past caregiving. While all chapters in this volume are, *in practice*, rigorous, some identify the importance of this requirement directly. For example, Doat (Chap. 17) emphasises the responsibility of researchers to be constantly aware of, and account for, the influence of personal values and potential resulting bias in their analyses; Roberts (Chap. 6) and Conlogue et al. (Chap. 8) are explicit in arguing the need for conservatism in assessment of disease impact and interpretation of this impact; and Wilson et al. (Chap. 16) present the online application *Digitised Diseases* as an aid for increased accuracy in visualising disease impact in bioarchaeology of care research.

A third theme is that of 'care in the context of violence'. How do we approach a situation in which the probable caregivers may well have perpetrated the violence causing the injury that required care? Gowland (Chap. 12) discusses this paradox in relation to the elderly as a demographic group, and Willett and Harrod (Chap. 4) and Worne (Chap. 5) identify this as a possible issue in their respective case studies. Wesp (Chap. 13) notes that the indigenous patients cared for in the *Hospital Real San José de los Naturales* likely suffered injuries as a result of enforced participation in dangerous work projects mandated under colonial rule; these patients might be characterised as victims of structural rather than interpersonal violence (Klaus, 2012). In their case study of one individual surviving multiple incidents of trauma, Jolly and Kurin (Chap. 9) broaden discussion to specifically address the intersection between violence and care.

A fourth theme – perhaps a better term might be 'emerging practice' – is the use of ethnographic, ethnohistoric and historic sources of information where these are available. Most of the bioarchaeological studies into past care provision undertaken prior to those featured in this volume have centred on individuals from prehistoric contexts. The chapters by Willett and Harrod (Chap. 4), Worne (Chap. 5), Roberts (Chap. 6), Conlogue et al. (Chap. 8), and in particular those by Matczak and Kozłowski (Chap. 7) and Nystrom and Piombino-Mascali (Chap. 10), demonstrate the valuable contribution that ethnographic and historic materials can make to a bioarchaeology of care analysis, both by helping to elaborate a detailed and convincing context and by enriching the scope of interpretation.

A fifth and final example of a recurrent theme is that of 'using the past to inform the present'. In that this is one of the intrinsic goals of all (bio)archaeological and historical research, once again *all* chapters qualify for mention here. However, some chapters address this concern explicitly. For instance, Mennear (Chap. 18) puts this goal front and centre of his chapter; Doat (Chap. 17) and Gowland (Chap. 12) are almost equally as explicit in promoting this aim; and Roberts (Chap. 6) is unambiguous in drawing links between past and current healthcare philosophy and practice.

This volume is an important resource for all scholars interested in how health and disease are conceptualised, experienced and managed, whatever their discipline and in whatever period of time their interests lie. Together with *Theory and Practice in the Bioarchaeology of Care* (Tilley, 2015), it provides a springboard for future research into past disability and care.

References

Buikstra, J. E. (1977). Biocultural dimensions of archaeological study: A regional perspective. In R. L. Blakely (Ed.), *Biocultural adaptation in prehistoric America* (pp. 67–84). Georgia: University of Georgia Press.

IHME. (2016). Institute for Health Metrics and Evaluation—Global Burden of Disease 2010 Study. Retrieved January 2016, from http://www.healthdata.org/results/research-articles

Klaus, H. D. (2012). Bioarchaeology of structural violence: Theoretical model and case study. In D. L. Martin, R. P. Harrod, & V. R. Pérez (Eds.), *The bioarchaeology of violence* (pp. 29–62). Gainesville: University Press of Florida.

Rakita, G. F. (2014). Bioarchaeology as a process: An examination of bioarchaeological tribes in the USA. In B. O'Donnabhain & M. C. Lozada (Eds.), *Archaeological human remains: Global perspectives* (pp. 213–234). New York: Springer.

Sen, A. (2002). Why health equity? *Health Economics, 11*, 659–666.

Tilley, L. (2012). The bioarchaeology of care. *The Archaeological Record, 12*, 39–41.

Tilley, L. (2015). *Theory and practice in the bioarchaeology of care*. New York: Springer.

Tilley, L., & Cameron, T. (2014). Introducing the Index of Care: A web-based application supporting archaeological research into health-related care. *International Journal of Paleopathology, 6*, 5–9.

Tilley, L., & Oxenham, M. F. (2011). Survival against the odds: Modeling the social implications of care provision to seriously disabled individuals. *International Journal of Paleopathology, 1*, 35–42.

World Health Organization. (2004). *The global burden of disease*. Geneva: World Health Organization.

Chapter 2
Showing That They Cared: An Introduction to Thinking, Theory and Practice in the Bioarchaeology of Care

Lorna Tilley

Introducing the Bioarchaeology of Care Approach

Eleven thousand years ago Romito 2, born with acromesomelic dysplasia (a rare and particularly limiting form of dwarfism), lived to early adulthood in a hunter-gatherer community in the mountains of southern Italy. Seven thousand years later, around 4000BC, Man Bac Burial 9 (M9) survived with juvenile-onset quadriplegia for around a decade while living in a sedentary coastal community in northern Vietnam. These young men came from different social, economic and physical environments, and experienced different challenges, but both required health-related care – albeit very different forms of care – in order to achieve their corresponding age at death (Frayer, Horton, Macchiarelli, & Mussi, 1987; Frayer, Macchiarelli, & Mussi, 1988; Tilley, 2015a, 2015b; Tilley & Oxenham, 2011).

When examining archaeologically recovered remains it is common to discover evidence indicating that an individual experienced one or more episodes of disease – short or long-lasting, congenital or acquired, acute or chronic, resolved or unresolved – during their lifetime. Such findings are unsurprising, given the ubiquity of disease throughout human history. Sometimes, however, this evidence speaks to a lived experience of pathology likely to have seriously compromised an individual's ability to function independently or to participate appropriately within their physical and cultural setting. In such circumstances it is justifiable to infer that, over a period of time, this person received a level of health-related care to assist them in managing the impacts of disease.

Looking after those who are affected by illness or injury is one of the most common of human behaviours. It can also be one of the most complicated, physically

L. Tilley, Ph.D. (✉)
School of Archaeology and Anthropology, Australian National University, Canberra, ACT, Australia
e-mail: lorna.tilley@anu.edu.au

© Springer International Publishing Switzerland 2017
L. Tilley, A.A. Schrenk (eds.), *New Developments in the Bioarchaeology of Care*, Bioarchaeology and Social Theory, DOI 10.1007/978-3-319-39901-0_2

demanding and psychologically stressful. Moreover, the characteristics of the care given (and the willingness to give this care in the first place) reflect not only the motivations and commitment of the carers themselves, but also the values, traditions, experience, knowledge, beliefs, skills, resources, politics, economy and organisation of the society in which care occurs (Hofrichter, 2003; Pol & Thomas, 2001). An instance of caregiving can be envisioned as a narrative with a beginning, which is the onset of the condition that elicits care, a middle, which comprises the activities that make up the care itself, and an end – the point at which, for whatever reason, this care ceases. If an archaeological focus on care practice allows us to read just a portion of this narrative, then it may offer insights into past lifeways that are otherwise inaccessible.

The bioarchaeology of care is an approach developed to tease out the broader implications of health-related care provision. It provides a framework for case study-based research into past care, built on a foundation of theory that combines elements drawn from a range of archaeological sub-disciplines and schools of thought (including post-processualist, social, cognitive and mortuary archaeologies, and palaeopathology), with additional elements borrowed from non-archaeological disciplines relevant to consideration of caregiving behaviours (such as nursing, clinical medicine, philosophy, sociology and psychology) and adapted to the demands and limitations of archaeological – more specifically, ***bio***archaeological – method.

This framework also offers a clearly defined and systematic process for identifying, ordering, analysing and interpreting information. The bioarchaeology of care methodology divides analysis into four stages, each building on the contents of the one(s) preceding it and creating a structure that encourages logic, rigour and transparency. In Stage 1, the researcher assembles information about the individual, their disease and their lifeways; in Stage 2, the researcher examines possible clinical and functional impacts of the individual's disease within the lifeways described in Stage 1, and decides whether an argument for disability requiring care provision can be made; in Stage 3, the researcher develops a model of the care likely provided in response to the impacts posited in Stage 2 and within the lifeways context established in Stage 1; and in Stage 4, the researcher attempts to deconstruct the rationale for the proposed 'model of care' and then reconfigure the components of this reasoning, juxtaposing what is reasonably well established against what has been inferred in seeking to gain a new understanding both of the community providing care and of the person receiving it.

This chapter provides a background for the chapters that follow, introducing some of the thinking behind the early development of the bioarchaeology of care approach and outlining what a bioarchaeology of care analysis entails. It is written from the perspective of research undertaken on skeletal materials from prehistoric contexts, but theory and method are equally relevant to research using preserved soft tissue remains (see Nystrom and Piombino, this volume) and to research using remains from historic periods (see Roberts, Matczak and Kozłowski, Conlogue et al., Wesp, and Critcher, various chapters this volume).

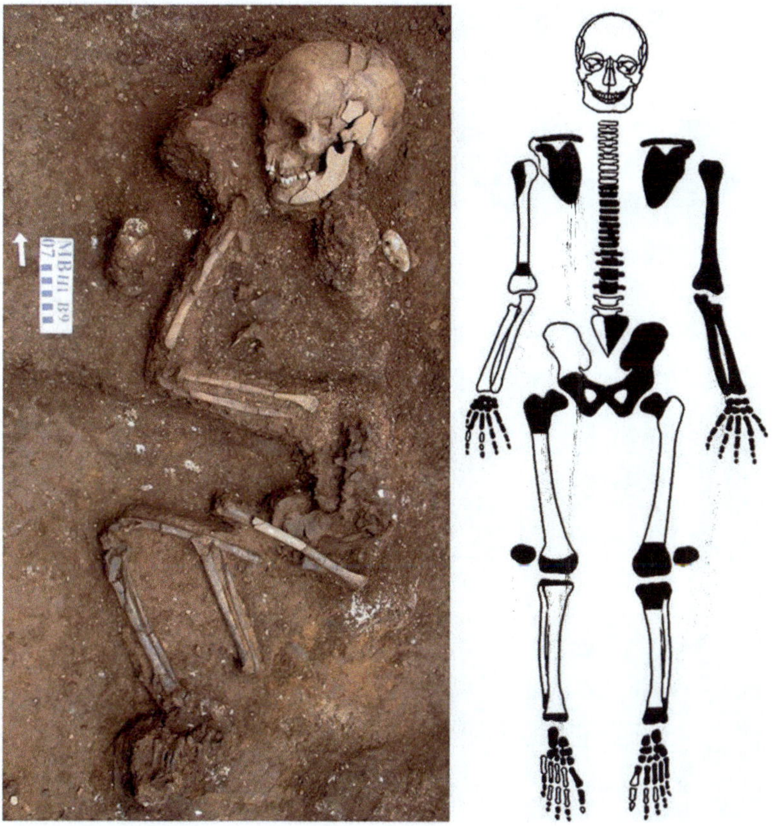

Fig. 2.1 M9 remains in situ (*left*), and schematic summarising M9's skeletal preservation (*right – black* represents missing portions – adapted from Oxenham et al., 2009) (Image by Lorna Tilley)

The remainder of this section of the chapter briefly describes the role and format of the Index of Care, an instrument developed to support application of the bioarchaeology of care methodology. The chapter then proceeds to identify some of the principles and parameters defining the bioarchaeology of care approach, before walking the reader through the four stages of the bioarchaeology of care methodology, using material drawn from the case studies of M9 (Fig. 2.1) (Tilley, 2015a; Tilley & Oxenham, 2011) and Romito 2 (Fig. 2.2) (Tilley, 2015b) to demonstrate how analysis works in practice. (For full details of the bioarchaeology of care approach, including development of the Index of Care, see *Theory and Practice in the Bioarchaeology of Care* – Tilley, 2015a).

The final section of the chapter briefly raises two fundamental philosophical questions arising from a focus on care: how might research into past caregiving behaviours contribute to our knowledge of self and society, and what ethical considerations should be observed when undertaking bioarchaeology of care research?

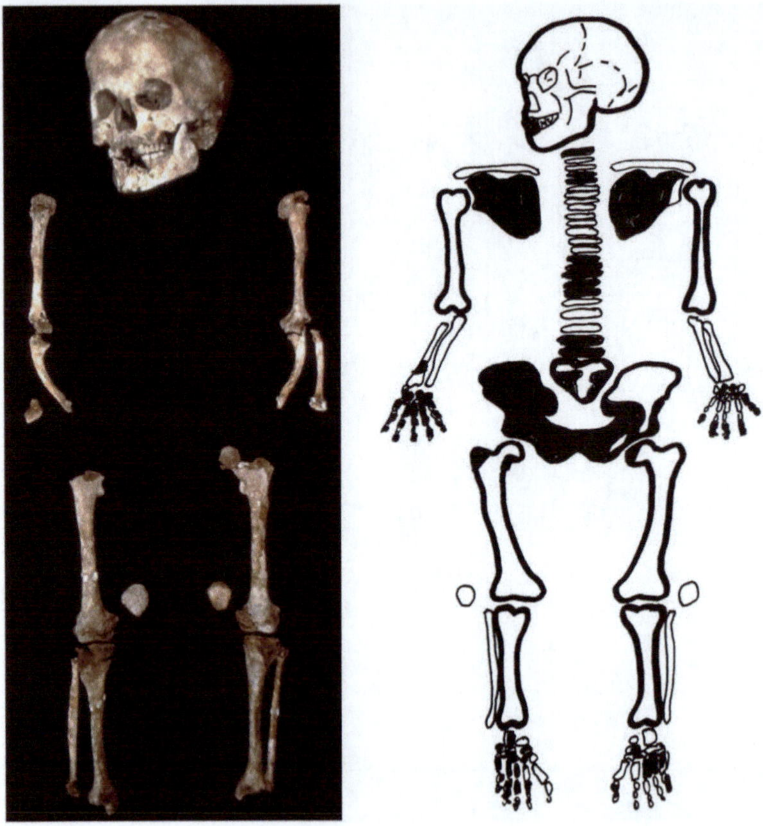

Fig. 2.2 Romito 2 remains (*left*) (image courtesy of David Frayer), and schematic by the author (*right*) summarising skeletal preservation, based on the description of Romito 2 by Mallegni and Fabbri (1995):100, 125–127 – *black* represents missing portions. Frayer et al. (1987, 1988) were unable to access certain elements of Romito 2's remains, explaining the discrepancy between photograph and schematic (Tilley, 2015b). Fragments of 4 right and 6 left ribs were also recovered but are not included in the graphic

The Index of Care

The Index of Care is an instrument designed to help researchers work through a bioarchaeology of care case study, and in form and content it encompasses the theory on which the bioarchaeology of care approach is based (Tilley & Cameron, 2014). It is an open-access, non-prescriptive, web-based application (www.indexofcare.org) divided into four linked modules, or 'Steps', which correspond to the four stages of the bioarchaeology of care methodology; each Step contains a series of worksheets designed to assist in identifying and evaluating information relevant to these stages. (Appendix 1 contains the Index of Care web application workflow diagrams for reader ease of reference.) The Index provides a means of recording information, observations, inferences and conclusions in a systematic manner that facilitates a continuous review of research procedure and its underlying rationale.

The Index of Care can be conceived of as 'operationalising' the bioarchaeology of care methodology, but it is *not* a join-the-dots formula for analysis. Every individual receiving care, and every circumstance in which care is given, are unique, and this is clearly illustrated in the examples of M9 and Romito 2. The evidence considered in deciding on the likely presence of disability requiring care, the likely care given and the likely significance of this care will often be open to competing interpretations. It will be up to the researcher to decide which interpretation is the most plausible and, where interpretation is disputed, to justify the choices made.

The Bioarchaeology of Care: Principles, Definitions, Caveats and Constraints

Principles

The core principle of research into past disability and care is that it is quintessentially bioarchaeological (Buikstra & Beck, 2006). Although the evidence that triggers a bioarchaeology of care analysis is bioanthropological, the full significance of this evidence cannot be realised without continuous reference to, and testing against, what is known about the archaeology – the material culture, social and economic practices, and physical setting – of the time and place in which care occurred. Some basic symptoms of a particular pathology may be biologically determined, but the concepts of 'health' and 'disease' are likely to be defined very differently in different cultures and at different times in history. At both a societal and an individual level, the experience of disability and the detail of the care response will derive much of their form, content and meaning from their context (e.g. Levin & Browner, 2005; Martin & Horowitz, 2003; Scheper-Hughes & Lock, 1987).

The second organising principle in bioarchaeology of care analysis is the acknowledgement of agency as central to all aspects of health-related care behaviours. Care provision typically consists of a sequence of actions taken over a period of time (however brief this period may be), and these actions always involve intent; both those giving care and those benefitting from care act on the basis of choices made and options rejected. Care is not a default response, which is precisely why it provides such a useful window into the past.

While most would concur that care*givers* exercise agency, the proposal that care recipients also exercise agency may be less intuitive. Bioarchaeology of care analysis approaches human remains displaying evidence of disability as representing both 'subject *and* object' or 'actor *and* artefact'. Actor, because these remains represent a once-living person challenged by disability, and artefact, because the disease indicators prompting inference of disability exist by virtue of that care which allowed the person to survive, minimally for the time taken for these disease indicators to register. But the person receiving care is not passive. Recipients' negotiation of, contribution to, and cooperation with their care is integral to its design and its outcomes.

Definitions

What the concept of disability comprises, and whether we can have confidence in the retrospective identification of disability, are central concerns for bioarchaeology of care analysis. For this reason it is important to define what is meant when talking about 'disability', and to acknowledge the historical debate surrounding use of this term in archaeology.

A quarter of a century ago, Dettwyler (1991) argued that disability cannot be identified in the archaeological record because it is, above all, a *social* phenomenon. Conflating care (behaviour) with compassion (motivation) she critiqued attempts to identify either of these on the basis of archaeological evidence alone, asserting that there can be no justification for

> *drawing conclusions either about the quality of life for disabled individuals in the past or about the motives or attitudes of the rest of the community from skeletal evidence of physical impairment* (Dettwyler, 1991, p. 375).

Dettwyler's (1991) position reflects one of the central tenets of western disability politics in the last decades of the twentieth century – rejection of a medical model of disability in favour of theorising disability as a predominantly sociopolitical creation – and her widely cited article was influential in discouraging (bio)archaeological research into disability and care for almost 20 years (Tilley, 2015a, pp. 43–48; for detailed refutation of Dettwyler's arguments see Doat, Chap. 17 this volume). The view of disability as a wholly social construct is now repudiated by most disability theorists. This stand 'fails to capture the complexity of disabled people's lives' (Shakespeare, 2008, p. 11), and by denying the very real physical or 'medical' impacts of disease it disempowers, and may even belittle, the person who is forced to confront these (Shakespeare, 2006, 2008; Vehmas, 2008), which was, of course, the very opposite of its intention. Disability is now accepted as resulting from a combination of biological, psychological and social factors, and in general this is reflected in present-day social policy, if not always in practice (Bickenbach, Chatterji, Badley, & Üstün, 1999; Shakespeare, 2006; WHO, 2003; 2011a; for further discussion see Doat, Chap. 17 this volume).

The bioarchaeology of care approach follows the World Health Organisation (WHO) in defining disability as a state arising from impairment in body function or structure, associated with activity limitations and/or participation restrictions, and given specific meaning in relation to the context in which disease is experienced (WHO, 2011a, 2011b). This definition establishes disability as produced through interaction between the physical features of pathology and the social and physical environments in which disease is experienced, and is the basis for Stage 2 bioarchaeology of care analysis.

'Health-related care' is defined in bioarchaeology of care research as the delivery of assistance to an individual experiencing short-, medium- or long-term disability arising from pathology. It is conceptualised along a continuum extending from 'direct support', which refers to the more labour-intensive forms of caregiving in circumstances where an individual is mostly or wholly reliant on others, to 'accommodation of difference' – the adoption of strategies that make it easier for someone to take their place in the community when disease renders what is viewed as 'normal' participation difficult or impossible. These forms of care are not mutually exclusive. While accommodation of difference is usually less hands-on than direct support it may be equally necessary for an individual's survival, and a person may require both forms of care either simultaneously or sequentially, in response to the same, or different, diseases. One of the important implications of this 'continuum' definition of care is that the disease experience suggested by skeletal evidence need not have resulted in total disability, nor have been lifelong and/or ultimately fatal, in order to qualify for bioarchaeology of care analysis.

The fine detail of care will always depend upon the nature of disability, features of the lifeways context in which disability occurs and individual care-recipient characteristics. However, as will be discussed in describing Stage 3 analysis, there are certain requirements in those caregiving practices that correspond to the 'direct support' end of the care continuum that are largely independent of contextual factors. Where evidence for survival suggests direct support it may be possible to infer some basic components of this care with a degree of confidence.

Caveats and Constraints

Many of the 'caveats and constraints' encountered in bioarchaeology of care research arise from reliance on osteological and/or dental indicators to identify the presence and nature of disease. Relatively few diseases (other than bone fracture, periodontal pathology and degenerative joint conditions) register in bone, and even those that do have this potential will do so, on average, only 10–20 % of the time (Ortner, 2009, p. 328). In many potentially debilitating diseases the average frequency of skeletal involvement may be even lower – for example, diagnostic markers occur in only 1–5 % of cases of leprosy, syphilis and tuberculosis (Ortner, 2003, pp. 112–115; see Roberts, Chap. 6 this volume, for further discussion in relation to leprosy). Skeletal responses to disease are generally limited in expression. In the absence of a distinctive pattern of response, diagnosis may be difficult or impossible, and the ability to identify a specific disease and/or stage of disease is further compromised when remains are incomplete or poorly preserved – as they so often are (Ortner, 2003; Waldron, 2009). Other than in cases of trauma, skeletal involvement usually occurs in advanced or chronic phases of disease; this means that those who experienced disease, but either recovered or died before bone was affected, cannot be identified from the archaeological record as having experienced pathology (Ortner, 2009; Wood, Milner, Harpending, & Weiss, 1992) – or as having required and received care, for that matter.

Furthermore, every individual responds to disease symptoms, even symptoms of the *same* disease, in their own way, reflecting individual biology, psychology, and personal, social and cultural life experience (Bowling, 2002; Jylhä, 2009; Roberts, Chap. 6 this volume). This variability in individual response means that in a bioarchaeology of care analysis there can be no presumption of an *in*variable relationship between pathology and its consequences for the subject; any impact claimed must be freshly argued in each case.

Finally, and in addition to the points made earlier, archaeology rarely provides us with a representative sample of a population – and this is especially the case when working with remains from prehistoric sites. Any assessment of the burden of disease within a particular community will almost inevitably be broad-brush at best – even under the most favourable conditions.

If we cannot achieve an accurate picture of disease prevalence then it is clearly impossible to estimate the need for care at a population level, but we can be confident that such need existed (see Oxenham and Willis, Chap. 11 this volume). There is evidence for human experience of systemic infection, trauma and congenital disease from Middle Palaeolithic times onwards (e.g. Berger & Trinkaus, 1995; Cohen & Armelagos, 1984; Cohen & Crane-Kramer, 2003; Roberts & Manchester, 2005; Steckel & Rose, 2002). Many of the incapacitating infectious diseases that we confront today date back thousands of years; for example, the first case of tuberculosis in humans has been dated to 9000 BP (Hershkovitz et al., 2008), experience of malaria may extend back 10,000 years (Ewald, 2003) and evidence for chronic respiratory tract infection is present in South American mummies dating from 8000 BP to colonial times (Allison, 1984). Ortner (2003) calculates that in 'typical archaeological human skeletal samples about 15 % of burials will show evidence of serious disease' (Ortner, 2003, p. 112).

Ethnographic studies of disease in pre-industrial communities may also be useful in considering past levels of need for health-related care provision. Sugiyama (2004), for example, records high rates of illness and injury in Amazonian hunter-gatherer communities, the majority of these conditions manifesting in soft tissue and, in 65 % of those reporting disease, resulting in an inability to participate in community activity for periods of over 30 days. He concludes that without care, many in this latter category would have died (Sugiyama, 2004, pp. 382–384). Comparable rates and levels of morbidity (and sometimes caregiving) have been reported in other pre-industrial communities in Africa, Papua New Guinea and Asia and South America (Frankel, 1986; Hewitt, 2003; Kaplan, Hill, Lancaster, & Hurtado, 2000; Lewis, 1975). Extending consideration to the global burden of disease also produces comparable findings (WHO, 2004, 2011b). In recent epidemiological analyses, the World Health Organization (2011b, pp. 27, 289) reported that, at any one time, approximately 15 % of adults worldwide experience significant difficulties in everyday functioning resulting from physical and/or psychological disease; as in Sugiyama's (2004) study, many of the diseases responsible primarily affect soft tissue and would therefore be invisible in the skeletal record. Caution is required when extrapolating from the present to the past, but it seems reasonable to assume a rough equivalence in levels of experience of disease (although not necessarily of the *same* diseases) and disability over time – and therefore most likely a similar equivalence in level of general demand for health-related care. We will never be able to quantify this demand with any precision, however.

The caveats and constraints identified earlier lead to three observations. First, bioarchaeology of care research, and particularly research involving prehistoric remains, will usually focus on case studies rather than address population-level healthcare practices. Second, individual variability in disease response means that, in assessing disease impact on a subject's ability to function, only the most conservative estimates of disability (and therefore care) consistent with the evidence can be hypothesised. And third, because we cannot accurately identify past levels of need for care, we will always *underestimate* the frequency of caregiving in the past.

Bioarchaeology of Care Stage 1: Describe, Diagnose, Document

In Stage 1 the researcher brings together information about the individual and their lifeways. At this point the data-gathering process is comprehensive and indiscriminate, because even seemingly unimportant information may later help shed light on aspects of caregiver and care-recipient behaviour and identity. The quantity and reliability of Stage 1 content will determine the quality, breadth and depth of bioarchaeology of care analysis and interpretation.

Step 1 of the Index of Care structures the search for, and recording of, this information. In relation to the individual, the information sought spans basic descriptors of age, sex, completeness and condition of remains; through nature and distribution of disease indicators, differential diagnoses and most *likely* diagnosis; to the detail of recovery context, disposition of remains, associated artefacts, and so on. Although in some studies no specific diagnosis may be possible, carefully described pathology indicators may still provide sufficient information for considering possible impacts on functioning capability (Stage 2 analysis). In documenting lifeways context, Step 1 first seeks descriptions of geography, topography and climate, independent variables which may influence what constitutes 'disability', what care is needed and what care is possible. It goes on to seek information about cultural, social, political and economic organisation and practice in the subject's community, including at variables such as group size and composition, food production and diet, domestic lifestyle arrangements, occupations, belief systems and/or ritual activities, gender and/or status differentials, technological development, artefact production, between-group trade or exchange, within or between-group violence and mortuary traditions. It asks for an assessment – or at least an impression – of general population health status, and looks at whether previous instances of possible healthcare provision can be identified.

In most studies undertaken to date, bioarchaeology of care analysis has been initiated following off-site examination of remains. In the case of M9, however, indicators of serious pathology were evident while the remains were still in situ and well before detailed analysis, allowing archaeologists present (and this author in particular) to contemplate the implications of survival with disability while still excavating the context in which this occurred. In contrast, the bioarchaeology of care study of Romito 2 was based solely on published materials, relying on skeletal description and analysis produced almost 30 years ago by Frayer et al. (1987, 1988), supplemented with a later description of elements unavailable to these researchers (Mallegni & Fabbri, 1995), and benefitting from wide-ranging archaeological research at the Romito site from the early 1960s to the present day (reviewed in Tilley, 2015b).

The Stage 1 descriptions of M9, Romito 2 and their respective lifeways are summarised in Fig. 2.3.

Stage 1: describe, diagnose, document

<u>**Man Bac Burial 9**</u>: ~4000 BP; male, ~20-25 yrs.; northern Vietnam. Cemetery burial (two small pots), flexed, N-S orientation.
Description: ~75% complete; C1-T3 vertebrae fused; atlantoaxial rotary fixation; occipitalisation; extreme bone atrophy; fusion right sacroiliac joint; TMJ arthritis. No evidence of infection or trauma.
Diagnosis: quadriplegia, acquired ~12-14yrs, (likely trauma-related) complication of congenital Klippel-Feil Syndrome.
Lifeways (general): Estuarine environment (Red River delta); cool winters, hot humid summers; hunter-gatherer (fishing) economy (fish >50% of dietary protein), no evidence for agriculture; no settlement traces - thought small group, sedentary; no evidence for hierarchy (but some graves 'richer' than others); regional trade. Morphology mix of Australo-Melanesian and NE Asian - reflects start of Asian 'demic diffusion'? **Lifeways (mortuary)**: ~100 burials, male and female, infant-adult; standard disposition supine, extended, E-W orientation; grave goods pots, shells, beads, bracelets. **Lifeways (health)**: high levels dental disease + cribra orbitalia; osteoarthritis; no evidence of serious trauma or violence (1 healed forearm fracture).

<u>**Romito 2**</u>: ~11000 BP; male 17-20 yrs, ~110-120 cms (male mean 166 cms); Calabria, Italy. Double burial with female ?35+yrs, (2 auroch horns), supine, extended, N-S orientation.
Description: ~85-90% complete. Long bones disproportionately short (45-58% of mean), particularly forearm bones; limited forearm extension and rotation; wrist + hand anomalies (Madelung's deformity?); cranial anomalies; spinal pathologies.
Diagnosis: acromesomelic dysplasia (very rare dwarfism syndrome).
Lifeways (general): Mountainous terrain; temperate; highly mobile, hunting, small group economy, targeting middle-upper altitude, medium-large game - mainly meat diet, periods of scarcity; manufacture in stone, bone, shell; little/no sexual dimorphism; no evidence of hierarchy.
Lifeways (mortuary): 8 adult burials - 5 males, 3 females from 2 double + 4 single interments; all supine, extended, N-S orientation, (different) grave goods.
Lifeways (health): frequent nutritional stress; Romito 8 (male) lived with disability likely requiring care following trauma (no further information available).

Fig. 2.3 Summary of Stage 1 bioarchaeology of care analysis for M9 (Oxenham et al., 2009; Tilley, 2015a; Tilley & Oxenham, 2011) and Romito 2 (Frayer et al., 1987, 1988; Tilley, 2015b)

Bioarchaeology of Care Stage 2: Assess Disability and Need for Care

Stage 2 is divided into two sections. In the first of these, the researcher identifies the range of clinical symptoms known to be associated with the nature and extent of pathology indicated by the skeletal evidence, and considers which of these were probably, or possibly, experienced by the individual. In the second section, the researcher examines the likely impact of these possible and probable clinical symptoms on the subject's ability to function successfully in their everyday environment. Based on the results of analysis, the researcher makes an assessment of whether – *on the balance of probability* – the subject experienced a level of disability that required the provision of care.

Clinical Impacts

On the assumption that basic human biological responses to particular disease stimuli are more or less constant over time and culture, the first part of Stage 2 analysis uses modern medical literature to consider possible primary and secondary clinical impacts of the individual's pathology.

Step 2 of the Index of Care provides researchers with a list of body systems and functions, adapted from the International Classification of Functioning, Disability and Health (ICF) (WHO, 2003) and reproduced in Table 2.1. In linked worksheets, the researcher is asked to nominate which of these domains have the *potential* to be affected by the disease in question, which domains *were likely* involved in the subject's case (on a scale from 'not involved/impossible to tell' to 'probable'), the symptoms the subject may have experienced in each domain rated 'possible' or 'probable', and the likely severity and duration of each symptom ('symptom severity' is operationalised using descriptors adapted from those in the ICF (WHO, 2003, pp. 2–4)). Certain diseases may be commonly associated with specific complications

Table 2.1 Body systems/functions potentially affected by pathology[a]

1. (Neuro)musculoskeletal and movement-related systems/functions	7. Sensory functions/nervous system (i): pain (e.g. acute, chronic, intermittent)
2. Mental functions (e.g. intellectual, consciousness, attention, language)	8. Sensory functions/nervous system (ii): other (e.g. sight, hearing, balance)
3. Cardiovascular system/function	9. Haematological system/function
4. Respiratory system/function	10. Immune system/function
5. Digestive, metabolic, endocrine system/function	11. Genitourinary, reproductive system/function
6. Integumentary system/function	12. Other [name/describe]

[a]Adapted from the ICF (WHO, 2003, pp. 2–4)

and/or co-morbidities that are unlikely to leave a skeletal signature. In some circumstances, it may be valid to factor these impacts into Stage 2 (and Stage 3) analyses, as in the case of M9 (see later), and the decision to do this should be thoroughly explained.

Where an individual's remains display evidence for more than one disease, or where there are competing diagnoses, the above exercise is repeated for each pathology.

An assessment of individual experience of disease symptoms on the basis of bone lesions must obviously be approached with utmost caution and conservatism (see earlier discussion of 'caveats and constraints'), and researchers can only ever postulate the minimum level of clinical impact suggested by the skeletal evidence. However, minimum level of impact may be enough to justify considering how the disease may have operated on the individual's ability to perform 'normally' within their community.

Functional Implications

The second part of Stage 2 analysis addresses possible activity limitations and participation restrictions affecting the individual as a consequence of pathology. It examines the functional implications of clinical impacts in terms of the individual's potential to perform '*essential* activities of daily living' and '*instrumental* activities of daily living', and the Index Step 2 protocol adapts content from widely used modern health assessment measures to assist in this.

'Essential activities of daily living' refer to those basic tasks in which competency is a prerequisite for enabling a minimum level of self-maintenance. The items included in the corresponding Index worksheet to help assess competence are largely derived from work by Katz, Downs, Cash, and Grotz (1970) and deal with six activities. These involve the ability to access food and water placed in close proximity, eat and drink without assistance, manage personal hygiene, manipulate objects in the immediate vicinity (including self-dressing), achieve mobility over limited distance (e.g. moving from bed to chair) and control body position (e.g. moving from a resting to a sitting position). If any one of these tasks is beyond an individual's capability then, regardless of context, that person will, to some extent, be dependent on others for their survival.

In contrast, assessment of likely functional capability in performing 'instrumental activities of daily living' is almost entirely context dependent. 'Instrumental activities' refer to those tasks making up the fabric of everyday economic, social, domestic and interpersonal living within a community; tasks considered normal and appropriate for members of a particular cohort. An individual experiencing disease may remain capable of performing essential activities of daily living, yet find it impossible to participate in the full range of instrumental aspects of community life at a level that meets community needs and/or expectations.

The Index of Care adapts material from modern measures of instrumental activities (Australian Department of Veterans' Affairs, 1998; Chong, 1995; Lawton & Brody, 1969), including the ICF (WHO, 2003), to identify seven 'instrumental activity' domains: basic lifestyle (e.g. settlement practices), economic activities, domestic activities, mobility patterns, community life (social and cultural activities not covered previously), interpersonal relations and learning/applying knowledge (domains are fully explained in the Index of Care). The Index asks the researcher to use the context established in Stage 1 to describe, against each domain, activities typically undertaken and the physical, social and economic lifeways factors likely to affect, positively or negatively, the subject's performance of these. It then prompts the researcher to assess the subject's ability to participate in domain tasks at an appropriate level. Based on the results of this, the researcher must consider whether the effects of disease compromised the subject's ability to undertake instrumental activities to the extent that direct or indirect assistance was needed – remembering that only minimum likely impact on functioning capability can be posited.

At the end of Stage 2, the researcher makes a judgement as to whether the individual most likely required a form of health-related support to secure their survival with disability. Where a case for care provision cannot be made, bioarchaeology of care analysis ceases. In the case of M9, disease impacts place him in the category of those unable to perform essential activities of daily living, and his need for care over an extensive period is indisputable. The situation of Romito 2 is more nuanced. Although capable of all essential activities of daily living, he was likely significantly restricted in many of the instrumental activities intrinsic to the hunting-based subsistence economy of his group. Romito 2's survival with limitations in physical capability would almost certainly have required some degree of 'accommodation' from childhood onwards. Stage 2 analyses for M9 and Romito 2 are summarised in Fig. 2.4.

Bioarchaeology of Care Stage 3: Develop a 'Model of Care'

Having concluded that the individual most likely received care, Stage 3 analysis asks the researcher to position what has been inferred about clinical and functional impacts of pathology (Stage 2) within the subject's lifeways context (Stage 1), and to examine what responses, along the envisioned continuum of 'direct support' to 'accommodation of difference', may have been adopted to address the effects of these impacts. Stage 3 then asks the researcher to consider the likely duration of caregiving, possible changes in care practice over time, likely effort and resources involved in care provision, and how effective this care might have been.

The results should provide material for constructing a plausible model of the applied aspects of care received by the subject, although of course this can never be complete. It will be impossible to identify the individual's psychological or spiritual needs, although without doubt these existed and helped to determine the shape and content of their care (e.g. Lewis, 1975; Scheper-Hughes & Lock, 1987; see Wesp,

Stage 2: assess disability and need for care

<u>**Man Bac Burial 9**</u>
Clinical impact: total lower body paralysis; partial (at best) upper body paralysis; loss of mineral bone density; head 'fixed' in tilted position; possible problems with mastication; possible muscle contracture lower limbs (leg flexure). Almost inevitable complications of immobility include (at some level): depressed immune system; respiratory, cardiovascular, gastrointestinal dysfunction; kidney failure; pressure sores; pain; depression.
Functional impact: no lower body/very limited upper limb control - unable to perform most/all <u>essential</u> activities of daily living (i.e. unable to access food; likely limited self-feeding; unable to manage hygiene; no mobility; limited object manipulation and/or control over body position). Automatically excluded from all physically demanding <u>instrumental</u> activities of daily living (likely able to participate at some level in non-physical social/cultural activities with assistance).
On the balance of probability, was care required? **YES** - Care in the form of 'direct support' essential for survival.

<u>**Romito 2**</u>
Clinical impact: developmental delays in infancy. From childhood on, mobility and endurance compromised by abnormal gait; forearm extension restricted to 130°; restrictions on pronation and supination of forearm and wrist, with deformities in hand bones, suggest reduced grip strength and manipulation skills. Likely neuropathic pain. (Common impacts include cardiovascular sensory, respiratory, endocrine dysfunction.)
Functional impact: independent in all <u>essential</u> activities of daily living. Restricted participation in <u>instrumental</u> activities: hunting in mountainous terrain impossible; mobility over distance compromised (slower, difficulties in transporting loads); exclusion from tasks requiring manual strength, dexterity, and precision (e.g. tool making); *but* likely able to forage for plants, and participate in most social activity - i.e. could contribute to group, but *not* conform to 'normative expectations' for demographic.
On the balance of probability, was care required? **YES** - Care required in the form of 'accommodation of difference'.

Fig. 2.4 Summary of Stage 2 bioarchaeology of care analysis for M9 (Tilley, 2015a; Tilley & Oxenham, 2011) and Romito 2 (Tilley, 2015b)

Chap. 13 this volume). We usually have little or no insight into *how* a particular disease was comprehended within a particular cultural context, yet this understanding influences both the way the individual is regarded by their community and the type of treatment offered (e.g. Garro, 2006; Leininger, 1988). Finally, the conservatism mandatory in interpreting likely clinical and functional implications of disease will frequently result in underestimating even practical requirements of the subject's care.

Despite these provisos, earlier discussion foreshadowed the potential to identify a number of basic components of care practice with a high level of probability. This assertion rests on the contention that, just as there is a general uniformity in physiological responses to particular disease stimuli that allows Stage 2 analysis of clinical impact, there is an equivalent uniformity in the basic measures necessary to address these disease responses that transcends cultural and individual imperatives. If we can identify these measures, then we have the beginnings of the subject's plan of care.

Table 2.2 'Constants of care' (direct support) for a bioarchaeology of care analysis[a]

1.	*Provision of food and water* (may include special diet, assistance with eating/drinking)	6	*Monitoring health status* (to allow timely response to physiological needs, and to avoid health crises – see [7], [8] and [9] in particular)
2.	*Maintaining body temperature within normal range* (may include protection from elements – provision shade/shelter)	7.	*Maintaining personal hygiene/protection of integument* cleanliness is essential for skin integrity and preventing and treating infection
3.	*Facilitation of rest and sleep* (may include postural adjustment, provision of pain relief)	8.	*Physical manipulation* (turning, lifting, stretching and massage essential maintain/improve body system and organ function in cases of immobility [9])
4.	*Ensuring physical safety* (may include protection from self-harm, domestic and wider environmental (e.g. human, animal, reptile) hazards – may require regular monitoring [see 6])	9.	*Maintaining physiological functioning* (involves timely response to metabolic, respiratory, gastrointestinal, circulatory and urinary, etc. dysfunction – includes physical manipulation, temperature control, diet and hydration)
5.	*Maintaining/assisting mobility* (integral to management of/recovery from disease as immobility can be fatal – see also [8])e	10.	*Specific intervention(s)/technologies* (includes invasive/non-invasive surgery, e.g. orthopaedic, trepanation, amputation, control of haemorrhage; pharmaceuticals; practical aids, e.g. prosthetics)

[a]This table borrows from and adapts Henderson's (1964) components of nursing practice

The bioarchaeology of care approach nominates ten possible 'constants of care', drawing heavily from the work of the nursing theorist Virginia Henderson (Henderson, 1964, 1966). These constants, presented in Table 2.2 provide the structure for the first part of Stage 3 analysis, which focuses on possible provision of care in the form of direct support.

The corresponding set of worksheets in Step 3 of the Index of Care first lists the constants of care identified earlier, asking the researcher to indicate whether one or more of these were 'probably' or 'possibly' an element in the subject's care; to elaborate on what this component of care provision may have comprised in practice; to estimate the period over which this form of care was provided and how it may have changed over this period; and to consider the likely 'costs' incurred in carrying out this care component, in terms of resources employed and additional work involved, directly or indirectly, in caring for the subject.

Stage 3 consideration of accommodation of difference – caregiving at the opposite end of the spectrum to direct support – centres on the instrumental activities of daily living domains introduced in Stage 2. The focus at this point in analysis is different, however. Stage 3 asks the researcher to refer to the Stage 2 assessment of the individual's likely functioning capability in relation to activities in each instrumental activities domain. Where the subject is deemed unlikely to have been able to function 'normally', the researcher is asked to attempt to identify possible adjustments to group expectations and practices necessary to accommodate, or adapt to, the subject's disability. This unarguably involves speculation. We may be able to generate a variety of suitable adjustments and alternative activities appropriate for an individual with a particular disability, but we will never be certain exactly *which* strategies were implemented. Notwithstanding, this exercise allows the researcher to identify a range of options for care provision, and reference to context (Stage 1) may justify these being ranked in order of likelihood. The very act of doing this encourages the researcher to consider the nature of both the care given and the community giving it, and is good preparation for Stage 4 analysis.

The corresponding set of Step 3 worksheets repeats the format adopted in looking at 'direct support' options. It lists instrumental activity domains; invites commentary on necessary, possible and probable 'accommodation' strategies; and asks for estimates of the period over which these strategies were applied and of the costs incurred.

Although level of detail achieved will depend on the quality of the bioanthropological and archaeological evidence available, on completion of Stage 3 analyses the combination of identified 'possible' and 'probable' components of caregiving should allow the researcher to construct a model of care unique to the individual and specific to their context.

Stage 3 'models of care' generated for M9 and Romito 2 are summarised in Fig. 2.5.

Stage 3: develop a 'model of care'

Man Bac Burial 9
Long-term care (~10 years, from acquisition of injury to death); likely involved most/all group members (directly in giving care, or indirectly in making it possible for others to do so). Care for an immobilised person is resource intensive, and includes most 'constants': provision of food (special diet) + water, help with eating and drinking, and maintaining hydration; regulating body temperature inc. shelter, bedding; ensuring hazard-free environment; constant monitoring of health status; managing hygiene and protecting integument (removal of wastes, bathing, elevation off ground); maintaining physiological function through massage, manipulation, positioning, nursing/other therapeutic care (as needed). Care likely encompassed inclusion in social activity - a psychological requirement.
(N.B. *Long-term survival and lack of evidence for either pressure sores or bone fracture reflect consistent, skilled care.*)

Romito 2
Extended 'normal nurturing' during infancy and early childhood to compensate for developmental delays. Care from childhood onwards takes form of 'accommodation' - acceptance of, and adjustment to, Romito 2's differences in functioning capability, including revision of 'normative' expectations. Provisioning (in nutritionally stressed society) was most costly aspect of care - isotope evidence shows Romito 2 received the same 'meat-rich' diet as others. He likely received special consideration in relation to other typical lifeways demands (e.g. those relating to mobility, possibly artefact manufacture, etc.); group 'adjustment' may have meant (re)division of general tasks to ensure allocation of those the subject was capable of performing. 'Accommodation' of Romito 2 would require behavioural adaptation/agreement from all members of the small group.

Fig. 2.5 Summary of Stage 3 bioarchaeology of care analysis for M9 (Tilley, 2015a; Tilley & Oxenham, 2011) and Romito 2 (Tilley, 2015b)

Bioarchaeology of Care Stage 4: Interpretation: Agency and Identity

To recapitulate: health-related care provision is conceived as a sequence of actions taking place over time. These actions are enacted through a series of choices, made by caregivers and care-recipients, which reflect the opportunities, constraints, values and beliefs of the cultural, social, physical, personal and emotional contexts in which these choices were made. The evidence in human remains that allows the inference of care is the product of these choices, and in this sense the individual receiving care quite literally embodies the decisions that helped prolong survival from age of disability onset to age at death.

Stage 4 analysis is based on the premise that the behaviours involved in both giving and receiving care express the agency of those concerned, and that this agency has the potential to illuminate aspects of group and individual identity. It asks the researcher to interrogate the model of care produced over Stages 1–3, taking various elements and (re)combining these to explore what a particular case of caregiving may reveal about social relations, organisation and practice in the community in which care took place, and about the life experience and personality of the person who was cared for. Stage 4 asks: 'If, in *this* lifeways environment, *this* form of care was provided, or survival occurred in relation to a pathology with *that* impact, what does it suggest about the context for providing care and/or the group giving this care and/or the subject receiving it?'

All Stage 4 analysis involves interpretation of inferred behaviours, and is therefore, by definition, open to accusations of subjectivity. Most of what emerges in the Stage 4 process is undeniably speculative – although it is speculation built on a solid, defensible platform of reason. Some researchers will be uncomfortable with this, and may choose to cease bioarchaeology of care analysis at Stage 3. However, as long as the potential for subjective bias is openly acknowledged, and speculation is identified as such, interpretations can be accepted or rejected on their merits. Where Stage 4 interpretation can withstand scrutiny, it can enrich academic *and* public engagement with the past – an observation revisited at the end of this chapter.

Collective Agency and Identity

The first part of Stage 4 analysis focuses on the question of collective agency: it asks what the decision to provide care may have entailed and how this decision may have been reached, what care options were likely available and implemented, and what the answers to these questions may suggest about the way the community operated more generally. It hypothesises a generic decision path, summarised in Fig. 2.6, and asks the researcher to think about the choices made at each point in a journey beginning with recognition of an individual's disability and need for care and ending with

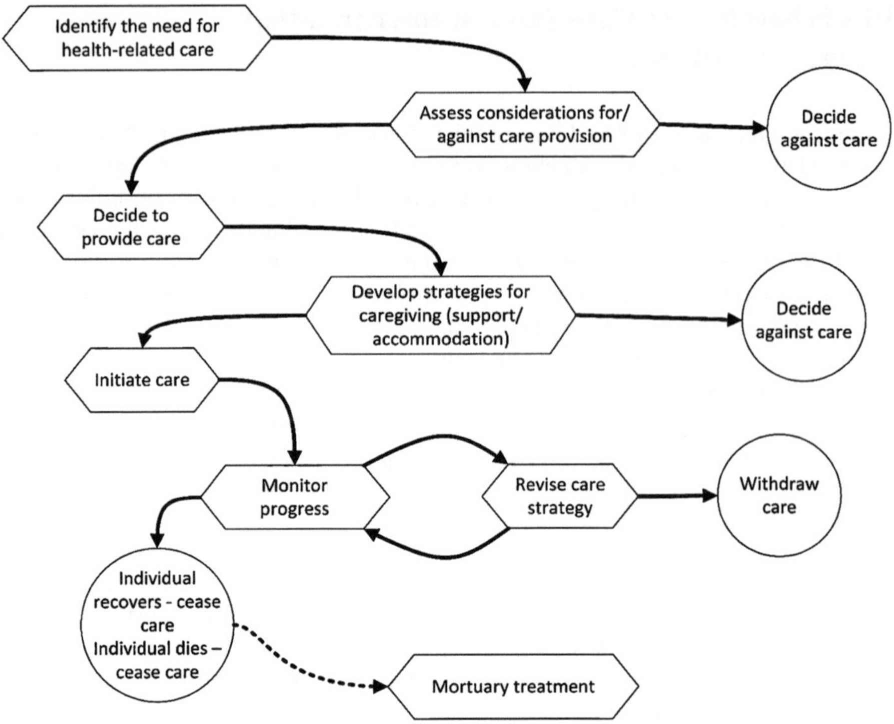

Fig. 2.6 Generic 'decision path': decision-making points in the health-related caregiving process

the cessation of care and, possibly, with the subject's treatment after death (treatment after death is *not* an automatic extension of treatment during life, but may sometimes throw light on this latter; see Matczak and Kozłowski, Chap. 7 this volume, also e.g. Carr, 1995; Hodder & Hutson, 2003; Parker Pearson, 1999). What do the decisions made along this path allow us to infer about the aims and motivations of the people involved? From these decisions can we deduce details of lifestyle, environment, skills and traditions for which we have no direct archaeological evidence?

Despite the deceptively neat visualisation of sequential actions and responses in the decision path proposed earlier, there is no blueprint for identifying what underlies behaviours in any example of past caregiving. Aspects of motivation for care provision might possibly be approached obliquely, through consideration of the costs caregivers were willing to bear. Yet caregiving is a sophisticated behaviour, and there are typically so many, and sometimes contradictory, motives for giving care that a simplistic, economically inspired equation can never satisfactorily capture these. On similar lines, 'aims' might be approached in terms of 'primary purpose or anticipated results of care', but coming to terms with the goal(s) of caregiving is usually far more complicated than this. Initial goals may reflect what is perceived as achievable in practice and/or culturally desirable, but will often (and sometimes rapidly) evolve to reflect improvement or deterioration in the subject's physical health status, the presence of people willing and able to provide care and the nature of their relationship with the care recipient, variability in the care-recipient's psychological state, changes in the physical environment, availability of resources, and so on. Regardless of these provisos, the 'decision path' offers a rudimentary map for researchers taking on the interpretive quest.

The corresponding Index of Care Step 4 protocol converts the seven points in the postulated decision path (Fig. 2.6) into enlarged 'decision domains', asking the researcher to use the content produced in Stages 1–3 to address the implications of the most likely decision made in each domain for understanding aspects of community. What might a decision to undertake a particular action, in a particular lifeways context, signify about the way that the community was organised and the relationships between community members? How might this decision reflect the aims and motivations (see above) driving care, and what might these hypothesised aims and motivations suggest about group social identity?

This process establishes the groundwork for the task that follows, in which researchers are asked to devise case study-specific questions with the aim of producing the most complete picture possible of the community in which care was given. For example, what might the decision to care for a particular subject in a lifeways with evidence of frequent interpersonal violence suggest about cultural practice, values and identity – where does care fit? (Chap. 9, by Sarah Jolly and Danielle Kurin, deals directly with this seeming paradox.) In a subsistence environment, what might the decision to provide long-term care to a severely disabled subject imply about group social relations?

While the identification of many of the influences and most of the reasoning behind decisions made in past care provision is beyond our scope, the process of reflecting on these is intrinsically valuable – not least because it raises awareness of how complex – and how fundamentally *human* – past societies were.

Individual Agency and Identity

Seeking the individual identity of the subject of care is an even harder proposition than attempting to tease out the collective identity of the community that provided it.

Archaeology is a blunt instrument for undertaking this job. In a bioarchaeology of care case study, a care-recipient is identified solely on the basis of skeletal indicators of lived-with pathology, but no one is simply the product of their disease. To pretend that we can 'know' a person on the basis of disability alone would be ridiculous. On the other hand, there are few things as immediate as living with a disability serious enough to require care. The response to experience of this state is likely to reflect, and, in a recursive relationship, to *shape*, aspects of personal identity.

The second part of Stage 4 analysis attempts to build up an impression of the individual around whom the case study revolves. To expand on earlier observations, while the nature of pathology and the environment in which it occurs to a great extent determine the nature of the care response, the individual *also* shapes their care – through negotiation with carers, by force of character, by virtue of group role and status, and so on. The subject of care possesses agency, even if this is limited to choosing between 'cooperation' and 'non-cooperation' with the care on offer.

If we can get some sense of how this agency was expressed it may suggest facets of personality, although it goes without saying these will never be amenable to proof. Important qualifications apply here. As the examples of M9 and Romito 2 reveal (see Fig. 2.7), it is much easier to justify the search for identity when the individual concerned required direct support for a seriously incapacitating disability over a lengthy period of time. In cases such as that of M9, survival can be construed as a personal achievement as much as an outcome of care quality, arguably providing clues to the subject's social persona and even to their private self. Where the individual has received care in the form of accommodation, as in the case of Romito 2, the task will be much harder. Where does community adjustment to accommodate disability end and personal achievement begin (or vice versa)? How can this possibly be discerned from the archaeological evidence available?

'Individual identity' comprises biological, behavioural and social characteristics that combine to create a person distinct from all others. Supported by Index Step 4 worksheets, Stage 4 begins by asking the researcher to construct a comprehensive osteobiography of the subject covering physical characteristics, familial and social identities; possible experiences of disability and care; and lifeways variables potentially influencing performance in social, economic and cultural spheres. The researcher is then asked to think about the subject as agent or actor, adapting as appropriate generic questions focusing on aspects of experience of, and response to, their care, and generating new questions specific to the case. Sample questions might include: 'What does survival with this particular disability suggest about personality and motivation?', 'With this disability, what was required from the subject in terms of cooperation in their own care?' and 'What does cooperation suggest in terms of level of functioning and personality traits?'. Material covered in the osteobiography and the responses to such queries are brought together to answer one last question: '*Who* was the subject of care?'.

Stage 4 analyses for M9 and Romito 2 are summarised in Fig. 2.7.

Issues and Ethics in Bioarchaeology of Care Analysis

Undertaking a bioarchaeology of care study comes with responsibilities, and two issues were singled out for consideration in the introduction to this chapter. First, how might research into past caregiving behaviours contribute to our knowledge of self and society, and second, what ethical issues should be taken into account in planning and undertaking bioarchaeology of care research?

Addressing the first question, as earlier observed, bioarchaeology of care research has the potential to enrich academic and public engagement with the past.

Stage 4: interpretation - agency and identity

Man Bac Burial 9
Social relations, social practice, and group identity: successful long-term intensive care in Man Bac context suggests ingenuity, experience, knowledge, skills in caregiving; behavioural flexibility, organisational skills in managing demands; cooperative community willing/able to incur costs of care; committed/non-fatalist outlook (care provided when no hope of recovery); inclusive of 'difference' (M9 involvement in social activity? - see 'care model'). Absence of fracture supports 'sedentary' lifestyle; quality of care supports peaceful community (suggests demic diffusion not marked by violence?). 'Deviant' burial in main cemetery suggests social inclusion *but also* recognition of difference - reflects beliefs about achievement of 'passage to afterlife'?
Individual identity: possible traits: strong will to live; adaptable; engaged with community; positive attitude (attractive personality?); patience; healthy self-esteem; and resilience. *(N.B. Refusal to cooperate with care due to depression is, in modern times, the third most frequent cause of death in the first years after quadriplegia onset.)*

Romito 2
Social relations, social practice, and group identity: maintaining a member unable to make 'equal' economic contribution in small, stressed group suggests strong internal cohesion, willingness and ability to juggle labour availability, task allocation, and often scarce resources. Unlikely (this form of) dwarfism encountered before; Romito 2 delayed development in infancy, increasing physical constraints and unusual appearance likely difficult to make sense of, yet subject accepted and cared for appropriately into young adulthood (n.b. burial treatment equal to others), so clearly some narrative developed. Integration may reflect 'dividual' social relations - i.e. those born to group part of indivisible 'whole', with *in*dividual 'differences' secondary. Possible care for Romito 8 may indicate caregiving a 'norm'.
Individual identity: limited potential for identity speculation. As a child, Romito 2 likely saw differences as 'normal'; maturity possibly brought comparison of his role and capabilities with those of peers. Demanding lifeways mean he likely developed non-normative ways to contribute to economy.

Fig. 2.7 Summary of Stage 4 bioarchaeology of care analysis for M9 (Tilley, 2015a; Tilley & Oxenham, 2011) and Romito 2 (Tilley, 2015b)

Both scholars and members of the general public have given an overwhelmingly positive reception to the bioarchaeology of care approach, and this has been gratifying and sometimes surprising. For many scholars, the appeal resides in the approach's clearly structured framework for analysis. The methodical, incremental approach to assessing level and impact of disability, and the ability to use these results as the basis for identifying likely components of a care response, allows extraction of additional meaning from descriptive skeletal data. Some scholars have gone further, embracing the more reputationally risky, but rewarding, adventure of interpretation.

For the lay public, it was the idea that, in the past, people looked after disabled community members which struck a chord. In December 2012, an article on M9 appeared in the *New York Times* (Gorman, 2012) and was reproduced in international print and electronic media, stimulating wide-ranging debate. Much of the commentary compared this example of behaviour in the past to usually unflattering examples of behaviour in the present, touching on issues ranging from the deficiencies of modern healthcare policy and practice, the need for greater social justice, the politics of access to medical care for the poor, through to vindication of economic rationalism, validation of the precepts of atheism, proof of the existence of God and support for the principles of evolution (Tilley, 2015a, pp. 294–298).

David Mennear (Chap. 18, this volume) urges the importance of communicating archaeological research as widely as possible. That there is an enormous appetite for information about the past is obvious from the success of television series, documentaries, films, magazines and blogs about archaeology, and when archaeology focuses on human remains this appetite seems even more voracious, perhaps reflecting the human ability to empathise with others of our species. When it comes to an archaeology that focuses not only on human remains, but on a distinctively human situation with which most people are personally familiar – in being either a provider or a receiver of health-related care – the prospects for empathy and identification are magnified.

The vast majority of people responding to the *New York Times* article on M9 had only the vaguest notion of the theoretical and methodological niceties of the original research. But does this matter from the perspective of encouraging reflection on self and society? Probably not. The main points of the study were communicated effectively: a young man in a low technology, subsistence-level community in the prehistoric past survived with devastating disability for far longer than anyone would have thought possible, because he was cared for. One of the primary reasons for studying archaeology, enunciated in all major codes of professional practice, is to help the public understand how society has become what it is today. Bioarchaeology of care research can make a significant contribution to this conversation, and, anticipating the discussion that follows, has a moral responsibility to do so.

Turning to the second question raised, it is a given that the ethical responsibilities implicated in planning and undertaking a bioarchaeology of care case study are, at the very least, commensurate with those found in any research with human remains that seeks to evoke both the individuals represented by their remains and the community in which these individuals resided. In other words, we are under an obligation to treat the individuals studied *as* individuals, with dignity, and we need to ensure that any re-creation of 'community' does not go beyond the available evidence. David Doat (Chap. 17, this volume) discusses these and related ethical concerns at length (see also Scarre, 2006; Tarlow, 2001, 2006).

There may be an extra level of responsibility involved in analysing disability and care, however. It has been argued that although human remains no longer retain a sentient existence, when subjected to archaeological study the individual whose remains we analyse (re)gains a form of *social* existence in the public sphere, and that this transformation must be respected (Tarlow, 2006, p. 202). The bioarchaeology of care approach goes further than most research undertaken with human remains. It does this initially by seeking access to experiences that, in a living individual, are often intensely private, and then in attempting to reproduce, for public consumption, a personal history of a no-longer-living person based on interpretation of what has been elicited in the first part of this exercise. The importance of responding to this difference may be more emotional than rational, but arguments for an awareness of the implications of this difference when performing bioarchaeology of care analysis have resonance.

The appropriate ethical response may be to do exactly what the bioarchaeology of care theory and methodology emphasise – to attempt the most complete and transparent account possible of the individual life and lifeways under study. To take the alternative route, to avoid or minimise interpretation for fear of 'getting it wrong', may be to abuse our privileged access to the remains of those who, though now mute themselves, can teach us so much. The bioarchaeology of care allows the capture of some of this richness and, to return to the first question raised at the beginning of this section, this may be how it best contributes to wider public discourse.

Conclusion

Bioarchaeology of care research provides entry into some of the most detailed and intimate aspects of life in the past. Focusing on the experience of one individual confronted with a range of health-related challenges, each case study opens up features of a community and its lifeways to the analytic gaze – and what we learn in this process allows a deeper understanding of one small segment of the past than was previously available to us. The bioarchaeology of care methodology, operationalised in the Index of Care, does not claim to provide categorical answers to the complex questions arising from past experiences of disability and caregiving – this would be impossible. But it *does* provide an easily navigated architecture that guides and supports efforts to think through the evidence for care (and the wider implications of this evidence) systematically; that has the flexibility to take account of, and manage, the ambiguities and uncertainties that are inescapable in any archaeological interpretation of inferred behaviour; and that allows an open and continuous review of results *and* of the rationale behind these. The bioarchaeology of care approach is continuously evolving and can be a powerful tool in the bioarchaeologist's research armoury. Nowhere is this more apparent than in the following chapters of this volume.

Acknowledgements All the contributors to this volume have been magnificent colleagues and collaborators, and I thank them from the bottom of my heart. This book grew from a symposium at the 2015 Society for American Archaeology annual meeting; the person who originally proposed the symposium was my co-editor, Alecia A. Schrenk, and I am very grateful for this brainwave – and her comradeship in making things happen. I would like to thank the two anonymous reviewers of this chapter for their helpful suggestions, and those colleagues, in particular Robyn Longhurst, who have read and commented on early drafts. I have thanked David Frayer previously for providing me with images and information in relation to Romito 2, and I thank him again. Finally, and as usual, I want to thank Tony Cameron for his help in producing my images, for his work on the Index of Care, and for his unwavering support in general.

Appendix 1

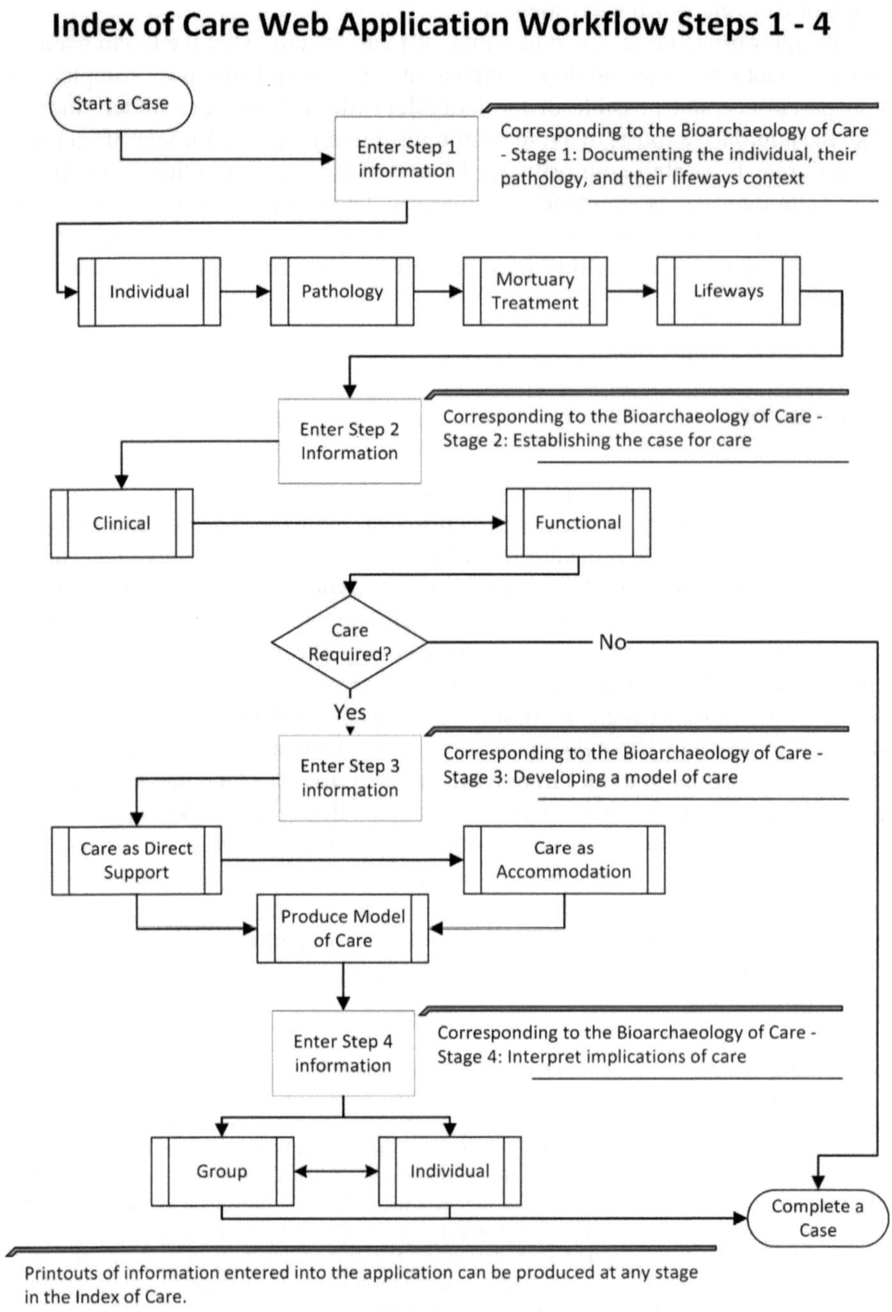
Index of Care Web Application Workflow Steps 1 - 4
Start a Case
Enter Step 1 information
Corresponding to the Bioarchaeology of Care - Stage 1: Documenting the individual, their pathology, and their lifeways context
Individual
Pathology
Mortuary Treatment
Lifeways
Enter Step 2 Information
Corresponding to the Bioarchaeology of Care - Stage 2: Establishing the case for care
Clinical
Functional
Care Required?
No
Yes
Enter Step 3 information
Corresponding to the Bioarchaeology of Care - Stage 3: Developing a model of care
Care as Direct Support
Care as Accommodation
Produce Model of Care
Enter Step 4 information
Corresponding to the Bioarchaeology of Care - Stage 4: Interpret implications of care
Group
Individual
Complete a Case
Printouts of information entered into the application can be produced at any stage in the Index of Care.

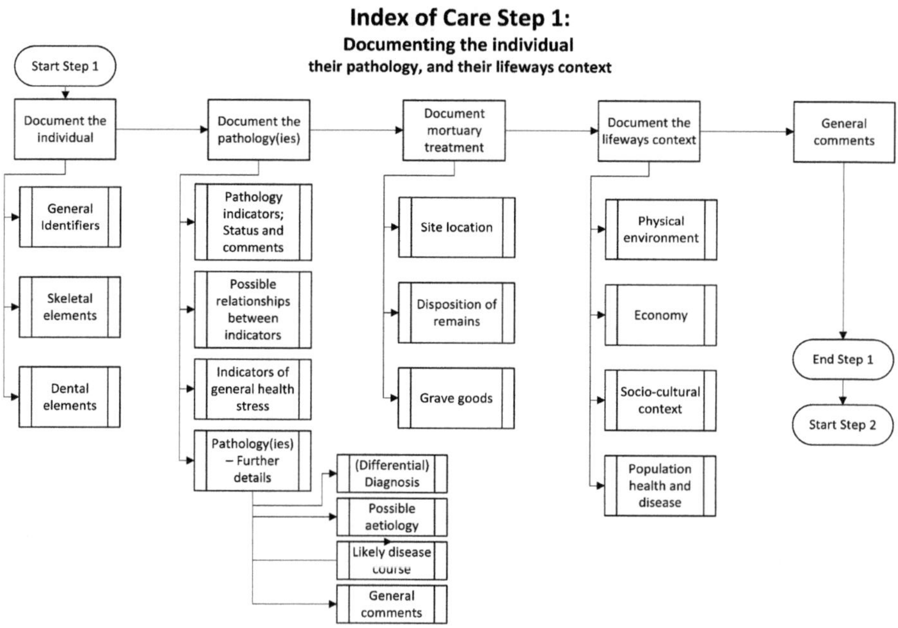
Index of Care Step 1:
Documenting the individual
their pathology, and their lifeways context
Start Step 1
Document the individual
General Identifiers
Skeletal elements
Dental elements
Document the pathology(ies)
Pathology indicators; Status and comments
Possible relationships between indicators
Indicators of general health stress
Pathology(ies) – Further details
(Differential) Diagnosis
Possible aetiology
Likely disease course
General comments
Document mortuary treatment
Site location
Disposition of remains
Grave goods
Document the lifeways context
Physical environment
Economy
Socio-cultural context
Population health and disease
General comments
End Step 1
Start Step 2

Index of Care Step 2:

Establishing the case for care

Section 1 - The clinical implications of pathology

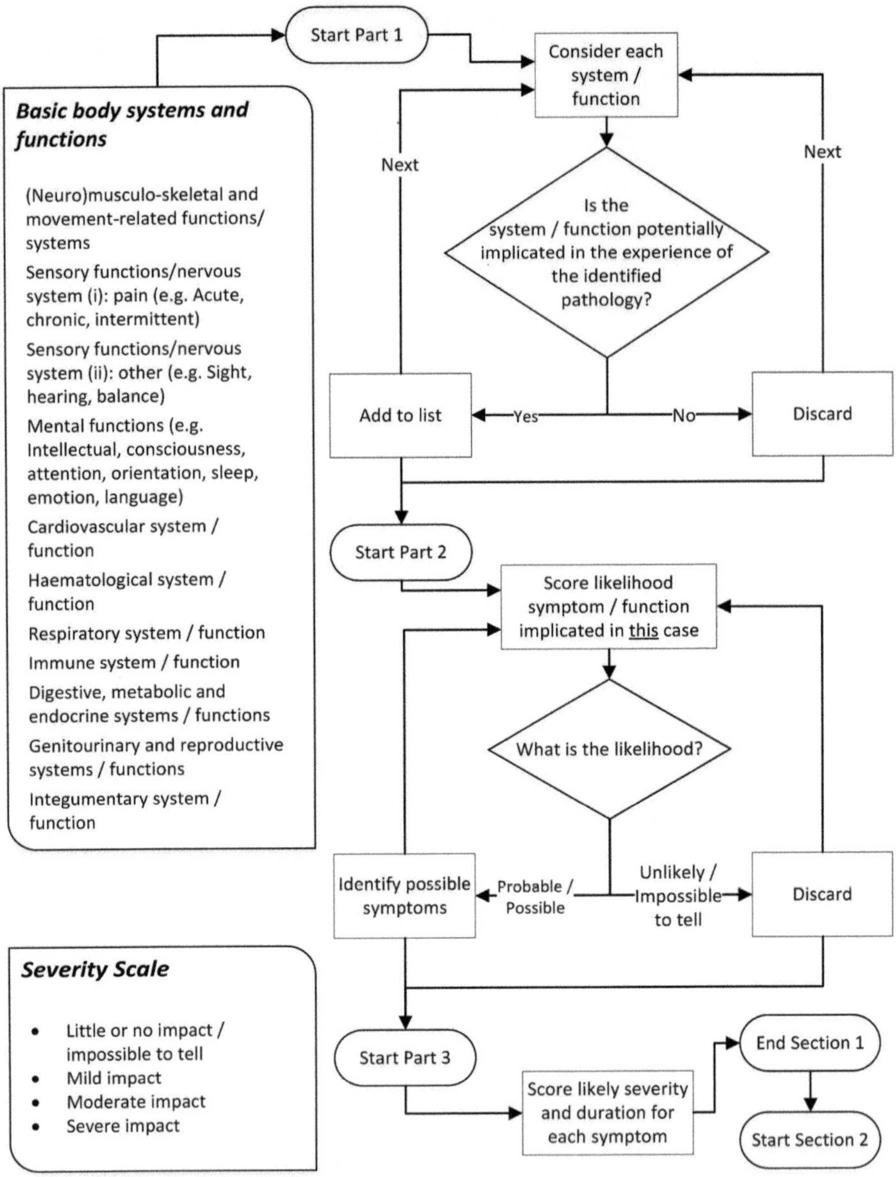

Index of Care Step 2:
Establishing the case for care
Section 2 - The functional implications of pathology

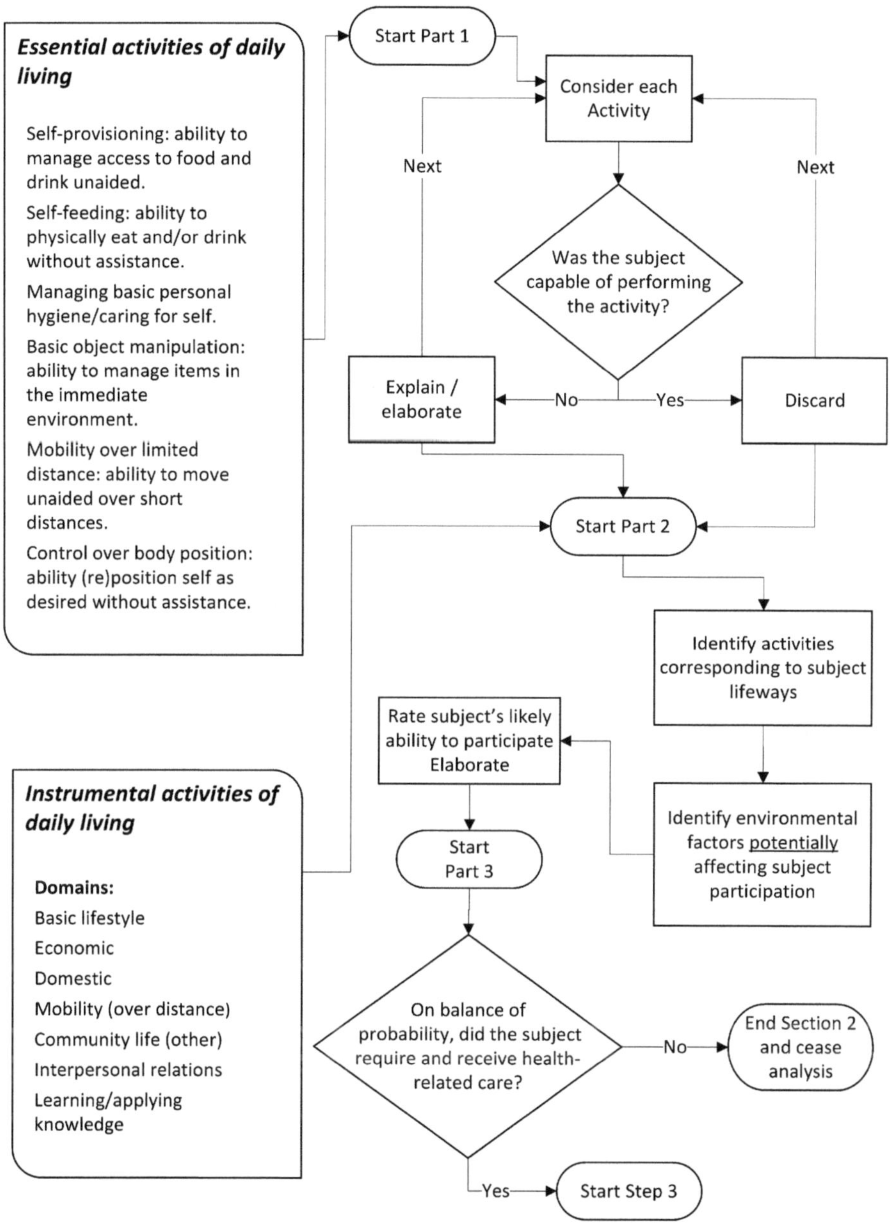

Index of Care Step 3:

Developing a Model of Care

Section 1 – Care as Direct Support

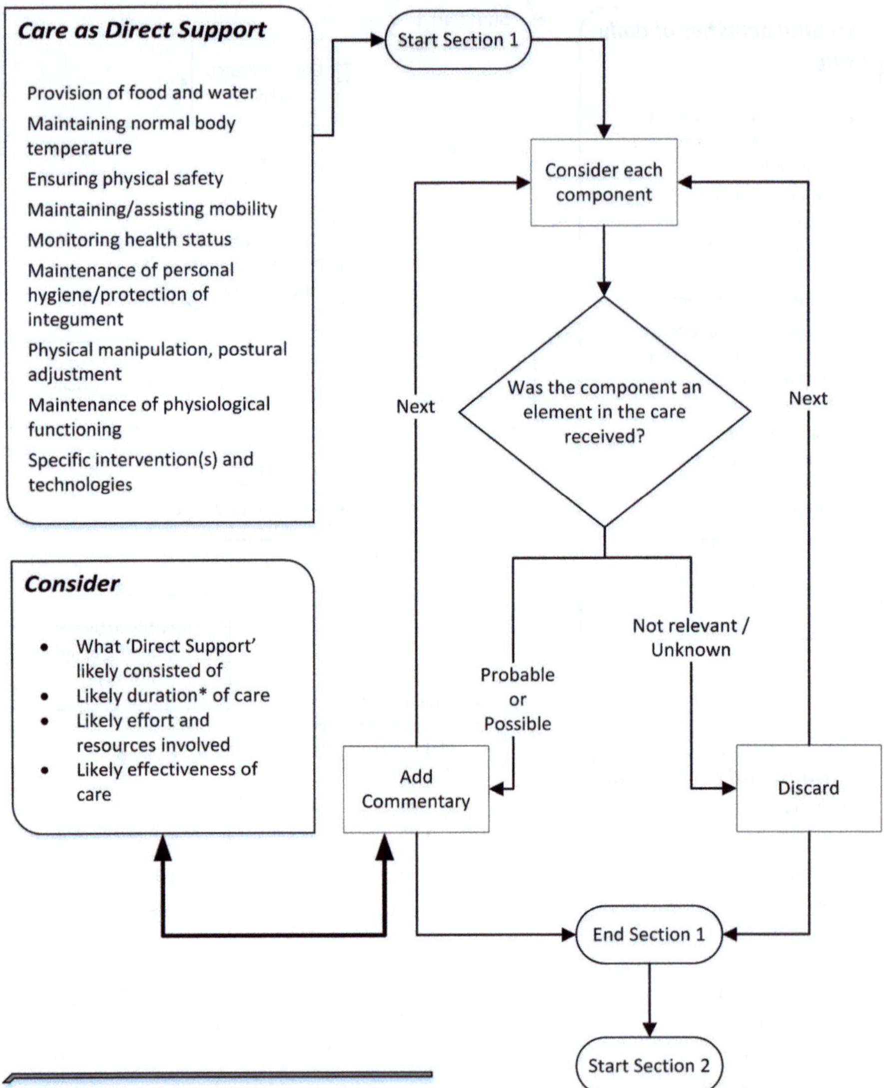

*'***Duration***' operationalised as:

- Short term = < 3 months
- Medium term = 3 – 6 months
- Long term = > 6 months

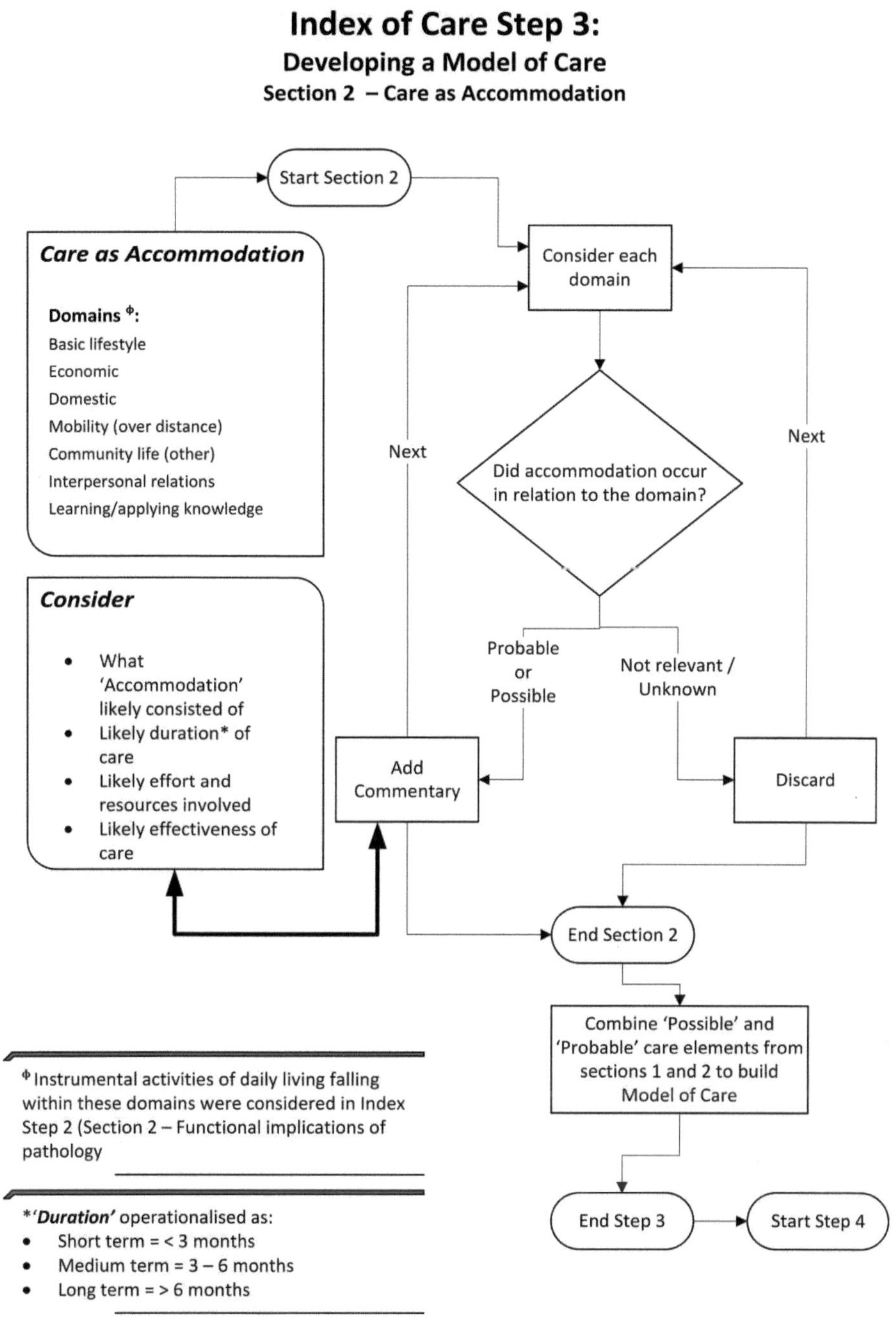
Index of Care Step 3:
Developing a Model of Care
Section 2 – Care as Accommodation
Start Section 2
Care as Accommodation
Domains ᶲ:
Basic lifestyle
Economic
Domestic
Mobility (over distance)
Community life (other)
Interpersonal relations
Learning/applying knowledge
Consider each domain
Next
Did accommodation occur in relation to the domain?
Next
Consider
• What 'Accommodation' likely consisted of
• Likely duration* of care
• Likely effort and resources involved
• Likely effectiveness of care
Probable or Possible
Not relevant / Unknown
Add Commentary
Discard
End Section 2
Combine 'Possible' and 'Probable' care elements from sections 1 and 2 to build Model of Care
End Step 3
Start Step 4
ᶲ Instrumental activities of daily living falling within these domains were considered in Index Step 2 (Section 2 – Functional implications of pathology
*'Duration' operationalised as:
• Short term = < 3 months
• Medium term = 3 – 6 months
• Long term = > 6 months

Index of Care Step 4:

Interpretation

Section 1 – Group Agency

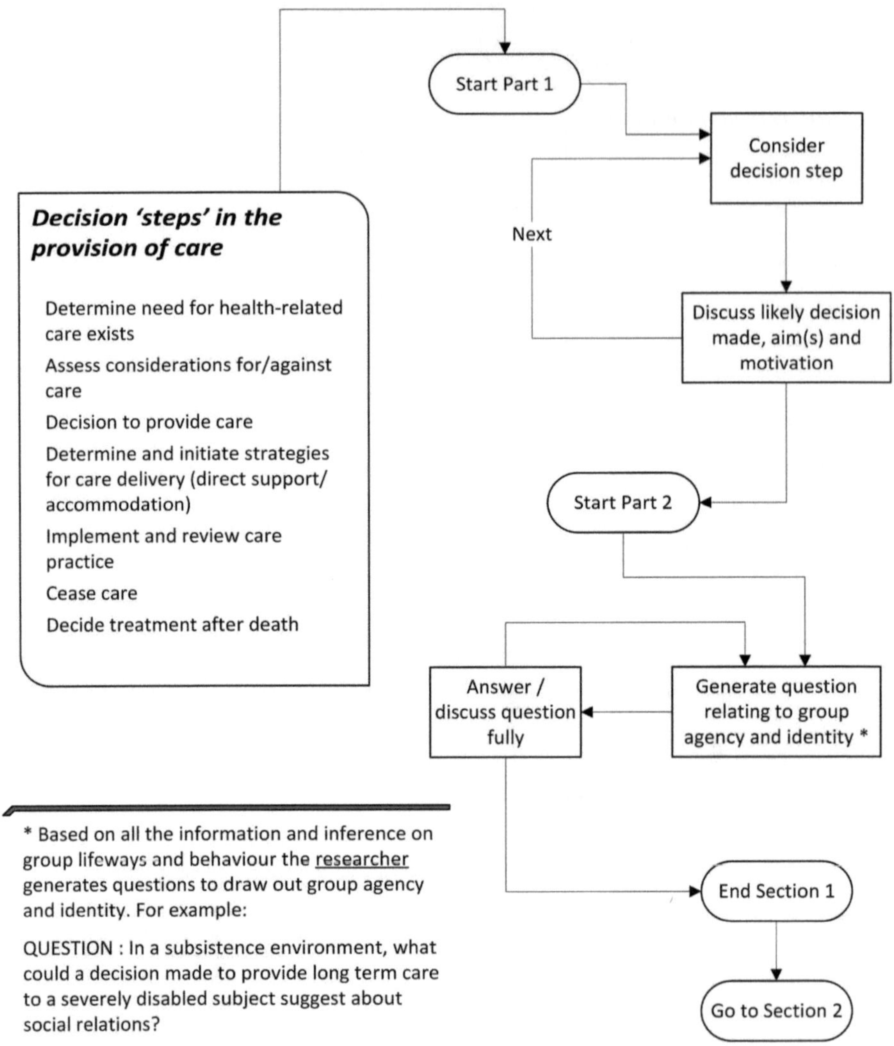

* Based on all the information and inference on group lifeways and behaviour the researcher generates questions to draw out group agency and identity. For example:

QUESTION : In a subsistence environment, what could a decision made to provide long term care to a severely disabled subject suggest about social relations?

DISCUSSION : Reflects cohesive community with strong collective identity - all members 'belonging' and given value? Normative behaviour - duty of care owed regardless of cost - 'dividual' versus 'individual'? and so on ...

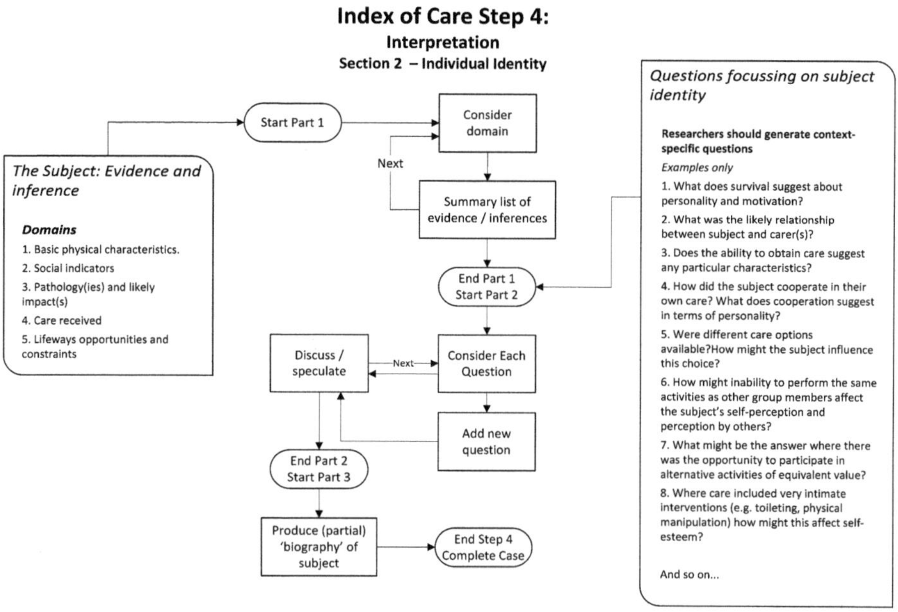

References

Allison, M. J. (1984). Palaeopathology in Peruvian and Chilean populations. In M. N. Cohen & G. J. Armelagos (Eds.), *Paleopathology at the origins of agriculture* (pp. 515–529). Orlando: Academic.

Australian Department of Veterans' Affairs. (1998). *Guide to the assessment of rates of veterans' pensions*. Canberra: Commonwealth of Australia (Department of Veterans' Affairs).

Berger, T. D., & Trinkaus, E. (1995). Patterns of trauma among the Neandertals. *Journal of Archaeological Science, 22*, 841–852.

Bickenbach, J. E., Chatterji, S., Badley, E. M., & Üstün, T. B. (1999). Models of disablement, universalism, and the international classification of impairments, disabilities and handicaps. *Social Science and Medicine, 48*, 1173–1187.

Bowling, A. (2002). *Research methods in health: investigating health and health services* (2nd ed.). Buckingham: Open University Press.

Buikstra, J. E., & Beck, L. A. (Eds.). (2006). *Bioarchaeology: The contextual analysis of human remains*. Amsterdam: Academic.

Carr, C. (1995). Mortuary practices: Their social, philosophical-religious, circumstantial, and physical determinants. *Journal of Archaeological Method and Theory, 2*, 105–200.

Chong, D. K. H. (1995). Measurement of instrumental activities of daily living in stroke. *Stroke, 26*, 1119–1122.

Cohen, M. N., & Armelagos, G. J. (Eds.). (1984). *Paleopathology at the origins of agriculture*. Orlando: Academic.

Cohen, M. N., & Crane-Kramer, G. (2003). The state and future of paleoepidemiology. In C. L. Greenblatt & M. Spigelman (Eds.), *Emerging pathogens: The archaeology, ecology, and evolution of infectious disease* (pp. 79–91). Oxford: University Press.

Dettwyler, K. A. (1991). Can paleopathology provide evidence for "compassion"? *American Journal of Physical Anthropology, 84*, 375–384.
Ewald, P. W. (2003). Evolution and ancient diseases: The roles of genes, germs, and transmission modes. In C. L. Greenblatt & M. Spigelman (Eds.), *Emerging pathogens: The archaeology, ecology and evolution of infectious disease* (pp. 117–124). Oxford: University Press.
Frankel, S. (1986). *The Huli response to illness*. Cambridge: University Press.
Frayer, D. W., Horton, W. A., Macchiarelli, R., & Mussi, M. (1987). Dwarfism in an adolescent from the Italian late Upper Palaeolithic. *Nature, 330*, 60–62.
Frayer, D. W., Macchiarelli, R., & Mussi, M. (1988). A case of chondrodystrophic dwarfism in the Italian late Upper Palaeolithic. *American Journal of Physical Anthropology, 75*, 549–565.
Garro, L. C. (2006). Cultural meaning, explanations of illness, and the development of comparative frameworks. In E. Whitaker (Ed.), *Health and healing in comparative perspective* (pp. 296–315). Upper Saddle River, NJ: Pearson Prentice Hall.
Gorman, J. (2012). Ancient bones that tell a story of compassion. *New York Times*. Retrieved 17 Dec, 2012, from http://www.nytimes.com/2012/12/18/science/ancient-bones-that-tell-a-story-of-compassion.html?_r=1&.
Henderson, V. (1964). The nature of nursing. *The American Journal of Nursing, 64*, 62–68.
Henderson, V. (1966). *The nature of nursing: A definition and its implications for practice, research, and education*. New York: Macmillan.
Hershkovitz, I., Donoghue, H. D., Minnikin, D. E., Besra, G. S., Lee, O. Y.-C., Gernaey, S. M., et al. (2008). Detection and molecular characterization of 9000-year-old *Mycobacterium tuberculosis* from a Neolithic settlement in the eastern Mediterranean. *PLoS One, 3*(10), 1–6.
Hewitt, B. R. (2003). Mortality in traditional hunter-gatherer, pastoralist and agriculturalist communities: The validity of longevity studies based on mobility and subsistence strategies. *Nexus, 16*, 27–49.
Hodder, I., & Hutson, S. (2003). *Reading the past: Current approaches to interpretation in archaeology* (3rd ed.). Cambridge, England: Cambridge University Press.
Hofrichter, R. (Ed.). (2003). *Health and social justice: Politics, ideology and inequity in the distribution of disease*. San Francisco: Wiley.
Jylhä, M. (2009). What is self-rated health and why does it predict mortality? Towards a unified conceptual model. *Social Science and Medicine, 69*, 307–316.
Kaplan, H., Hill, K., Lancaster, J., & Hurtado, A. M. (2000). A theory of human life history evolution: Diet, intelligence and longevity. *Evolutionary Anthropology, 9*, 156–185.
Katz, S., Downs, T. D., Cash, H. R., & Grotz, R. C. (1970). Progress in development of the index of ADL. *The Gerontologist, 10*, 20–30.
Lawton, M. P., & Brody, E. M. (1969). Assessment of older people: Self-maintaining and instrumental activities of daily living. *The Gerontologist, 9*, 179–86.
Leininger, M. M. (1988). Leininger's theory of nursing: Cultural care diversity and universality. *Nursing Science Quarterly, 1*, 152–160.
Levin, B. W., & Browner, C. H. (2005). The social production of health: Critical contributions from evolutionary, biological, and cultural anthropology. *Social Science and Medicine, 61*, 745–750.
Lewis, G. (1975). *Knowledge of illness in a Sepik society: A study of the Gnau, New Guinea*. London: The Athlone Press, University of London.
Mallegni, F., & Fabbri, P. F. (1995). The human skeletal remains from the Upper Palaeolithic burials found in Romito cave (Papasidero, Cosenza, Italy). *Bulletins et Mémoires de la Société d'Anthropologie de Paris, 7*(3), 99–137.
Martin, D. L., & Horowitz, S. (2003). Anthropology and alternative medicine: Orthopaedics and the other. *Techniques in Orthopaedics, 18*, 130–138.
Ortner, D. J. (2003). *Identification of pathological conditions in human skeletal remains*. New York: Academic.
Ortner, D. J. (2009). Issues in paleopathology and possible strategies for dealing with them. *Anthropologischer Anzeiger, 67*, 323–340.
Oxenham, M. F., Tilley, L., Matsumura, H., Nguyen, L. C., Nguyen, K. T., Nguyen, K. D., et al. (2009). Paralysis and severe disability requiring intensive care in Neolithic Asia. *Anthropological Science, 117*, 107–112.

Parker Pearson, M. (1999). *The archaeology of death and burial*. College Station: Texas A&M University Press.
Pol, L. G., & Thomas, R. K. (2001). *The demography of health and health care* (2nd ed.). New York: Kluwer Academic/Plenum Press.
Roberts, C. A., & Manchester, K. (2005). *The archaeology of disease* (3rd ed.). New York: Cornell University Press.
Scarre, G. (2006). Can archaeology harm the dead? In C. Scarre & G. Scarre (Eds.), *The ethics of archaeology: Philosophical perspectives on archaeological practice* (pp. 181–198). Cambridge: Cambridge University Press.
Scheper-Hughes, N., & Lock, M. M. (1987). The mindful body: A prolegomenon to future work in medical anthropology. *Medical Anthropology Quarterly, 1*, 6–41.
Shakespeare, T. (2006). *Disability rights and wrongs*. London: Routledge.
Shakespeare, T. (2008). Debating disability. *Journal of Medical Ethics, 34*, 11–14.
Steckel, R. H., & Rose, J. C. (Eds.). (2002). *The backbone of history: Health and nutrition in the western hemisphere*. Cambridge: University Press.
Sugiyama, L. S. (2004). Illness, injury and disability among Shiwiar forager-horticulturalists: Implications of health-risk buffering for the evolution of human life history. *American Journal of Physical Anthropology, 123*, 371–389.
Tarlow, S. (2001). The responsibility of representation. In M. Pluciennik (Ed.) *The responsibilities of archaeologists: Archaeology and ethics. Lampeter Workshop in Archaeology (4)* (pp. 57–64). BAR International Series 981.
Tarlow, S. (2006). Archaeological ethics and the people of the past. In C. Scarre & G. Scarre (Eds.), *The ethics of archaeology: Philosophical perspectives on archaeological practice* (pp. 199–216). Cambridge: Cambridge University Press.
Tilley, L. (2015a). *Theory and practice in the bioarchaeology of care*. New York: Springer.
Tilley, L. (2015b). Accommodating difference in the prehistoric past: Revisiting the case of Romito 2 from a bioarchaeology of care perspective. *International Journal of Paleopathology, 8*, 64–74.
Tilley, L., & Cameron, T. (2014). Introducing the index of care: A web-based application supporting archaeological research into health-related care. *International Journal of Paleopathology, 6*, 5–9.
Tilley, L., & Oxenham, M. F. (2011). Survival against the odds: Modeling the social implications of care provision to seriously disabled individuals. *International Journal of Paleopathology, 1*, 35–42.
Vehmas, S. (2008). Philosophy and science: The axes of evil in disability studies? *Journal of Medical Ethics, 34*, 21–23.
Waldron, T. (2009). *Palaeopathology*. Cambridge: Cambridge University Press.
Wood, J. W., Milner, G. R., Harpending, H. C., & Weiss, K. M. (1992). The osteological paradox: Problems of inferring prehistoric health from skeletal samples. *Current Anthropology, 33*, 343–370.
World Health Organization. (2003). *International classification of functioning, disability and health (Version 2.1)*. Geneva: World Health Organization.
World Health Organization. (2004). *The global burden of disease*. Geneva: World Health Organization.
World Health Organization. (2011a). *Fact sheet: Health topics: disability*. Geneva: World Health Organization. Retrieved from http://www.who.int/topics/disabilities/en.
World Health Organization. (2011b). *World report on disability*. Geneva: World Health Organization.

Part I
Case Studies: Applying and Adapting the Bioarchaeology of Care Methodology

Chapter 3
Applying the Index of Care to the Case Study of a Bronze Age Teenager Who Lived with Paralysis: Moving from Speculation to Strong Inference

Alecia A. Schrenk and Debra L. Martin

Introduction

Although we may never know if ancient people suffered and felt pain or discomfort, the Index of Care provides a guide for approximating the larger contexts within which disease was experienced in ancient populations. The Index of Care operationalizes the bioarchaeology of care methodology and guides researchers in testing their hypotheses regarding care provisioning. This is done by offering a systematic, rigorous four step process for describing pathologies, assessing disabilities, constructing a care model, and examining the implications of caregiving. This methodology leads researchers to look at the evidence of disease from every possible angle and to reconstruct (to the extent possible) the lived cultural experiences. However, the Index of Care works best when a diagnosis of a particular disease can be made. When this is not possible to do, as in the case study offered here, the Index is still invaluable for providing a framework for exploring multiple possible disease experiences, and distinguishing among those that may need more or less care.

This study applies the Index of Care to the case of a previously published 18-year-old female whose remains were recovered from the communal tomb at the Bronze Age site of Tell Abraq (UAE). Using the Index of Care in this re-analysis provided a more nuanced and complete interpretation of this young woman's experience of disease and care. This study, where a single diagnosis could not be made, still uses the Index of Care but modifies how the final interpretation is produced given the inability to identify a single pathology. Using the Index aided in moving the interpretation from being mere speculation to providing strong inference about two possible ways to think about this teenager's paralysis.

A.A. Schrenk, M.A. (✉) • D.L. Martin, Ph.D.
Department of Anthropology, University of Nevada, Las Vegas, Las Vegas, NV, USA
e-mail: schrenk.alecia@gmail.com

© Springer International Publishing Switzerland 2017

L. Tilley, A.A. Schrenk (eds.), *New Developments in the Bioarchaeology of Care*, Bioarchaeology and Social Theory, DOI 10.1007/978-3-319-39901-0_3

Materials and Methods

Tell Abraq is a Bronze Age site from the Umm an-Nar period that is located near Sharjah in the United Arab Emirates (UAE) approximately 50 km northeast of Dubai. Tell Abraq was occupied continuously from 2200 BC to 300 AD. It was situated in a coastal desert environment and access to the coast allowed the people of Tell Abraq to take advantage of marine food sources such as fish, dugong, mollusks, and turtle (Martin & Potts, 2012; Potts, 1990, 2001; Uerpmann, 2001). During the period that the tomb was in use (circa 2200–2000), the inhabitants of Tell Abraq practiced desert farming. Date palms were grown to provide shade for other agricultural crops (Gregoricka, 2013; Potts, 2001). Uerpmann (2001) notes that faunal evidence suggests sheep, goats, and cattle were able to graze on local flora, and these animals likely provided both meat and milk for the population. Likewise, local non-domesticated animals such as deer were also hunted to provide additional meat for the population (Baustian, 2005).

The Um an-Nar period is associated with a shift from nomadic herding to a sedentary agricultural economy based on oasis settlements that consisted of fortifications established around a water source and surrounded by small dwellings (Cleuziou, 2009; Martin & Potts, 2012; Potts, 2001). This period is associated with the inhabitants of the historically attested region known as Magan (Sumerian) or Makkan (Akkadian) and is identified with distinct styles of ceramics, metal weaponry, and softstone vessels (Potts, 2001). The site of Tell Abraq is typical of this period, containing a tomb that was associated with the Tell and fortress (Fig. 3.1). The fortress tower of Tell Abraq was constructed of mud brick and surrounded a

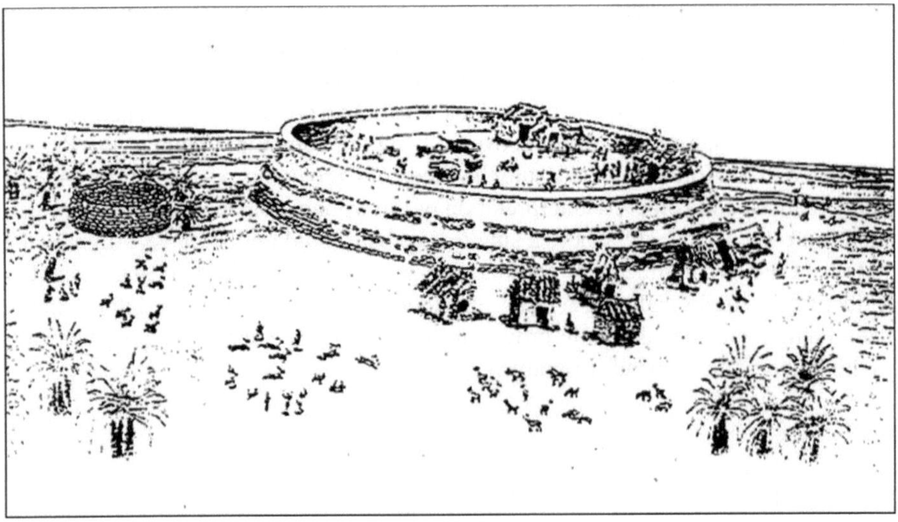

Fig. 3.1 Tell Abraq site sketch. The tomb (on the *left*) is 10 m from main fortress tower. Post holes suggest house structures were likely located outside the fortress tower. The habitation area covers 4 ha

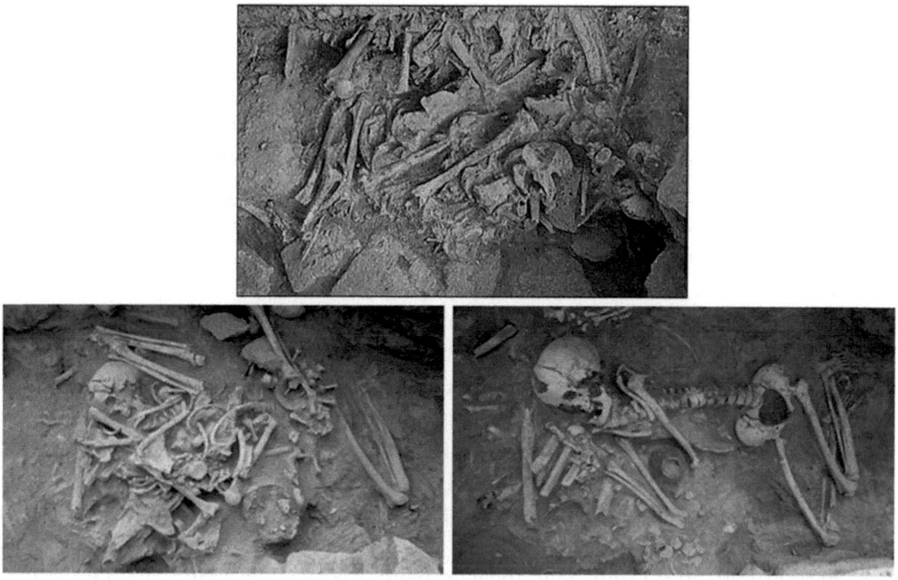

Fig. 3.2 *Top*: Dense bone bed of commingled and disarticulated remains found in Tell Abraq tomb, *Bottom Left*: Lesley in situ surrounded and covered by commingled and disarticulated remains, *Bottom Right*: Lesley in situ uncovered, fully articulated

solitary fresh water source. Magee (1996) and Potts (2000a, 2000b) argue that post holes found at the site are consistent with barista-like huts which were constructed outside the fortress from palm fronds and posts. Excavations of the settlement revealed rich material evidence of trade connections in the form of ceramics from Mesopotamia, southwestern Iran, ancient Dilmen, Baluchistand, and Central Asia. Ivory combs, softstone vessels, cubicle weights, and gold beads indicate further contact with Iran, Troy, Pakistan, and the Indus Valley (Potts, 1990, 2000a, 2000b, 2009, 2012). The abundant diversity of trade goods found within the tomb and settlement suggest that Tell Abraq was a principle Magan settlement.

The Tell Abraq tomb is located 10 m west of the tower, roughly 6 m in diameter, and comprises beach rock and limestone (Martin & Potts, 2012). Radiocarbon dates derived from charcoal indicate that the tomb was used during the end of the Umm an-Nar period, from c. 2200–2000 BC. The tomb is circular in shape and divided into two chambers by a bisecting wall that runs through the center of the tomb. This wall provided support for the stone ceiling and it stopped short of the entrance (Martin & Potts, 2012). The tomb comprised a dense bone bed of disarticulated, fragmentary, and commingled skeletal remains includes those of individuals of all ages and both sexes (Fig. 3.2). The excavated remains represent a minimum of 405 individuals interred over approximately 100 years (Osterholtz, Baustian, Martin, & Potts, 2014). The tomb is unusual in that it was not robbed in antiquity, nor otherwise disturbed, except for a small part at the back of the tomb which is missing part of the outer wall. No other tombs have been found near the site. The remains recovered from the tomb are currently housed at the University of Nevada, Las Vegas.

"Lesley"

Burial 1, dubbed "Lesley" by the excavation crew because she was so complete, was the only fully articulated individual in the tomb (Martin & Potts, 2012) (Fig. 3.2). Her estimated age-at-death is 18–20 years old, based on evidence of long bone fusion, dental eruption, and pubic symphysis morphology (Buikstra & Ubelaker, 1994). Lesley's estimated sex is female based on the characteristics of her right sciatic notch, subpubic angle, and other dimorphic features of the right pelvis and cranium (Buikstra & Ubelaker, 1994).

Martin and Potts (2012) published a full description of Lesley and using standard differential diagnosis techniques they published that Lesley had some form of neuromuscular condition. Although poliomyelitis was one of the possibilities presented, the authors suggested that the morphological changes on Lesley's bones could not differentiate between various more specific neuromuscular conditions. We decided to undertake a complete re-analysis of Lesley's remains using the Index of Care (Tilley & Cameron, 2014) as a guide so that a more complete interpretation might result. Paleopathological changes in the skeleton were observed macroscopically and radiographically. Long bone measurements were taken using standard osteological methods (White, Black, & Folkens, 2012). Dental pathology was observed macroscopically and radiographically.

The Index of Care is used to further explore the diagnosis of Lesley's underlying condition as well as to clarify whether it is likely that care and/or accommodation was necessary for Lesley's survival to the age of 18. The results of the differential diagnosis re-analysis suggest two plausible candidates for Lesley's condition. The Index of Care does not provide specific advice about how to develop a model of care when two pathologies, each associated with different clinical and functional implications, are equally likely. This study therefore extends the way that the Index is normally applied by developing two possible models of care and then exploring the implications of each one.

First, differential diagnosis is used to narrow the condition that may have led to Lesley's paralysis. Second, modern clinical literature is used to construct a possible model of care for the two primary candidates for Lesley's health problems. At this juncture the analysis becomes more challenging because the two potential but different conditions have different impacts on health. This study contends with this by treating the pathologies independently and examining the clinical impact and likely need for care for each of these. Third, the identified need for care in relation to each pathology is then placed within the reconstructed cultural context for the Bronze Age and for the site of Tell Abraq to determine what sort of care (if any) was necessary for this individual to survive. Finally, information from the cultural context and medical literature is combined to explore the agency of both the caregivers and the care-receiver with regard to each of the likely pathologies identified. While using the Index of Care to produce separate models of care and agency is more laborious, it does allow for the exploration of care in cases where differential diagnosis fails to distinguish a single condition creating the health problem.

Paleopathological Analysis

Martin and Potts (2012) note that during the excavation of the tomb that Lesley was unique for being the only articulated burial in the tomb and for presenting noticeably thin and fragile long bones. In addition to this, the first analysis of her complete skeleton revealed a calcaneo-cavo valgus deformity of her left foot; periosteal reactions at the growth plates of her long bones; raised and inflamed sites of muscle attachment; hypertrophy of the humeri, radii, and ulnae; poor dental health; a healed cranial depression fracture; and hyperplastic reconfiguration of the nasal aperture (Martin & Potts, 2012) (Fig. 3.3). These indicators suggested that Lesley suffered a neuromuscular disease at some time during her development, but that is as far as the authors could go with their analysis at that time.

A re-analysis of Lesley's skeletal remains using the Index of Care as an additional guide revealed more details about her pathological condition, including limb length discrepancy. Lesley's left arm is 5 mm shorter than the right when combining the asymmetry found in both the humerus and radius. The left tibia is 2 mm shorter than the right (Table 3.1). Unfortunately, her left femur and fibula were broken in situ, making a comparison of total leg length impossible. While these limb length asymmetries are admittedly small, they are potentially important in that they are consistent with other asymmetries on Lesley's left side. For example, the sciatic notch on her left os coxa is narrower than that on her right. As mentioned above, Lesley's left foot also exhibited a calcaneo-cavo valgus deformity which could have caused further asymmetry on the left leg. The slight asymmetry of Lesley's left limbs, combined with these other observations, leads the authors to conclude that the condition causing these was developmental and likely originated from neuromuscular problems affecting her left side.

Other noticeable anomalies on her skeleton include the sacrum, which is both concavely and convexly pronounced (Fig. 3.3E). There is reactive bone suggesting inflammation of the muscle attachments on the radius, ulna, and clavicle that point to sustained use of the upper body (Fig. 3.3A). Poor oral health for an 18-year-old was notable. Lesley had multiple large caries, abscesses, and antemortem tooth loss (Fig. 3.4). A dental radiograph revealed severe mandibular and maxillary abscesses at the time of death (Fig. 3.4A).

Step 1: Differential Diagnosis

The noticeably thin, long, and smooth leg bones (femora, tibiae, and fibulae) are consistent with paraplegia (Martin & Potts, 2012; Novak, Cavka, & Slaus, 2014; Colonna & Vom Saal, 1941). Morphological characteristics of her upper and lower limbs suggest that paralysis set in during growth and development of the long bones. With this in mind, we focused differential diagnosis on childhood diseases that cause paralysis and influence limb asymmetry. These include tuberculosis, paralytic poliomyelitis, and cerebral palsy.

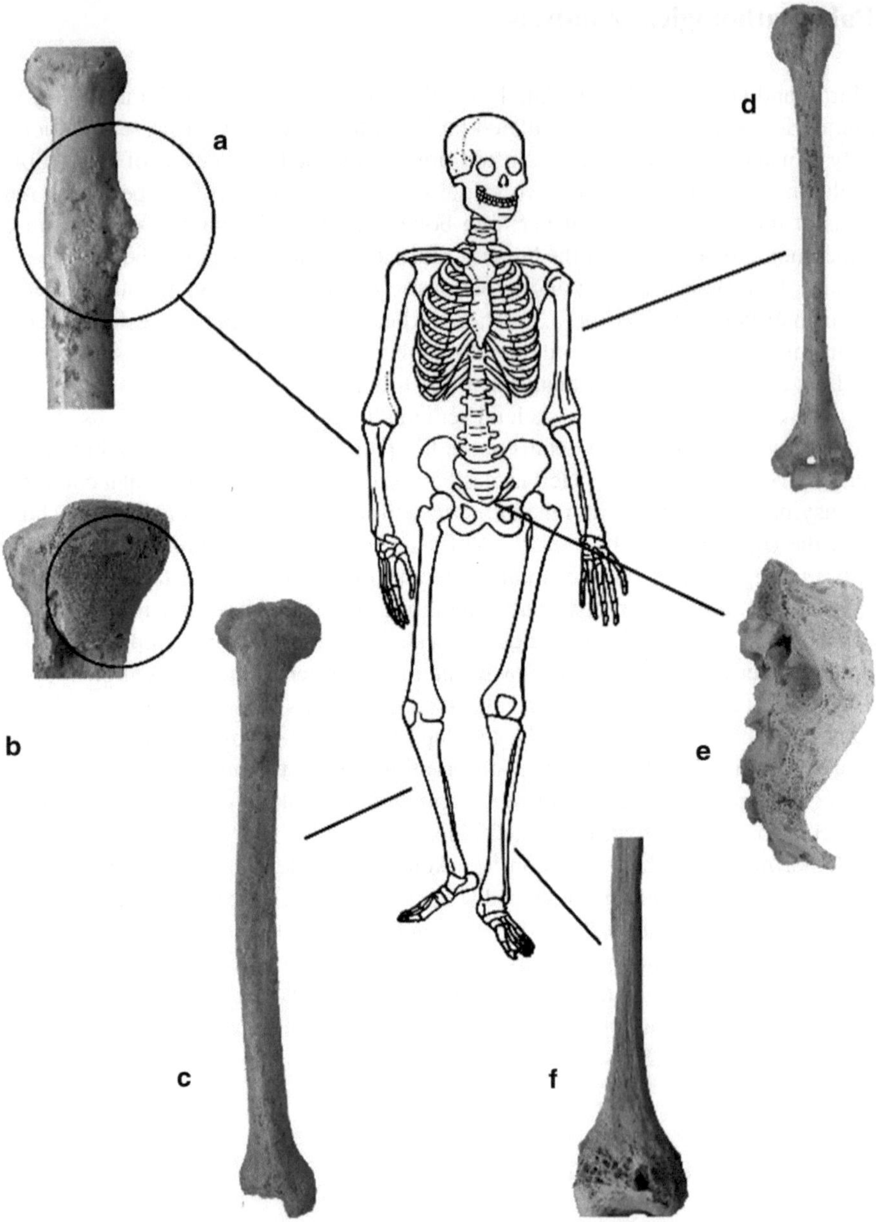

Fig. 3.3 *A*: Inflammation of the radial tuberosity; *B*: Periosteal reaction along the growth plate of the tibia; *C*: Thin and elongated tibia; *D*: Gracile humerus; *E*: Concave curvature of the lower sacrum; *F*: Thin and gracile fibula

Although extreme cases of tuberculosis can result in paralysis, it is unlikely that this was the cause of Lesley's paraplegia. While her nasal aperture, conchae, and septum show signs of destruction and hyperplastic activity, skeletal indicators

Table 3.1 Long bone measurements (mm) for the right and left long bones. Right-left asymmetry is noted in the final column

	Length by side (mm)		
	Right	Left	Asymmetry
Humerus	312	308	4
Radius	255	256	1
Ulna	275	275	0
Femur	–	444	–
Tibia	377	375	2
Fibula	357	358	1

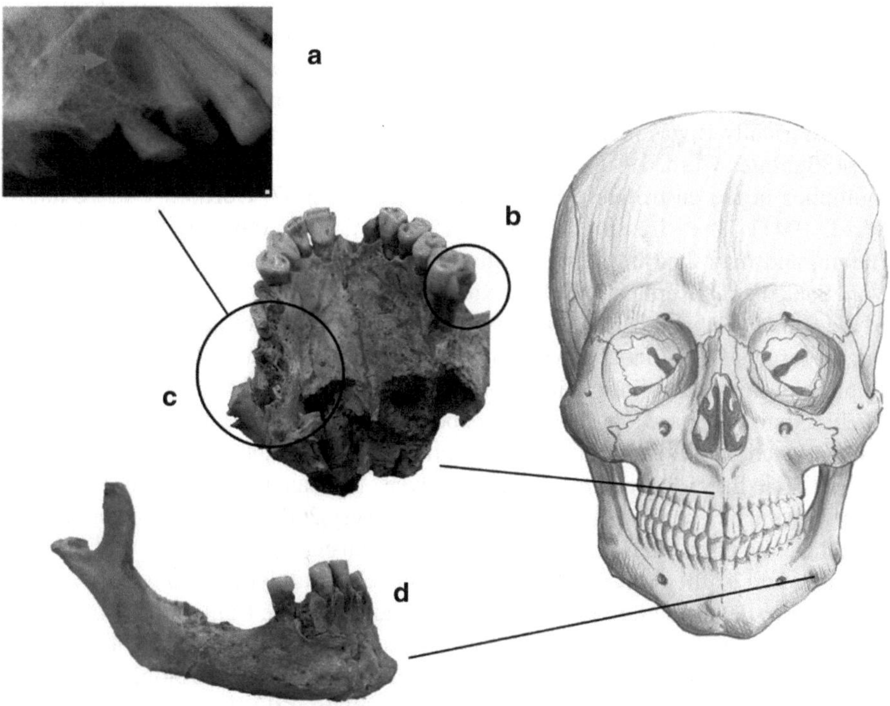

Fig. 3.4 *A*: Radiograph revealing active abscess in right maxilla, *B*: Carious lesion on left maxillary first molar, *C*: AMTL and abscesses on right maxilla, *D*: AMTL on right mandible

frequently associated with tuberculosis (Ortner & Putschar, 1981, p. 228), they do not exhibit the erosion characteristics of this disease. Furthermore, there are no other signs of cranial tuberculosis, such as sieve-like perforations of the vault, lesions with exposed diploe, and vascular lesions along the inner table of the cranial vault (Ortner & Putschar, 1981, p. 228). The most common cause of paralysis as a result of tuberculosis is destruction of vertebral bodies (Ortner & Putschar, 1981, p. 228). Lesley's vertebrae show no sign of lytic activity, cavitation, or collapse associated with tuberculosis. Finally, other skeletal indicators of tuberculosis, such as arthritis in the knee and hip joint and destruction of the carpals and tarsals, are not present in Lesley's remains. The differential diagnosis for this study therefore concentrates on the diseases of paralytic poliomyelitis and cerebral palsy.

Paralytic Poliomyelitis

Poliomyelitis is a highly contagious viral infection that enters the body through a fecal–oral route. It is sometimes associated with contaminated water or food; however, it can also be contracted through contact with an infected individual (Jesus, 2007; Hargreaves, 1948; Gordon, 1941). Although there is, to date, no unequivocal evidence for active poliomyelitis in Bronze Age Arabia, its presence is widely inferred in nearby northern Africa from possible descriptions of this disease from dynastic Egypt (Minor, 2012). Humans are the only known reservoir of poliomyelitis and historically it was most prevalent in densely settled populations (Novak et al., 2014; Sabin & Ward, 1941). The virus enters the body through the oral cavity and multiplies in the gastrointestine or pharynx (Jesus, 2007; Gordon, 1941; Sabin & Ward, 1941). The virus then infects lymphoid tissues, traveling into the bloodstream, and may then invade the central nervous system (Jesus, 2007; Colonna & Vom Saal, 1941). Replication of the virus in the motor neurons of the anterior horn of the spinal cord and brain stem results in the destruction of nervous tissue resulting in paralysis (Colonna & Vom Saal, 1941; Hargreaves, 1948; Gordon, 1941). Initial symptoms of poliomyelitis are similar to those of a cold, and most individuals likely remain unaware that they have experienced this disease. However, 1 in every 100 infected individuals experiences more severe symptoms, such as extreme fatigue, limb flaccidity, and temporary paralysis. Permanent paralysis, usually in the form of paralysis of the legs, results in 1 out of every 200 cases (as calculated by the World Health Organization, 2014). Gawne and Halstead (1995) argue that the older an individual is, the more likely they are to develop paralytic poliomyelitis. Adults also tend to develop more severe cases of paralysis in the trunk and all four limbs than children, as well as being more likely to develop lung paralysis (Young, 1989). It is possible that Lesley contracted poliomyelitis later in her development, placing her at greater risk of developing the paralytic version of the disease.

The most compelling evidence of this condition in Lesley's remains are her extremely thin, elongated femora, tibiae, and fibulae. These are distinct indicators of paraplegia, which is the most common form of paralytic poliomyelitis (Novak et al., 2014). The skeletal indicators of paralytic poliomyelitis also include scoliosis (30 % of cases), hip dysplasia, femoral neck anteversion, and foot deformities (Colonna & Vom Saal, 1941; Ebnezar, 2003). While there were no obvious indications of scoliosis, the spine of T6 curves drastically to the right, indicating that the disease may have had a slight effect on the vertebral column. Poor preservation of the superior and inferior borders of the vertebral bodies prevented a full assessment of spinal curvature. Lesley's left os coxa shows signs of asymmetry, in that the sciatic notch is much smaller and more curved than its counterpart. Martin and Potts (2012) also noted that a reconstruction of Lesley's left foot by a physician in the 1990s using modeling clay indicated a calcaneo-cavo valgus deformity, in which the tendons of the foot tightened causing it to twist inward. Considering all of the above, a compelling but not conclusive case for paralytic poliomyelitis can be made.

While the literature on the dental effects of poliomyelitis is scant, Haberle, Van Stewart, Staat, Gettleman, and Sleamaker (2001) point out that stiffening and paralysis of the neck muscles during and following poliomyelitis may cause difficulty in swallowing. The connection between this and oral health is compelling. Caries are the result of fermented carbohydrates that create an increased acidity and production of proteolytic enzymes in the oral cavity (Tayles, Domett, & Nelson, 2000, p. 77). The "clearance rate," or the period in which food is removed from around the teeth, disrupts this process. Salivary flow rate then is one factor in removal of food particles and bacteria from the oral cavity, and salivary flow rate corresponds to the amount of chewing as well as swallowing involved in the consumption of food (Thylstrup, 1994). Therefore, it is possible that difficulties in swallowing as a result of paralysis could lead to an increase in caries.

While not ruling out other possible diagnoses, the suite of skeletal and dental conditions present is consistent with a diagnosis of paralytic poliomyelitis.

Cerebral Palsy

Cerebral palsy is defined as a "static neurological condition resulting from brain injury occurring before cerebral development is complete" (Krigger, 2006, p. 91). Generally, cerebral palsy is used as an umbrella term for motor and developmental dysfunctions. Cerebral palsy is most commonly attributed to a lack of oxygen to the perinate at the time of birth, usually when the umbilical cord is compressed during labor (Novak et al., 2014). However, the condition can also be caused by premature birth, low birth weight, intrauterine growth, intracranial trauma, and general trauma to the fetus (Krigger, 2006, p. 91). In mild cases of cerebral palsy, subtle motor impairment is the most common symptom. More severe cases exhibit total paralysis as well as possible mental problems and refractory seizures. In 23–25 % of cases, the individual suffers urinary incontinence (Krigger, 2006, p. 91). Muscle imbalance across the joints can cause shortening of the limbs, joint contracture, bone deformity, and joint subluxation or dislocation (Krigger, 2006, p. 2021). Cerebral palsy can cause flexion of the joints, such as the shoulder girdle, humerus, radius, ulna, metatarsals, tarsals, knee joint, hips, carpals, and metacarpals.

Scoliosis, kyphosis, and lordosis are also symptoms of this condition. The patient's gait is often described in medical literature as "toe walking, crouched gait, knee flexion, jump gait, scissoring, and windblown pelvis" based on the flexion of the joints and severity of the condition (Koman, Smith, & Shilt, 2004, p. 2021). Only 25 % of individuals with cerebral palsy are unable to walk. Diplegia, or paralysis of two limbs, in which the legs are more affected than the arms, is the most common form of paralysis in cerebral palsy. This is in contrast to hemiplegia, where only one side is affected and often occurs on the left side of the body (Koman et al., 2004; Novak et al., 2014). In cases of cerebral palsy, multiple movement disorders often coexist, and their impact can range from limited mobility to paralysis.

Lesley exhibits several boney changes consistent with cerebral palsy. Her paraplegia, combined with the asymmetry of the left side of her body, is indicative of multiple mobility disorders. Furthermore, in cerebral palsy some skeletal systems may be more affected than others, in that the left side of the body is often more affected than the right (Koman et al., 2004; Novak et al., 2014). In Lesley's case, disease-related impact to the left os coxa, foot, and sacrum appears greater than that to left upper and lower limbs. The skeletal features of Lesley do not demonstrate the full range of symptoms associated with cerebral palsy, but the disease is highly variable in individual expression and therefore remains a possible diagnosis.

Since neither paralytic poliomyelitis nor cerebral palsy can be ruled out as the cause for Lesley's paraplegia, a care model was constructed for each disease to allow the authors to fully explore the possibilities for care at Tell Abraq.

Step 2: Clinical Impact

Paralytic Poliomyelitis: Late Onset Symptoms to Paraplegia

Paralytic poliomyelitis can be contracted at any time of life. However, the relatively small extent of asymmetry in Lesley's limbs suggests that if she experienced poliomyelitis then she may have contracted this disease at the stage of adolescent development when limb growth is almost complete, around 12–16 years of age. This is also the age range in which the risk for developing the paralytic version of poliomyelitis is heightened but survival prospects are reasonably good (Gawne & Halstead, 1995; Hargreaves, 1948; Gordon, 1941; Smallman-Raynor, Cliff, Trevelyan, Nettleton, & Sneddon, 2006; Young, 1989). Adults who contract the paralytic version often die, as the virus quickly progresses to their lungs, while subadults under the age of 10 years old are less likely to contract the paralytic version (Colonna & Vom Saal, 1941; Smallman-Raynor et al., 2006; Young, 1989).

The Index of Care prompts consideration of changes in symptoms of disease and the impacts of these changes on functional ability over time, but researchers are inevitably limited in this regard when considering pathologies where the timing and progression of the disease are unclear. However, despite the difficulty in determining the precise age at which Lesley contracted poliomyelitis, we can still explore the lived experiences of paralytic poliomyelitis in the past.

The initial symptoms of poliomyelitis are stiffness, neck pain, fever, fatigue, headache, vomiting, and stiffness in the neck and limbs (Colonna & Vom Saal, 1941; Jesus, 2007; Sabin & Ward, 1941). Since these symptoms mimic those of the average cold or flu, most infected individuals are not aware they have contracted the virus (Robertson et al., 1994), and the non-paralytic version of poliomyelitis is only clinically confirmed with a fecal or tissue sample (Sabin & Ward, 1941).

Often poliomyelitis is not suspected until the patient develops acute flaccid paralysis (AFP) of the limbs with no other apparent cause (Sabin & Ward, 1941; Robertson et al., 1994). The onset of AFP from poliomyelitis varies from person to person based on individual immunocapacity; however, AFP usually develops within the first few days of contracting the virus (Bodian, 1952; Gordon, 1941; Smallman-Raynor et al., 2006). The dental pathologies caused by problems with swallowing and the viscosity of the saliva can create a great deal of pain and provide additional routes for staphylococcal or streptococcal infection. Paralytic poliomyelitis usually affects the lower limbs first, sometimes one at a time, and can then progress to the upper limbs (Bodian, 1952). If Lesley's experience followed this pattern, she most likely first experienced paralysis of her legs, and then possibly paralysis or impaired movement of her left arm, while her right arm appears relatively unaffected (Sabin & Ward, 1941; Robertson et al., 1994).

If Leslie contracted the disease between 12 and 16 years of age, then she survived the virus for a minimum of 2 years and a maximum of 8 years. Depending on her immunocapacity, she would likely have recovered from the virus itself within 3 months to 1 year, since longer periods tend to see the poliovirus spread into the lungs which would have proven fatal (Bodian, 1952; Gordon, 1941; Sabin & Ward, 1941; Smallman-Raynor et al., 2006). Quick recovery might also explain the very minor limb length discrepancy as any disruption to development caused by disease would have been relatively brief. The result of the disease would have been permanent paraplegia most likely from Lesley's early to mid-teens up to her death (Bodian, 1952; Hargreaves, 1948). To an observer Lesley would have appeared to have a common cold that progressed into a severe illness, accompanied by a loss of control over voluntary movement that ultimately became an established paraplegia.

Cerebral Palsy: Onset from Birth

As stated earlier, cerebral palsy is used as an "umbrella term" for motor and developmental dysfunctions, and it manifests itself differently from person to person depending on which parts of the brain were deprived of oxygen or damaged in utero (Koman et al., 2004; Krigger, 2006). The extent of damage to the brain can also result in variation of the severity of this condition. Finally, as an individual develops from infancy into childhood, their condition can improve or deteriorate and multiple disorders may emerge (Krigger, 2006).

If the diagnosis of cerebral palsy is correct, Lesley's condition would have been apparent soon after birth, with signs of impairment in her motor (and possibly mental) functions manifesting within the first year of life (Krigger, 2006). It is possible that she was paraplegic for her entire life; however, paraplegia as a result of cerebral palsy tends to develop over time, because the condition produces increasing muscle imbalance across the joints and this affects motor skills (Koman et al., 2004; Krigger, 2006, p. 2021). It is possible that she may have had a motor impairment in early childhood that later developed into paraplegia. A complication of cerebral palsy is urinary incontinence which effects 23–25 % of cases (Krigger, 2006, p. 91). If Lesley experienced these complications, it would have emphasized her difference as she grew out of infancy. It is impossible to know at what age limb asymmetry first became apparent, and whether limb length discrepancy was present from birth or whether it was the product of a period of growth disruption affecting only one side of her body. However, the slightness indicates that growth was only halted for a short period. Once she began to develop the calcaneo-cavo valgus deformity of her left foot, causing her to have a “toe walking” or “crouched gait” posture, she would have been visibly different from others (Koman et al., 2004). The effect cerebral palsy had on her sciatic notch and sacrum indicates that giving birth, walking, and possibly even sitting would have been very difficult. Thus, Lesley would have appeared as a motor impaired infant who became increasingly less mobile and eventually paraplegic as she grew older.

Step 3: Identifying a “Model of Care”

In this step, there are two complications inherent in a differential diagnosis with multiple possible pathologies. First, there is the difficulty in discussing the type of care needed and how it is provided, since regardless of similarity in terms of pathological impact on bone, disease complications and their expressions may vary widely. Second, if it is not possible to determine the subject’s age at pathological onset, which is the case in this study, then constructing a possible history of care provision along with age-appropriate forms of care is challenging.

This study addressed these issues by constructing a model of care for each pathology independently of the other. While this creates two hypothetical care models that in some ways overlap, it also allows for the full exploration of the range of care responses necessary for each pathology. This study also considered multiple possibilities based on the different ages that the pathology could have affected the individual.

Paralytic Poliomyelitis: Short-Term Intensive Care and Long-Term Accommodation

Paralytic poliomyelitis requires two phases of healthcare: intense short-term care that typically develops into long-term accommodation. During the acute phase of disease the patient needs to be given nourishment and kept hydrated. The health status of the patient needs to be continuously monitored, and body temperature needs to be managed to counteract high fever (Smallman-Raynor & Cliff, 2006). Postural adjustments may be necessary to prevent development of bedsores and/or to facilitate the healing of these. Muscle massages can alleviate pain from muscle spasms, prevent muscle atrophy, and prevent the tearing of tendons (Smallman-Raynor & Cliff, 2006). In cases of extreme difficulty in swallowing or throat paralysis, the patient needs assistance with eating and drinking to prevent choking (Ebnezar, 2003; Smallman-Raynor & Cliff, 2006).

After surviving the acute phase of paralytic poliomyelitis, the patient may require the ongoing provision of sustenance, facilitated access to household and daily use items, and possible help with personal hygiene. If Lesley had contracted paralytic poliomyelitis, she would have been transformed from a fully functioning individual into one who was paralyzed from the waist down. She would also have needed short-term intensive care during the initial stages of the disease, followed by long-term accommodation afterwards.

In the immediate stages of poliomyelitis, the virus causes extreme fever, nausea, and paralysis. During this period, Lesley would have required intensive care in the form of temperature control, provision of food and water, and posture adjustment along with hygiene maintenance. Lesley may also have needed assistance with ingesting food and water, with possible limb massages and postural manipulation to counter the impacts of muscle spasms and to avoid pressure sores. This care could have been provided by multiple individuals sharing tasks and responsibilities, or equally by one or two individuals devoted to temporary intensive care. Both options would require substantial investments of time and resources, either by those providing care and/or by those supporting them in this task.

Although left with paraplegia following recovery from the virus, Lesley may still have been capable of providing for her basic needs. Entheseal activity visible on the radii, ulnae, and clavicles suggests that she was using her arms extensively in the period before her death. It is possible that Lesley was moving within her domestic setting and even around the immediate village confines. Despite postulating this level of independent mobility, she may still have needed continued assistance with postural adjustments and managing the full range of hygiene requirements (from toileting, through maintaining bodily cleanliness, to provision of clean clothing and a clean sleeping and living environment). Similarly, it is unlikely that she would have been able to gather food from the agricultural fields surrounding the area on her own, resulting in the need for food provisioning. On the other hand, she may have been able to prepare her own meals so long as the means for doing so were placed within reach. The life-changing results of poliomyelitis would have been dramatic and required Lesley to make considerable adjustments to her expectations of life and likely to her very perception of aspects of self. The complications of disease may have affected her dental health, possibly altering other aspects of her personhood such as appearance and smell. Thinking about her status and habitus in life, she would be a quite different person before and after contracting paralytic poliomyelitis. Adjustment to and acceptance of her new personhood may have been an important element of the caregiving she received.

The care required by Lesley in order to manage the long-term impacts resulting from poliomyelitis might include hands-on "direct support" (such as physical therapies and help with hygiene maintenance), but would certainly include adoption of everyday strategies to accommodate her wants and needs by those in her community. This accommodation would likely require very little alteration to the normal daily practices of most community members, but would probably place a greater demand on close family members.

Cerebral Palsy: Long-Term Care and Accommodation

Cerebral palsy is an ongoing neuromuscular condition present from birth. Due to the variability in disease impact, the care required will differ in accordance with the severity of the condition. As previously noted, if paraplegia is an outcome of cerebral palsy, then onset may be gradual. During this process the patient may progressively require assistance in walking, through the use of a walking stick or crutch. Once paraplegia is established, it is probable that the patient will require the same model of care as that canvassed above in relation to the long-term care (accommodation) for paraplegia resulting from paralytic poliomyelitis.

However, the Lesley born with cerebral palsy would have had a very different experience of life (and disease) to the Lesley who contracted polio around her early teens. There are some important differences in aspects of the care likely to be required in response to the impacts of cerebral palsy, and these are briefly raised here and in the following section.

If Lesley did have cerebral palsy, she may have begun to require care additional to standard parental nurturing a few months after her birth, with need for special attention becoming more apparent with delay or failure in achieving early developmental milestones. The skeletal evidence suggests she suffered from a severe version of cerebral palsy, which may have resulted in paraplegia early in life. She may never have been able to walk or crawl. She would likely have required an intensification of caregiving as her condition deteriorated, but this need would probably plateau if her condition stabilized. At this stage, care may then have consolidated into "care as accommodation" once Lesley had learned to negotiate around the functional limitations resulting from her disease.

It was hypothesized earlier that the care offered to the Lesley paralyzed following a brief period of acute illness would require the community to make a conceptual adjustment to one member's disability. The Lesley with cerebral palsy would be "different" to her peers in functioning capability and physical appearance from early infancy onwards, and so her condition would not suddenly pose a challenge for her family and community. The behavior of caring for Lesley was likely an integral part of her growing up within the community, and accommodation of her needs was likely automatic by the time paralysis became complete.

Step 4: Care and Agency

Tell Abraq was a primary trading center for the Magan, providing goods for trade and possibly generating surplus, which may have lessened any economic burden involved in caring for Lesley (Potts, 2000b). While there has been some exploration of who the people living at Tell Abraq were, because of the great antiquity of the site there is no cultural continuity with people living in the region today (Potts, 2000b). The Bronze Age is not well understood in terms of basic demographic configurations or in terms of cultural lifestyle and ideology. Therefore we can only try to provide the most basic assessment for each scenario of what care might have comprised. Generating information on individual personhood and agency is likewise very challenging.

Paralytic Poliomyelitis

In the case of paralytic poliomyelitis, Lesley would have transformed from a fully functioning young teenager into an individual who was paralyzed from the waist down around age 15. As mentioned previously, the paralytic form of the poliovirus causes extreme fever, nausea, and paralysis during which the patient requires intensive care. Lesley would have needed care during the period in which she contracted the virus in the form of temperature control, provision of food and water, posture adjustment, and hygiene maintenance. She may also have needed care in the form of assisted swallowing and limb massages to alleviate pain from muscle spasms. This model of care could be provided by multiple individuals sharing the responsibility evenly to lessen the burden or by one individual devoted to intensive care. Either provision model would require substantial consideration in time and resources for the duration of the paralytic poliomyelitis by the individual or individuals providing care.

The paralysis as a result of paralytic poliomyelitis would have required a less intensive and long-term accommodation. After recovering from the virus, Lesley's paraplegia would not have left her incapable of providing for her basic needs. The inflammation of the entheses on the humeri, radii, ulnae, and clavicles suggests that she was extensively using her arms before she died. This indicates that Lesley may have been using her arms to move about in her daily life. She may have been able to cook and prepare her own meals provided that materials were placed within reach. She may have also needed assistance with posture adjustments and hygiene maintenance; however, it would have been possible for her to readjust her position and cleanse herself without assistance. This model of care suggests that accommodation could be provided by several individuals in the community with slight alteration of their normal daily practices.

Cerebral Palsy

The care model for cerebral palsy would require an ongoing commitment to Lesley's care from birth, with possible intensification as her condition developed. Lesley's skeletal pathologies indicate the possibility that she contracted the disease at birth and that it resulted in paraplegia early in her life. While some caretaking beyond what is normally provided for children may have been necessary, it is also possible that she may also have grown to be more or less independent as time passed. Lesley's condition would have been apparent within the first year of life (Koman et al., 2004; Krigger, 2006). The model of care suggests that a single individual could have provided care for Lesley, or several individuals could have shared the task among themselves to create a less intensive care model. Parents and siblings could easily accommodate taking care of a child with cerebral palsy.

Mortuary Context and Special Treatment

Lesley's placement in the tomb was unique in that she is the only fully articulated individual. She was placed in the passageway directly in front of the doorway. Carbon dating on Lesley suggests that she was placed into the tomb towards the end of its usage (circa 2000 BC). This could suggest that she was among the last individuals placed in the tomb, accounting for her placement at the entrance. Martin and Potts (2012) suggest that Lesley may have been wrapped or bound in an organic material, such as cloth or hide, which kept her remains from commingling with the rest of the tomb's commingled skeletons. Small pieces of flax linen were found in the tomb, but they could not be associated with any individual(s) due to poor preservation (Reade & Potts, 1993). Thus Lesley may have received unique treatment that both placed her within the communal tomb, but that kept her separate from the rest of the deceased. The reasons for this are pure speculation, but there is no doubt that she was accorded special treatment that may reflect her unique status within the community.

Conclusions

A bioarchaeology of care analysis is challenging when differential diagnosis is unable to rule out more than one possible disease. In examining how to approach this problem, the authors applied the Index of Care to the case of a young female with a lower limb paralysis most likely resulting from one of two conditions. The authors create parallel interpretations through the construction of two care models, providing a basis for strong inference regarding the experience of paralysis. This is a much more satisfying conclusion than all previous speculations. While this leads to alternative interpretations of past agency, the process illustrates how the characteristics of different diseases have different implications for thinking about the necessities of care. Different diseases can have comparable impacts on function, as seen here, so that elements of the care required will be similar.

This study deviated from the original Index of Care methodology during the third step, where care provisioning and agency of care are examined. For the third step this study noted two complications when multiple pathologies are equally likely: a difficulty in discussing care provision and a difficulty in constructing a care model when it is unclear how, and for what duration, the pathology affected the individual. This study addressed these by creating two care models and exploring how these would vary based on the age of onset. Despite the two diagnoses, the utilization of the Index of Care enabled us to provide a more robust interpretation regarding Lesley's experience of illness and offered two alternative hypotheses. It is possible that as stable isotope, radiocarbon dating, and other analyses are performed on the collection of which Lesley is a part, one of the alternative diagnoses may be ruled out.

References

Baustian, K. (2005). *Health status of infants and children from the bronze age tomb at tell Abraq, United Arab Emirates*. Las Vegas: University of Nevada, Las Vegas.

Bodian, D. (1952). Pathogenesis of poliomyelitis. *American Journal of Public Health, 42*, 1388–1402.

Buikstra, J. E., & Ubelaker, D. H. (1994). *Standards for data collection from human skeletal remains*. Research Series, no. 44. Fayetteville, AR: Arkansas Archaeological Survey.

Cleuziou, S. (2009). Extracting wealth from a land of starvation by creating social complexity: A dialogue between archaeology and climate? *Comptes Rendus—Géoscience, 341*(8), 726–738. doi:10.1016/j.crte.2009.06.005.

Colonna, P. C., & Vom Saal, F. (1941). A study of paralytic scoliosis based on five hundred cases of poliomyelitis. *Journal of Bone Joint Surgery, 23*, 335–353.

Ebnezar, J. (2003). *Essentials of orthopaedics for physiotherapist*. New Delhi: Jaypee Brothers Medical Publishers.

Gawne, A. C., & Halstead, L. S. (1995). Post-polio syndrome: Pathophysiology and clinical management. *Critical Reviews in Physical and Rehabilitation Medicine, 7*, 147–188.

Gordon, J. (1941). Constitutional types and susceptibility to paralysis in poliomyelitis. Preventative medicine and epidemiology. *Preventative Medicine and Epidemiology*, 456–468.

Gregoricka, L. (2013). Residential mobility and social identity in the periphery: Strontium isotope analysis of archaeological tooth and enamel from southeastern Arabia. *Journal of Archaeological Science, 40*, 452–464.

Haberle, C. B., Van Stewart, A., Staat, R. H., Gettleman, L., & Sleamaker, T. F. (2001). Special considerations for treating dental patients exhibiting the 'Post-polio Syndrome'. *Special Care Dentist, 32*(1), 167–171.

Hargreaves, E. R. (1948). Poliomyelitis: Effect of exertion during the pre-paralytic stage. *British Medical Journal, 2*(4588), 1021–1022.

Jesus, N. H. (2007). Epidemics to eradication: The modern history of poliomyelitis. *Virology Journal, 4*(70).

Koman, A. (2004). Cerebral palsy. *The Lancet, 363*, 1619–1631.

Krigger, K. (2006). Cerebral palsy: An overview. *American Family Physician, 73*(1), 91–100.

Magee, P. (1996). Excavations at Muweilah. Preliminary report on the first two seasons. *Arabian Archaeology and Epigraphy, 7*, 195–213.

Martin, D., & Potts, D. (2012). Lesley: A unique bronze age individual from southeastern Arabia. In A. L. W. Stodder & A. M. Palkovich (Eds.), *The bioarchaeology of individuals* (pp. 113–126). Gainsville: University Press of Florida.

Minor, P. D. (2012). The polio-eradication programme and issues of the end games. *Journal of General Virology, 93*, 457–474.

Novak, M., Cavka, M., & Slaus, M. (2014). Two cases of neurogenic paralysis in medieval skeletal samples from Croatia. *International Journal of Paleopathology, 7*, 25–32.

Ortner, D., & Putschar, W. (1981). *Identification of pathological conditions of human skeletal remains*. San Diego, CA: Academic.

Osterholtz, A. J., Baustian, K. M., Martin, D. L., & Potts, D. T. (2014). Commingled human skeletal assemblages: Integrative techniques in determination of the MNI/MNE. In A. J. Osterholtz, K. M. Baustian, & D. L. Martin (Eds.), *Commingled and disarticulated human remains: Working toward improved theory, method, and data* (pp. 35–50). New York: Springer.

Potts, D. T. (1990). *A prehistoric mound in the Emirate of Umm al-Qauwain: Exavations at Tell Abraq in 1989*. Copenhagen: Munksgaard.
Potts, D. T. (2009). The archaeology and early story of the Persian Gulf. In L. Potter (Ed.), *The Persian Gulf in History* (p. 2753). New York: Pallgrave Macmillan.
Potts, D. T. (2012). *In the land of the Emirates: The archaeology and history of the UAE*. London: Trident Press.
Potts, D. (2000a). Arabian time capsule. *Archaeology, 53*(5), 44–48.
Potts, D. (2000b). *Ancient magan: The secrets of tell Abraq. United Arab Emirates*. London: Trident Press.
Potts, D. (2001). Before the emirates: An archaeological and historical account of developments in the region c. 5000 BC to 679 AD. *Perspectives on the United Arab Emirates*, 28–69.
Reade, W. J., & Potts, D. T. (1993). New evidence for late third millennium linen from Tell Abraq, Umm Al-Qaiwain, UAE. *Paléorient, 19*, 99–106.
Robertson, S. E., Suleiman, A. J., Mehta, F. R., Al-Dhahry, S. H., & El-Bualy, M. S. (1994). Poliomyelitis in Oman: Acute flaccid paralysis surveillance leading to early detection and rapid response to a type 3 outbreak. *Bulletin of the World Health Organization, 72*(6), 907.
Sabin, A. B., & Ward, R. (1941). The natural history of human poliomyelitis: I. Distribution of virus in nervous and non-nervous tissues. *Journal of Experimental Medicine, 73*, 771–793.
Smallman-Raynor, M. R., Cliff, A. D., Trevelyan, B., Nettleton, C., & Sneddon, S. (2006). Poliomyelitis. A world geography: Emergence to eradication. Oxford: Oxford University Press.
Tayles, N., Domett, K., & Nelson, K. (2000). Agriculture and dental caries? The case of rice in prehistoric southeast Asia. *World Archaeology, 32*(1), 68–83.
Thylstrup, A. (1994). *Textbook of clinical cariology*. Copenhagen: Munksgaard.
Tilley, L., & Cameron, T. (2014). Introducing the index of care: A web-based application supporting archaeological research into health-related care. *International Journal of Paleopathology, 6*, 5–9.
Uerpmann, M. (2001). Remarks on the animal economy of tell Abraq (Emirates of Sharjah and Umm al-Qaywan, UAE). *Proceedings of the Seminar for Arabian Studies, 31*, 227–233.
White, T. D., Black, M. T., & Folkens, P. A. (2012). *Human osteology*. San Francisco: Elsevier Academic Press.
World Health Organization. (2014). *Poliomyelitis: Fact sheet Ndegree114*.
Young, G. R. (1989). Occupational therapy and the postpolio syndrome. *American Journal of Occupational Therapy, 43*, 97–103.

Chapter 4
Cared for or Outcasts: A Case for Continuous Care in the Precontact U.S. Southwest

Alyssa Y. Willett and Ryan P. Harrod

Human remains with evidence of severe traumatic injuries or other debilitating pathological conditions that limit mobility and decrease self-sufficiency logically lead to the discussion of whether or not somebody cared for this individual. Some researchers have argued (DeGusta, 2002; Dettwyler, 1991) that bioarchaeologists cannot identify care from skeletal remains because survival does not always necessarily indicate an individual received a significant amount of assistance from other individuals. The onus is on the researcher to go beyond the physical evidence of a healed fracture or lesion and gather additional evidence to identify if an injured person received care in the form of assisted healing and provisioning. Chapter 2 of this volume describes the bioarchaeology of care approach, which lists a series of analytical stages that researchers can work through to help determine whether there is evidence of care.

Stage 1 of the bioarchaeology of care approach involves the osteological description of the human skeletal remains; identification and differential diagnosis of the pathological conditions; and a detailed reconstruction of the cultural, social, economic, environmental, and mortuary context. Stage 2 promotes the use of clinical literature to determine if the pathological condition was sufficient to have caused either permanent or temporary disability. Establishing whether the individual was disabled (see Chap. 2 for a description of disability) is crucial for suggesting the individual required care. Stage 3 of analysis is where a researcher describes what other people, and the individual themselves, would have needed to do to facilitate the process of healing. Stage 4 attempts to reconstruct the individual's identity and how they would have been perceived by, and interacted with, the rest of the community. This final stage of analysis relies on the detailed descriptions provided about the individual, the pathological condition, and the approach to care identified in the first three stages. Taken together the four stages assist with the reconstruction of

A.Y. Willett (✉) • R.P. Harrod, Ph.D.
Department of Anthropology, University of Alaska Anchorage, Anchorage, AK, USA
e-mail: aywillett@alaska.edu

© Springer International Publishing Switzerland 2017
L. Tilley, A.A. Schrenk (eds.), *New Developments in the Bioarchaeology of Care*, Bioarchaeology and Social Theory, DOI 10.1007/978-3-319-39901-0_4

how the person's daily life would have been affected by the injuries and associated disability, both in the short and long term.

In 2014, Tilley and Cameron developed a web-based program called the Index of Care to provide researchers with a tool that walks them through the four stages of the bioarchaeology of care approach. In this chapter we used the Index of Care to examine whether or not care was necessary for the survival of a woman living in the precontact U.S. Southwest, who had osteological evidence of a severe traumatic injury.

Possible Disability and Care in the Precontact U.S. Southwest

The U.S. Southwest offers an excellent case study because it is characterized by fluctuating weather conditions, environmental hazards with residential areas that are difficult to navigate, and frequent nutritional concerns associated with an agrarian diet in an arid landscape (Dozier, 1970). Thus a severe injury acquired by an individual living here nearly a thousand years ago can tell us a great deal about how they were able to operate, given their particular disability, within this particular cultural and environmental context.

There are a number of cultures identified in the U.S. Southwest, but the focus of this chapter is on the Ancestral Pueblo living in northern New Mexico (Fig. 4.1).

The individual we chose to assess using the Index of Care was represented by a set of human skeletal remains recovered from the site known as Aztec Ruins. Located in northern New Mexico, Aztec Ruins consists of three village sites named West Ruin, East Ruin, and North Ruin that were occupied between *circa* A.D.

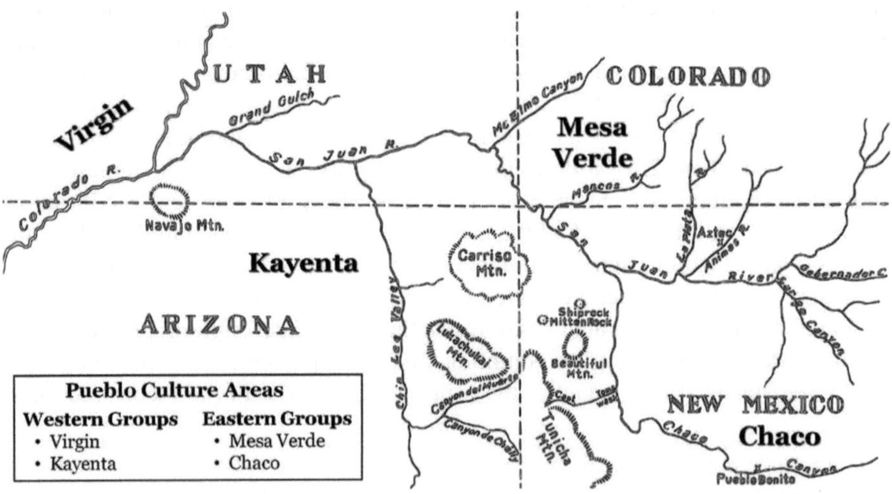

Fig. 4.1 Culture areas of the ancestral Pueblo. Adapted from Morris (1927, p. 134) and previously used in (Harrod, 2013, p. 34)

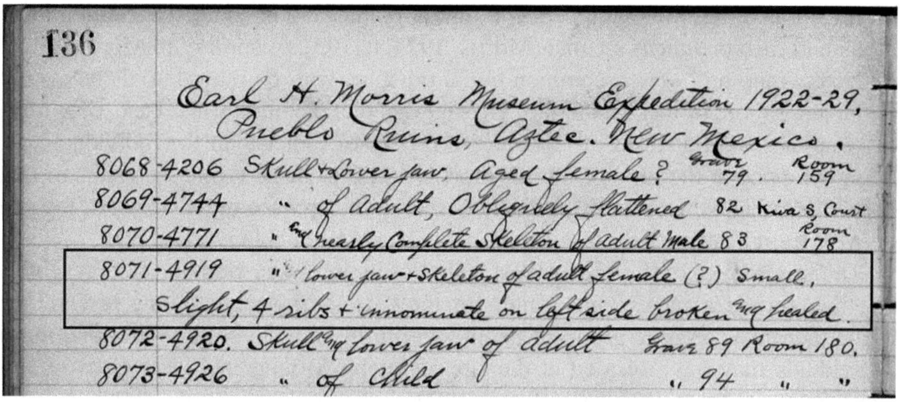
136
Earl H. Morris Museum Expedition 1922-29,
Pueblo Ruins, Aztec. New Mexico.
8068-4206 Skull+lower jaw, aged female? Grave 79. Room 159
8069-4744 " of adult, Obliquely flattened 82 Kiva 8, Court
8070-4771 " " nearly complete skeleton of adult male 83 Room 178
8071-4919 " lower jaw+skeleton of adult female (?) Small, slight, 4 ribs + innominate on left side broken & healed.
8072-4920. Skull & lower jaw of adult Grave 89 Room 180.
8073-4926 " of Child " 94 " "

Fig. 4.2 Notes about catalog number 99/8071 at Aztec Ruins. Courtesy of the Division of Anthropology, American Museum of Natural History

1100–1290 (Brown, Windes, & McKenna, 2008). The human remains were recovered from West Ruin between 1916 and 1922 and later curated at the American Museum of Natural History (AMNH) by Earl Morris (Lister & Lister, 1990). Cataloged as 99/8071 in the AMNH collection, the original notes about this burial (Fig. 4.2) do not list the grave and room numbers (as they do for other burials listed in the catalog).

Harrod (2013) used Morris's detailed description of the traumatic injuries to determine which, of the nearly two hundred burials described by Morris, this individual represented.

> *The eighth, ninth, tenth, and eleventh ribs on the left side had been broken about 2½ inches from their articulations with the vertebrae. These fractures had completely healed. The left innominatum had also been broken, the pubis having been driven somewhat forward from its normal position. In this case healing was not so thorough, and marked exostoses were present along the edges of the severed bone.* (Morris, 1924, p. 196)

The severe injuries described by Morris match the injuries Harrod (2013) found on the human remains cataloged as 99/8071 at AMNH, which suggests that the individual selected as a case study for the Index of Care is the individual known to Morris as "Burial 88."

Burial 88

Morris (1924) recovered Burial 88 from a room in the northern wing of West Ruin at Aztec Ruins buried below 20 in. of refuse composed of corncobs, ash, and wood debris (Morris, 1924, p. 195). His initial assessment suggested that these were the remains of a probable female. Interred in Room 182, she was found in the flexed position on her left side facing the east wall (Morris, 1924, p. 195). While no grave goods are mentioned, she was wrapped in a turkey feather cloth, some sort of additional cloth, and rush or *Juncus sp.* mat (Morris, 1924, p. 195). According to Morris (1924, p. 223), wrappings were a common burial practice, with 66 other burials recovered with one or more of these materials. He suggests that the burials that lack some form of wrapping were a result of taphonomic processes rather than the individuals not being wrapped at the time of burial (Morris, 1924, p. 223). While the status of this particular burial is not readily apparent based on the archaeological context, the site of West Ruin itself is fairly significant in the Ancestral Pueblo world.

The importance of the site of West Ruin lies in the suggestion that it represents a site that served as a regional center for the Ancestral Pueblo. Some researchers argue there was an elite group of people within the Pueblo culture, and that these individuals may have resided at the site of Pueblo Bonito in Chaco Canyon and West Ruin at Aztec Ruins (LeBlanc, 1999; Lekson, 1999, 2006, 2009; Wilcox, 1993, 2004). One hypothesis is that West Ruin seems to develop as a possible replacement for Pueblo Bonito as Pueblo Bonito begins to decline (Brown et al., 2008; Harrod, 2012; Lekson, 1999). Based on ceramic typology (Morris, 1924), which is supported by more recent dendrochronology (Brown et al., 2008), the primary occupation at West Ruin was in the A.D. 1200s, which is well after the height of occupation at Pueblo Bonito. Support for a temporal connection between the sites at Aztec Ruins and those in Chaco Canyon is based on similarities in the overall size of the sites, the architectural design, the material culture, and the alignment to cosmological and cardinal orientations (Judge, 1989; Lister & Lister, 1987; Munro & Malville, 2011; Stein & McKenna, 1988; Toll, 2008; Van Dyke, 2009).

Constructing a basic biological profile for Burial 88 using standard osteological techniques indicates she is a woman in her mid to late thirties (30–35 years old). Sex was assigned using anatomical features of the pubis (Phenice, 1969), the ilium (White, Folkens, & Black, 2012), and different regions of the cranium and mandible (Buikstra & Ubelaker, 1994), while estimation of age was based on morphological changes to the pubic synthesis (Brooks & Suchey, 1990; Todd, 1920) and auricular surface (Buckberry & Chamberlain, 2002; Lovejoy, Meindl, Pryzbeck, & Mensforth, 1985), and to a lesser extent the fusion of the cranial sutures (Mann, Jantz, Bass, & Willey, 1991; Meindl & Lovejoy, 1985).

As mentioned by Morris (1924), Burial 88 has a number of traumatic injuries on her body (see Fig. 4.3). Cranial injuries included a slight nasal fracture and antemortem tooth loss that may or may not have been trauma related. Postcranial injuries included a fractured pelvis and multiple broken ribs on both sides of the body (8th–11th ribs on the left and 2nd rib on the right). Additionally, there were morphological changes to some of the bones, including torsion or anteversion of the left femur and atrophy of the right clavicle, which may have traumatic etiology.

In a prior study, Harrod and Martin (2014) highlighted the injuries found on Burial 88 and an adult male from the same site displaying complete fusion of T12-L1 vertebra, moderate atrophy of the left humerus, and fractured left 2nd and 3rd ribs to discuss the possibility of captives, or at least of low status individuals, at Aztec Ruins. They compared the trauma found on these two individuals to the injuries found on women from a nearby site in the La Plata River Valley in northern New Mexico, who Martin (1997; 2008) argued were captives in a system of regional raiding.

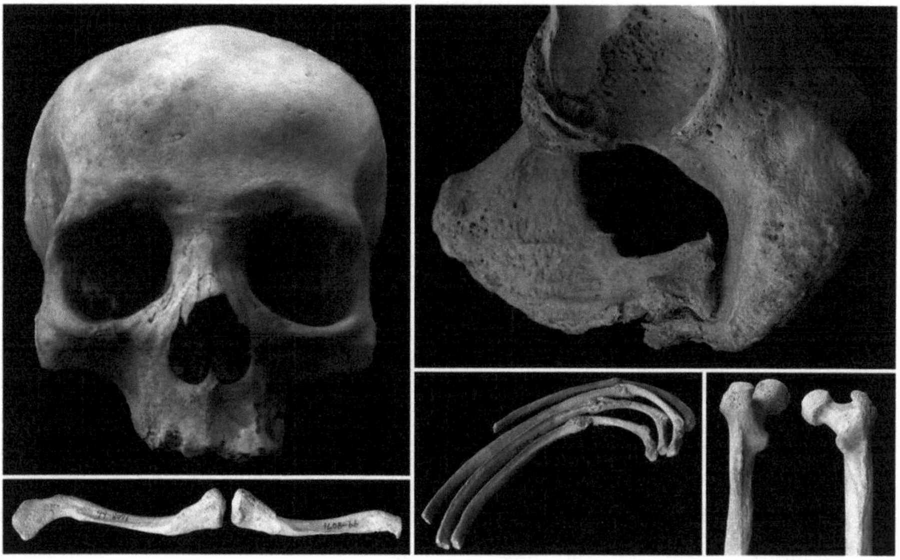

Fig. 4.3 Young female identified as Burial 88 from Aztec Ruins. *Top left*: cranium; *top right*: left *os* coxae; *bottom left*: left and right clavicle; *bottom middle*: left ribs; proximal left and right femur. Photo of the cranium (*top left*) taken by Avery Underwood, other photos taken by Ryan Harrod

The possibility of captivity in relation to the individuals from West Ruin was proposed because of the well-documented warfare in the region during the occupation at Aztec Ruins (Billman, Lambert, & Leonard, 2000; Haas & Creamer, 1996), and demographic research has suggested there are more women than expected at the site (Kohler & Kramer, 2006). The problem with regard to interpreting the status of Burial 88 is that there is insufficient context to definitively identify the cause of the cranial trauma. What is clear is that the postcranial trauma to the pelvis is unlikely to be a result of violence, and the left rib fractures are probably related to the pelvic trauma. Similar to the findings of Chap. 5 (this volume), the pelvic injuries are more consistent with an accidental injury (e.g., a fall). The cranial trauma and the fracture of the right 2nd rib and atrophy of the clavicle may be the result of a separate traumatic event, which could mean a pattern of repeated injury or injury recidivism.

The reality, however, is that even if we accept that this woman was a captive or subordinate member of the community this does not necessarily negate the possibility that she was cared for by other people at Aztec Ruins. Ethnographic and archaeological research suggests that the identity of being a "captive" can be liminal, and a person can transition from being a captive outsider to a community member over their lifetime (Cameron, 2011). Citing ethnographic data collected by Halbmayer (2001, 2004), who was working with the Yukpa, and Tooker (1962), who was working with the Huron, Harrod and Martin (2015) show examples where captives are eventually incorporated into the group as seemingly equal members of the society. Thus, regardless of the motivations behind the traumatic injury, the fact that the woman's most severe injuries (e.g., pelvic fractures) were well healed speaks to the presence of care.

Pelvic Trauma

The pelvic girdle forms a ring as the *os coxae* connect anteriorly at the pubic symphysis where the two pubic bones meet and posteriorly where the *os coxae* and sacrum meet at the sacroiliac joints (SIJ). Ligaments hold the entire pelvic ring together, and the interosseous sacroiliac ligaments associated with the posterior ring are crucial for maintaining pelvic stability (Tile, 1988, p. 2). Given the complex biomechanics associated with the pelvic girdle these fractures are some of the most challenging injuries to diagnose, but classification is the first step in planning the most successful treatment of a pelvic injury.

The classification of fractures types is based on the location, stability, mechanism of injury, integrity of the posterior sacroiliac complex, and degree of disruption (A = stable, B = rotationally unstable, and C = vertically and rotationally unstable) (Prevezas et al., 2009; Ruatti et al., 2015; Tile, 1988). Young and Burgess (1987) expanded on the classification system by adding more descriptions of compressive forces and a new category called Combined Mechanical Injury (CM), used when the injuries do not fit the original categories. The identification of the exact type of pelvic ring fracture on skeletonized human remains is problematic, because the mechanism of injury is unknown and soft tissue is not present. Báez-Molgado, Bartelink, Jellema, Spurlock, and Sholts (2015) discuss these limitations in a recent forensic article, and suggest that certain changes on the pelvis can be useful for identifying the classification type.

The recorded pelvic injuries on Burial 88 indicate she suffered a high impact injury that severely fractured her pelvis and may have resulted in some of the other postcranial injuries (Figs. 4.4 and 4.5). For example, clinical literature suggests rib fractures correlate with high-energy trauma, which might explain the fractures to ribs 8–11 on the left side. The pelvis was fractured at the ischiopubic ramus, the acetabulum, and the ischial spine. Additionally, there was fusion of the sacroiliac joint with osteophytic growth, which elevates the pelvic ring fracture classification from type A to type B (Tile, 1988).

Together these injuries are a classic example of a pelvic ring fracture where the integrity of structure is compromised (Stimson, 1899, p. 290). The injury may be elevated further from type B to type C because of the trauma to the ischial spine. We conservatively identified it as a type B fracture with the malunion at the ischiopubic ramus because we cannot determine if the ischial spine injury happened at the time of the initial trauma or as a result of subsequent insult (Tile, 1988; Young & Burgess, 1987). One caveat to consider is that if the ischial spine was injured at the same time as the rest of the pelvic ring it would have likely caused pelvic floor disruption and have been associated with puncture of viscera (i.e., bladder and nerve entrapment). This is due to the loss of integrity of the sacrospinous ligament, which inserts into the lateral border of the sacrum and attaches to the ischial spine (Fig. 4.6).

Associated with the pelvic ring fracture there was also an acetabular fracture and morphological changes to the femur. The acetabular fracture (see Fig. 4.4) on Burial 88 is characterized as an anterior wall fracture on the left *os coxae*, which occurs

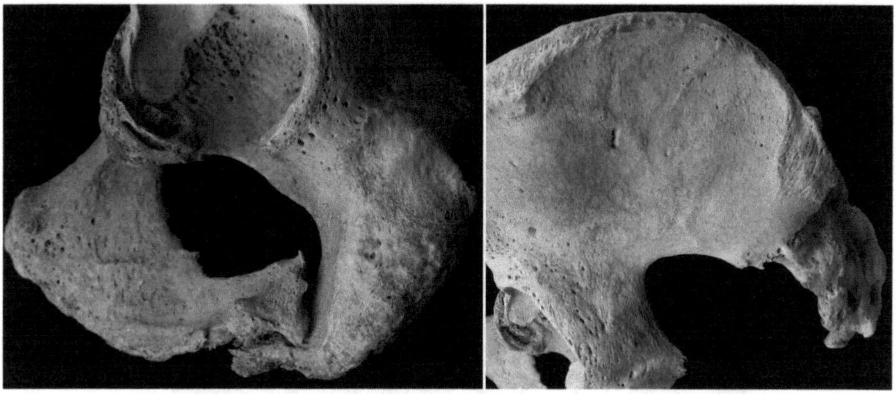

Fig. 4.4 Fractured left *os* coxae. Photos taken by Ryan Harrod

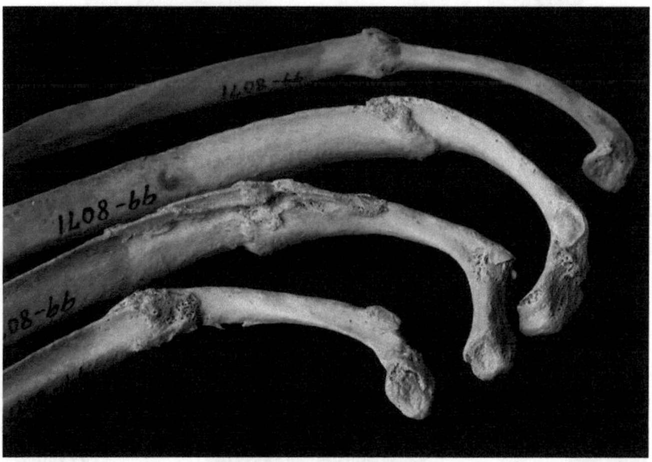

Fig. 4.5 Fractured left ribs 8–11. Photos taken by Ryan Harrod

less often than the posterior wall fracture (Letournel, 1970, 1980). On the same side of the body there was notable femoral anteversion or torsion of the femur (Fig. 4.7).

Femoral anteversion may be important for determining the age at when the fractures occurred, as research indicates that the morphological change of the axis of the femoral neck to the axis of the knee rapidly shifts between 12 and 16 years of age (Cibulka, 2004, p. 550; Gulan, Matovinović, Nemec, Rubinić, & Ravlić-Gulan, 2000, p. 523; Mudge et al., 2014, p. 23). Given the fracture pattern, involvement of the acetabulum, and femoral torsion, we suggest that Burial 88 may have still been growing when the injury occurred. According to Djukic, Milenkovic, Milovanovic, Dakic, and Djuric (2014, p. 300), problems with the biomechanics of the pelvis and femur during development can alter the femoral neck anteversion. If she injured her pelvis prior to the decrease in the angle between the femoral neck and the knee, then it is

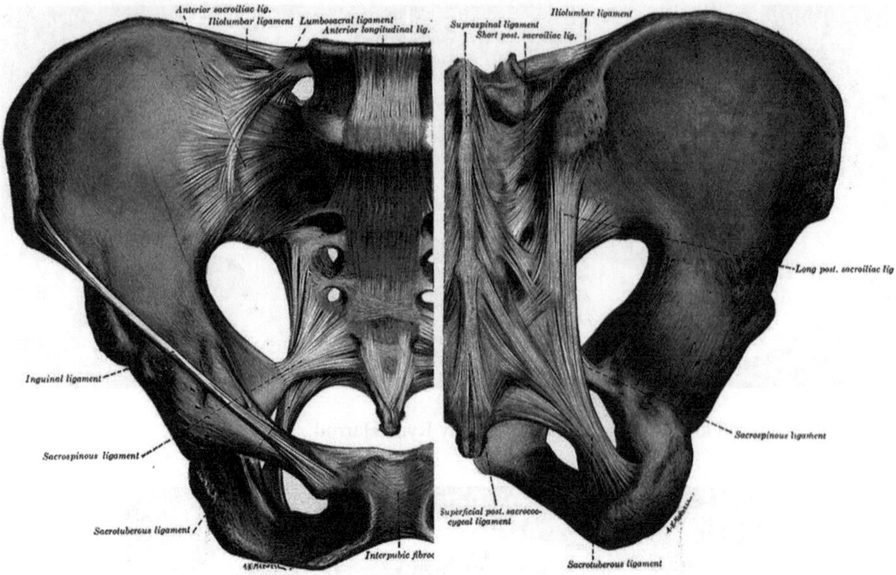

Fig. 4.6 Images of the pelvic ligaments. Compiled illustrations from Gray 1918 (Gray 2000: plate 320 and 321)

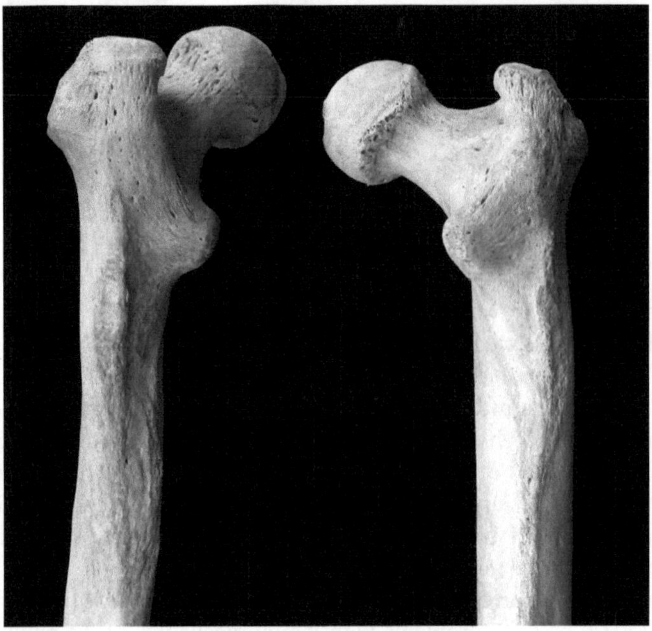

Fig. 4.7 Femoral anteversion (left femur). *Left* (on *left* of image) and right femora, posterior views. Photos taken by Ryan Harrod

possible that the differential use of one of her legs is responsible for the asymmetrical femoral anteversion because of involvement of the triradiate cartilage resulted in changes to the acetabulum which may increase the likelihood of dislocation and subluxation of the femur head. Subbu and Haddad (2015, p. 4) suggest that femur anteversion may be an adaptation to prevent future dislocations.

High-energy pelvic ring injuries like the one found on Burial 88 have numerous detrimental outcomes in residual dysfunction, even when treated with surgery (Vallier, Cureton, Schubeck, & Wang, 2012). Siegmeth, Müllner, Kukla, and Vécsei (2000) note that 47 % of individuals with type B fractures and 84 % of individuals with type C fractures exhibit poor outcomes and chronic pain. Even after being treated, 25 % of patients suffered long-term neurological dysfunction (Siegmeth, Müllner, Kukla, & Vécsei, 2000). There is a 28 % mortality rate for patients with high-energy pelvic ring injuries.

Considering these injuries in relation to the muscles, nerves, and arteries it is clear that multiple anatomical layers were involved, possibly including vital organs and even significant blood loss, all of which would have been associated with pain and disability (see Chap. 2 in this volume for a discussion of disability).

Traditional Care Among the Pueblo

The treatment of broken and dislocated bones by healers not trained in Western schools of medicine is found worldwide, in both industrial and preindustrial cultures, across time (Agarwal & Agarwal, 2010). Capener (1932, p. 1009) suggested that "… empirical methods, good and bad, have been used by bonesetters as long as medicine has existed." There are numerous ethnographic and historical accounts of individuals in preindustrial societies who were specialists at setting bones; these include reports from Africa (Eshete, 2005; Oyebola, 1980; Warren, 1974), Southwest Asia (Hatipoğlu & Tatar, 1995; Pillsbury, 1978), Southern Asia (Panda & Rout, 2015), East Asia (Katada, 1970; Ling, Aimin, Xihe, Xiaoshu, & Cummings, 1996; Yamauchi, 1996), Mesoamerica (Huber, 1990; Paul, 1976), and the U.S. Southwest (Parsons, 1936).

Pueblo Healers

There are also numerous accounts of healers among historic and modern-day Pueblo communities. An early ethnography by Parsons (1936) of Taos pueblo in New Mexico during the 1930s describes the presence of multiple healers among this Pueblo community. She discusses the activities of four healers in the community, one of whom, Lorenzo Martinez, was a "bonesetter" (Parsons, 1936, p. 58). Grant (1982, p. 300), looking at the healers among the Hopi in Arizona, also discusses the importance of being a bonesetter, which he says is evident in the presence of splints and other stabilization devices. The presence of splints is important for considering the possibility of care being provided for Burial 88. A different female recovered from West Ruin by Morris was found with an unhealed fracture of the arm and pelvis, but what was unique about her was the fact that her fracture arm was still splinted when she was found. While Parsons suggests the bonesetter is a specialist focused on body manipulation, Grant says a healer must be able to heal multiple ailments. Leeman (1986), documenting the experiences and community perceptions of healers at Taos in the mid 1980s, found that the specialized healers Parsons (1936) described were not necessarily so specialized. He notes that, based on accounts of Taos residents, the activities of these individuals do vary, and cautions that they were reportedly still engaged in holistic approaches to healing that included the use of body manipulation, herbal remedies, and ceremonial practices. It is crucial to realize that within any community there are likely to be multiple health practitioners, and that while individual caregivers may be better at one type of healing than another, health practitioners are usually trained in many methods.

Having people in the community trained in manual therapies such as massage and manipulation, as well as an expert guiding ingestion and application of medicinal plants, would have been a great benefit to this woman at Aztec Ruins. Clinical data show that simple adjustments, such as wearing a shoe lift to correct leg length discrepancy, wrapping the pelvis, or the use of a cane, can have a tremendous impact on an individual's recovery (Cooper, 2006; Gillespie, 2009; Letournel, 1980). Grant (1982) gives an account of a practiced healer attuned to his client's responses and concerned for his well-being.

> *When a fracture is to be set or sprain manipulated, the healer attempts to distract the client by calmly talking to him then suddenly and very methodically performing the procedure.* (Grant, 1982, p. 302)

This technique enables the practitioner to manipulate the client before he can tense up in anticipation of pain. Once the adjustment is made, the healer uses physical touch and massage to relieve pain, showing open concern for the client (Grant, 1982, p. 302).

Recent chemical analysis of one of the plants native to Aztec Ruins (*Artemisia tridentata*) supports claims that it possesses medicinal properties (Turi, Shipley, & Murch, 2014). This is important, because there is evidence for the use of *Artemisia tridentata*, also known as Basin Brush, that dates from at least 1869 to the present day (Fewkes, 1896). *Artemisia tridentata* is a well-documented and versatile medicinal plant, employed to treat a wide range of ailments from respiratory problems to gastrointestinal issues. It can be ingested, applied topically, or burned as an inhalant, and has been effectively used as an analgesic, anti-inflammatory, antiseptic, immunostimulant; it is also used in spiritual/ceremonial contexts (Rainey & Adams, 2004; Turi et al., 2014). The common plant is an effective insecticide, as well as possessing antimicrobial properties that aid in food preservation (Bora & Sharma, 2011; Turi et al., 2014). In addition, its use has been recorded by Fewkes (1896, p. 17) in "an infusion of its leaves drank by a person whose ailment is supposed to lie in his Ilium."

Two other plants found at Aztec Ruins that have traditionally been seen to have medicinal properties are globe mallow and juniper bark. Globe mallow can be made into a paste for casts, while the leaves may be rubbed on sore muscles and ingested to help heal broken bones (Rainey & Adams, 2004). Moreover, the root may be chewed to ease digestive irregularities. Juniper bark can be used for diapering, making it suitable for wound packing.

Traditional healing practices in bone setting, often involving use of medicinal plants and wrappings to alleviate pain, still persist in many parts of the world. One example of this is the development of the bone setting practice called the *Puttur kattu* by Kadallam Gopal Raju in 1881. A recent article on this type of traditional healing suggests that practitioners see between "200–300 patients per day with various fractures and dislocations" (Panda & Rout, 2015, p. 174).

Management and Care

The clinical literature suggests that in the case of Burial 88 care would have been required and that this would have been on a continuum (Cooper, 2006). Essential care would include emergency management such as controlling blood loss and stabilizing the pelvis. During this time constant monitoring of health status, pain management, infection prevention, and provisioning of food and water would have been required. If the bladder or bowel were impacted, a special diet and extensive help with hygiene would be necessary to control for infection. Special attention to the changing of bandages, sling position, and careful bolstering of the patient would decrease the chance of infection and pain. Pain would almost certainly be persistent, varying in intensity as the injury moved through acute, subacute, and chronic phases. Additionally, level and nature of activity would feed into type and duration of pain (Hessman, Rickert, Hofmann, Rommins, & Buhl, 2010).

Essential Management of Immediate Complications

It is important to note that all of the described sites of trauma in this example are healed. It is difficult to know if these injuries occurred simultaneously or throughout this woman's lifetime; however, ongoing research is attempting to establish a temporal order to the injuries. The fracture with malunion of the pelvis was old enough to have caused a change in the skeletal structure to the femur, and the fractured ribs show callus formation. Of the traumas recorded, the pelvic fracture would be most debilitating.

There are many complications that result from pelvic fractures, and these problems vary in degree of severity depending on whether or not proper treatment is received. The current case study exhibits malunion of the ischiopubic ramus and a lesion on the ischial spine, which indicates that it is likely that this women experienced, at the very least, a pelvic floor disorder, if not a complete disruption (Tile, 1988) (Fig. 4.4).

Baessler, Bircher, and Stanton (2004) found a wide range of pelvic floor dysfunction after pelvic fracture, with development of bladder, bowel, and sexual dysfunction common even in those who did not experience direct injury to urogenital organs at time of trauma. Pelvic floor disorders generally occur when normal anatomy is disrupted (Yount, 2013). Symptoms of pelvic floor disorders include urinary, bowel, and sexual dysfunction. These disorders can have a profound effect on a person's life, leading to social isolation, personal hygiene issues, and alteration of self-perception. Sexual health is associated with many emotional, physical, mental, and cultural factors. Physical evidence of a complete fracture with malunion of the ischiopubic ramus points, at a minimum, to difficulty in giving birth.

Another consideration is how the non-pelvic injuries would have impacted her recovery if they occurred at or around the same time as the pelvic fracture. Pain with inhalation and exhalation from the broken ribs would have further hindered mobility. Inability to inhale and exhale fully would contribute to respiratory infections (de Bruijn, 2015). Her other traumatic injuries may have meant even more difficulty functioning and require adjustments to be made in working and resting positions. Finally, recovery from major trauma often requires more rest and additional calories to heal (Stefanski & Smith, 2006, p. 296).

Instrumental Care of Long-Term Complications

Long-term increased morbidity, disability, or deformity associated with complex pelvic fracture includes bony malunion or nonunion, leg length discrepancy, sitting disturbance, gait disturbance, muscle weakness, disuse osteoporosis, obstetric issues, and chronic pain (Gillespie, 2009, p. 295). The current case study exhibits malunion of the ischiopubic ramus and leg length discrepancy which would lead to the abovementioned complications.

Compromised mobility is evidenced by structural changes to the skeleton in Burial 88. Leg length discrepancy and femoral torsion or internal rotation would have changed gait patterns, perhaps leading to difficulty transferring weight, sitting disturbances, foot drop, and obstetric issues. Ongoing efforts by caretakers would be intended to help the patient regain stability, strength, and mobility. This type of injury requires multiple modalities of care, if not multiple caregivers.

There would be pain with sitting and standing, and rotational instability (Cooper, 2006; Gillespie, 2009). Chronic pain is the most common cause of permanent disability after unstable pelvic fracture. Neurological injuries are a major source of chronic pain complaints, but can be difficult to treat as pain can also be due to chronic instability, malunion, and/or posttraumatic osteoarthritis of the sacral iliac joint (Hessman et al., 2010, p. 128). Burial 88 exhibits all of these complications, so it is highly probable she would have endured ongoing pain.

After surviving the immediate and intermediate phase of trauma, lasting morbidities and disability would become central to Burial 88's daily life. This individual would have dealt with chronic pain, gait change, and possible pelvic floor disorder on a daily basis (Vallier et al., 2012). Each of these complications pose a challenge not only physically, but also emotionally and mentally, unique to a woman within a larger community.

Reconstructing Daily Life

Social roles become more visible when disrupted by conditions such as chronic pain. Today in the USA, cultural and social norms include expectations of objective evidence of specific cause (injury) if pain exists. Improvement is expected when treated with traditional Western medicine (Monsivais, 2013). It is hard to say what sort of expectations a society had in the past, but a human reaction to stigmatized chronic pain may shed light upon behavior. Monsivais (2013) notes a tremendous stigma accompanying someone with chronic pain. Goffman (1963) defines stigma as an attribute that is deeply discrediting given a particular set of circumstances and relations. This stigma, or fear thereof, may lead to behavioral reactions and coping strategies for people anticipating negative social perceptions based on pain, possibly shaping behaviors that interfere with care. Internalized stigma has a negative relationship with self-esteem and pain self-efficacy (Monsivais, 2013; Waugh, Byrne, & Nicholas, 2014).

Looking to the ethnographic record, Leeman (1986) states that Puebloan people along the Rio Grande are communal societies in which the well-being of the individual is inextricably linked to the well-being of the community. Because an individual's health could be determined by his or her daily interaction with community members, outcomes in Burial 88's case may have been positive in terms of inclusivity and care. The problem with citing ethnographic accounts of the Pueblo communities that Leeman was working with is that Chaco Canyon and, to a lesser extent, Aztec Ruin, seem to be socially and politically distinct from these later post-Pueblo III cultures (Lekson, 1999; Mills, 2004; Nelson, 1995; Plog & Heitman, 2010). Harrod (2012), looking at patterns of violence, suggests that there is significant internal conflict during the height of Chaco Canyon, which in turn suggests that the culture had a more rigid sociopolitical organization. For the later cultures along the Rio Grande, Pueblo well-being is a state of balance in which extremes are avoided because disharmony will affect the health of the entire community (Leeman, 1986). Dozier (1970) states that welfare of the community rests on the proper, timely, and calendric observation and performance of religious ritual.

We would argue that even in societies where hierarchy and inequality are present, the need to carry out ritual or conduct specific performative activities is still important. For Burial 88 it would be important to regain the ability to participate not only in ceremony, but also in the pivotally important task of food processing. Corn is not only important as a food source but central to origin stories and ceremony. Given activities are run by calendric ceremonies having to do with subsistence and health, it is important for all members of the community to be part of this system to ensure successful crops. Thus, at Aztec Ruins, care may have been practiced out of necessity.

It is clear that an individual can experience sickness due to disruption of a community, but it is equally true that individuals affect others in the community when in pain or disabled. Gait change due to femoral torsion, leg length discrepancy, and pain would set this female apart from the others. Her injury would remain visible to the community, possibly serving as a reminder of the attributed cause of disharmony. In addition to her visible difference, she may have been dealing with the personal discomfort of changing her expectations of fulfilling a woman's role. While a loss of mobility can be seen as a burden and result in further harm to an individual, it can also lead some members of the community to be sympathetic, want to work to correct any wrong committed against the individual, or simply offer counsel as they heal. Perhaps the community saw this person as a burden or maybe they were more empathetic. Either way, the community would have been invested in helping this woman for the goal of bringing balance back to the pueblo.

The current understanding of traditional healing practices is that these largely work through encouraging patients' responsibility for their own health and well-being. Healers bring "healing energy" to treatments, with practices taking into account contributions made to this healing process by the individual, their family, their community, and even future generations. For the patient, a sense of responsibility for their own health may bestow a sense of empowerment. Attitudes about pain and the perception of pain are largely affected by an individual's awareness of the availability of aid and their belief in their ability to help themselves. Grant (1982) finds that when a Hopi healer treats a condition, such as a fracture or sprain, there is always some degree of improvement, ranging from decrease in pain to complete resolution of the problem. He states that this could, in part, be due to the level of confidence patients have in their healer, as faith serves as an effective healing force that leads to a subjective feeling of well-being.

Implications for Group and Individual Identity, Social Relations, and Social Practice

The physical environment at Aztec Ruins comprises irregular ground with many changes in level, and this is reflected in the design of the multistory pueblo buildings. Steps and ladders are used to enter living and working areas, and these would have posed an extra challenge for a person dealing with pelvic instability (Fig. 4.8).

Help with moving in and out of domestic and ceremonial spaces would be a necessary part of accommodating difference, enabling disabled members of the community to still be part of group practice. If individual injury can be attributed to imbalance in the community, conversely, the failure of an individual in life activities may have repercussions for the entire village. Health and sickness are not limited to the individual body; instead, the entire pueblo feels it. The small rooms and multiple floors of pueblo buildings would not have been easy structures for Burial 88 to navigate, at least for the first few months following her injury (Fig. 4.8).

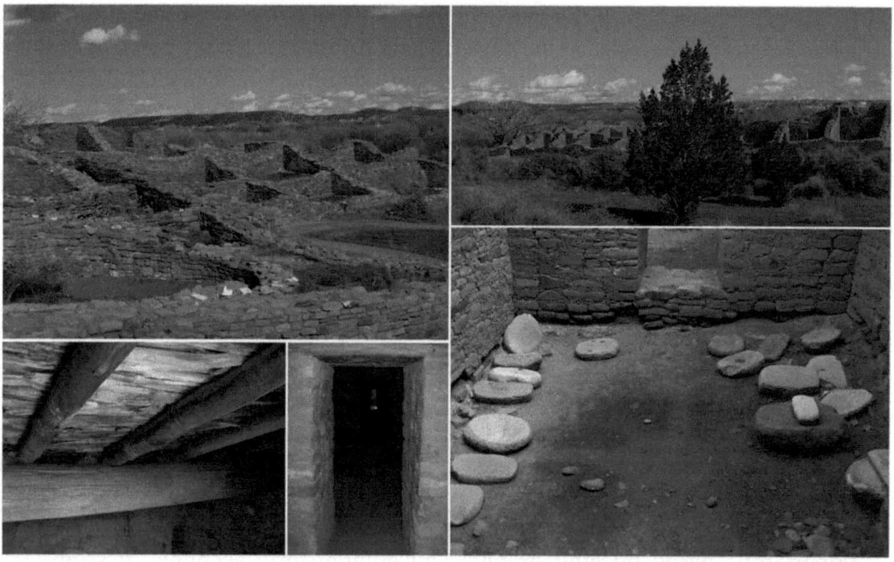

Fig. 4.8 Aztec Ruins. *Top left* and *right*: landscape views of Aztec Ruins; *Bottom left*: image of a room ceiling that also serves as the floor for the room above; *Bottom middle*: doorway; *Bottom right*: workspace with manos and metates. Photos taken by Stephanie Harrod

Physical ceremonial requirements, such as dance, contribute to identity by way of purposeful action.

> *Pueblos are well known for their communal ceremonial dancing. Dances are mandated by the Pueblo religion as essential to the maintenance of communal health and take place regularly lasting for 3–6 hours. The dances serve as a vehicle for healing the community body* (Leeman, 1986, p. 27).

Rotational instability of the pelvis may have excluded Burial 88 from participating in ceremonial activities (e.g., dance), leading to a lost sense of, or transition in, identity. We do not know how her society viewed disability, and the injury could have transformed her role in the community. While kivas are traditionally viewed as spaces exclusive to men, we use the following quote to illustrate how the community may have dealt with movement barriers so that all members could be included in ceremony.

> *We took crippled old Naquima into the kiva and had him smoke and pray with us...his prayers were better since he had a strong mind, and was single, handicapped, and less likely to be spoiled by lovemaking* (Simmons, 1942, p. 225).

Conservatively, Burial 88 would have had a decreased ability to contribute to "normal" physical labor demands, but could still have participated in the community in other ways, possibly through adjustments made specifically to enable this ("accommodation of difference" – see Tilley & Cameron, 2014). It is important to note that there would be a visible difference in the way this woman walked, as well as in her posture, which would have set her apart. It is not possible to know how the community would have perceived this difference, but the chance of exclusion in social settings is possible and may have added to the physical pain suffered on a daily basis. In addition to Burial 88's experience of chronic pain and continuing mobility challenges, the impact of pelvic injuries means she had a low chance of successfully giving birth. The potential for Burial 88 to embody her female identity may have been lost, or transitioned into a nontraditional role. Either way, there would be a period of uncertainty in the way Burial 88 felt about herself, the way she saw herself within the group, and the way the group envisioned her role within the community.

Conclusions

Burial 88's survival with reduced self-sufficiency and mobility suggests a community tolerance and understanding of disability as well as active care provision, and use of the Index of Care in assessing available evidence has helped to develop a possible and plausible account of her experience.

Importantly, based on ethnographic and ethnohistoric accounts, it seems the community would have had a vested interest in ensuring her care. This does not mean that caregiving was entirely altruistic. Both Leeman (1986, p. 11) and Grant (1982, p. 291) suggest that healers are chosen and that, because of the responsibility associated with ensuring the health of others in the community, the requirements involved in being a healer can be a burden. Care, or at least some aspects of care, may have been grudgingly provided rather than freely given. Stating that care was present in the past does not mean we are denying the reality that people were probably not always nice to one another.

Whether or not the injuries seen in Burial 88 were the result of a system of captivity (Harrod & Martin, 2014), the fact remains that one or more people almost certainly provided health-related care for her at various times during her life. This would have been in the form of "direct support" when her injuries were at the acute stage, and in the form of "accommodation of difference" as she adapted to coping with the lasting impacts of trauma. Bioarchaeological, archaeological, and ethnographic data combine to support the conclusion that Aztec Ruins was a community in which caregiving occurred.

References

Agarwal, A., & Agarwal, R. (2010). The practice and tradition of bonesetting. *Education for Health, 23*(1), 1–8.

Baessler, K., Bircher, M. D., & Stanton, S. L. (2004). Pelvic floor dysfunction in women after pelvic trauma. *BJOG: An International Journal of Obstetrics and Gynaecology, 111*(5), 499–502.

Báez-Molgado, S., Bartelink, E. J., Jellema, L. M., Spurlock, L., & Sholts, S. B. (2015). Classification of pelvic ring fractures in skeletonized human remains. *Journal of Forensic Sciences, 60*(S1), S171–S176.

Billman, B. R., Lambert, P. M., & Leonard, B. L. (2000). Cannibalism, warfare, and drought in the mesa Verde region in the twelfth century AD. *American Antiquity, 65*, 1–34.
Bora, K. S., & Sharma, A. (2011). The genus *Artemisia*: A comprehensive review. *Pharmaceutical Biology, 49*(1), 101–109.
Brooks, S., & Suchey, J. (1990). Skeletal age determination based on the Os pubis: A comparison of the Acsádi-Nemeskéri and Suchey-Brooks methods. *Human Evolution, 5*(3), 227–238.
Brown, G. M., Windes, T. C., & McKenna, P. J. (2008). Animas anamnesis: Aztec Ruins or Anasazi capital? In P. F. Reed (Ed.), *Chaco's northern prodigies: Salmon, Aztec, and the Ascendancy of the middle San Juan Region after AD 1100* (pp. 231–250). Salt Lake City: The University of Utah Press.
Buckberry, J. L., & Chamberlain, A. T. (2002). Age estimation from the auricular surface of the ilium: A revised method. *American Journal of Physical Anthropology, 119*(3), 231–239.
Buikstra, J. E., & Ubelaker, D. H. (1994). *Standards for data collection from human skeletal remains* (Research Series, No. 44). Fayetteville: Arkansas Archaeological Survey.
Cameron, C. M. (2011). Captives and culture change. *Current Anthropology, 52*(2), 169–209.
Capener, N. (1932). Sacro-Iliac displacements. *British Medical Journal (BMJ), 1*(3725), 1009.
Cibulka, M. T. (2004). Determination and significance of femoral neck anteversion. *Physical Therapy, 84*, 550–558.
Cooper, J. (2006). Pelvic ring injuries. *Trauma, 8*(2), 95–110.
de Bruijn, M. C. (2015). Chest injuries. In A. W. J. M. Glaudemans, R. A. J. O. Dierckx, J. L. M. A. Gielen, & J. Zwerver (Eds.), *Nuclear medicine and radiologic imaging in sports injuries* (pp. 245–255). Berlin: Springer-Verlag.
DeGusta, D. (2002). Comparative skeletal pathology and the case for conspecific care in middle Pleistocene hominids. *Journal of Archaeological Science, 29*(12), 1435–1438.
Dettwyler, K. A. (1991). Can paleopathology provide evidence for "compassion"? *American Journal of Physical Anthropology, 84*(4), 375–384.
Djukic, K., Milenkovic, P., Milovanovic, P., Dakic, M., & Djuric, M. (2014). The increased femoral neck anteversion in medieval cemetery of Pecenjevce. Aetiology and differential diagnosis in archaeological context. *Chungará (Arica), 46*(2), 295–303.
Dozier, E. P. (1970). *The pueblo Indians of North America*. New York: Holt, Rinehart and Winston.
Eshete, M. (2005). The prevention of traditional bone setter's gangrene. *The Journal of Bone and Joint Surgery, 87*(1), 102–103.
Fewkes, J. W. (1896). A contribution to ethnobotany. *American Anthropologist, A9*(1), 14–21.
Gillespie, P. (2009). Pelvic fracture. *Surgery, 27*(7), 292–296.
Goffman, E. (1963). *Stigma: Notes on the management of spoiled identity*. New York: Simon and Schuster.
Grant, R. E. (1982). The Hopi healer. *American Indian Quarterly, 6*(3/4), 291–304.
Gulan, G., Matovinović, D., Nemec, B., Rubinić, D., & Ravlić-Gulan, J. (2000). Femoral neck anteversion: Values, development measurement, common problems. *Collegium Antropologicum, 24*(2), 521–527.
Haas, J., & Creamer, W. (1996). The role of warfare in the pueblo III period. In M. A. Adler (Ed.), *The prehistoric pueblo world AD 1150–1350* (pp. 205–213). Tucson: The University of Arizona Press.
Halbmayer, E. (2001). Socio-cosmological contexts and forms of violence: War, vendetta, duels and suicide among the Yupka of north-western Venezuela. In B. E. Schmidt & I. W. Schröder (Eds.), *Anthropology of violence and conflict* (pp. 49–75). London: Routledge.
Halbmayer, E. (2004). 'The One Who Feeds has the Rights': Adoption and fostering of kin, affines and enemies among the Yukpa and other Carib-speaking Indians of lowland South America. In F. Bowie (Ed.), *Cross-cultural approaches to adoption* (pp. 145–164). New York: Routledge.
Harrod, R. P. (2012). Centers of control: Revealing elites among the ancestral pueblo during the "Chaco Phenomenon". *International Journal of Paleopathology, 2*(2–3), 123–135.
Harrod, R. P. (2013). *Chronologies of pain and power: Violence, inequality, and social control among ANCESTRAL Pueblo populations (AD 850–1300)*. Las Vegas: University of Nevada, Las Vegas.

Harrod, R. P., & Martin, D. L. (2014). Signatures of captivity and subordination on skeletonized human remains: A bioarchaeological case study from the ancient Southwest. In D. L. Martin & C. P. Anderson (Eds.), *Bioarchaeological and forensic perspectives on violence: How violent death is interpreted from skeletal remains* (pp. 103–119). Cambridge: Cambridge University Press.

Harrod, R. P., & Martin, D. L. (2015). Bioarchaeological case studies of slavery, captivity, and other forms of exploitation. In L. W. Marshall (Ed.), *The archaeology of slavery: A comparative approach to captivity and coercion* (pp. 41–63). Carbondale: Southern Illinois University, Center for Archaeological Investigations.

Hatipoğlu, S., & Tatar, K. (1995). The strengths and weaknesses of Turkish bone-setters. *World Health Forum, 16*(2), 203–205.

Hessman, M., Rickert, M., Hofmann, A., Rommins, P., & Buhl, M. (2010). Outcomes in pelvic ring fractures. *European Journal of Trauma and Emergency Surgery, 2*, 124–130.

Huber, B. R. (1990). The recruitment of Nahua Curers: Role conflict and gender. *Ethnology, 29*(2), 159–176.

Judge, W. J. (1989). Chaco Canyon-San Juan Basin. In L. S. Cordell & G. J. Gumerman (Eds.), *Dynamics of southwest prehistory* (pp. 209–261). Washington, DC: Smithsonian Institution Press.

Katada, K. (1970). Questions on the Judo-Seifukushi system [translated from Japanese]. *Seikeigeka [Orthopedic Surgery], 21*(13), 1092.

Kohler, T. A., & Kramer, T. K. (2006). Raiding for women in the pre-Hispanic northern pueblo southwest? *Current Anthropology, 47*(6), 1035–1045.

LeBlanc, S. A. (1999). *Prehistoric warfare in the American Southwest.* Salt Lake City: The University of Utah Press.

Leeman, L. M. (1986). *Pueblo health models and practices*. Berkeley: University of California, Berkeley.

Lekson, S. H. (1999). *The Chaco Meridian: Centers of political power in the ancient Southwest.* Walnut Creek: AltaMira Press.

Lekson, S. H. (2006). *The archaeology of Chaco Canyon: An eleventh-century pueblo regional center.* Santa Fe: School of American Research Press.

Lekson, S. H. (2009). *A history of the ancient southwest.* Santa Fe: School of Advanced Research Press.

Letournel, E. (1970). Pelvic fractures. *Injury: The British journal of accident surgery, 10*(2), 145–148.

Letournel, E. (1980). Acetabulum fractures: Classification and management. *Clinical Orthopaedics and Related Research, 151*, 81–106.

Ling, X., Aimin, L., Xihe, Z., Xiaoshu, C., & Cummings, S. R. (1996). Very low rates of hip fracture in Beijing, People's Republic of China: The Beijing osteoporosis project. *American Journal of Epidemiology, 144*(9), 901–907.

Lister, R. H., & Lister, F. C. (1987). *Aztec Ruins of the Animas: Excavated, preserved, and interpreted.* Albuquerque: University of New Mexico Press.

Lister, R. H, & Lister, F. C. (1990). *Aztec ruins national monument: Administrative history of an archaeological preserve* (Professional Papers No. 24). Santa Fe: Southwest Cultural Resources Center, National Park Service.

Lovejoy, C. O., Meindl, R. S., Pryzbeck, T. R., & Mensforth, R. P. (1985). Chronological metamorphosis of the auricular surface of the Ilium: A new method for the determination of adult skeletal age at death. *American Journal of Physical Anthropology, 68*(1), 15–28.

Mann, R. W., Jantz, R. L., Bass, W. M., & Willey, P. S. (1991). Maxillary suture obliteration: A visual method for estimating skeletal age. *Journal of Forensic Sciences, 36*, 781–791.

Martin, D. L. (1997). Violence against women in the La Plata River Valley (A.D. 1000–1300). In D. L. Martin & D. W. Frayer (Eds.), *Troubled times: Violence and warfare in the past* (pp. 45–75). Amsterdam: Gordon and Breach.

Martin, D. L. (2008). Ripped flesh and torn souls: Evidence for slavery in the prehistoric Southwest, AD 800–1500. In C. M. Cameron (Ed.), *Invisible citizens: Captives and their consequences* (pp. 159–180). Salt Lake City: The University of Utah Press.

Meindl, R. S., & Lovejoy, C. O. (1985). Ectocranial suture closure: A revised method for the determination of skeletal age at death based on the lateral-anterior sutures. *American Journal of Physical Anthropology, 68*(1), 57–66.

Mills, B. J. (2004). The establishment and defeat of hierarchy: Inalienable possessions and the history of collective prestige structures in the pueblo southwest. *American Anthropologist, 106*(2), 238–251.

Monsivais, D. B. (2013). Decreasing the Stigma burden of chronic pain. *Journal of the American Association of Nurse Practitioners, 25*(10), 551–556.

Morris, E. H. (1924). *Burials in the Aztec Ruin*. New York: Anthropological Papers of the American Museum of Natural History.

Mudge, A. J., Bau, K. V., Purcell, L. N., Wu, J. C., Axt, M. W., Selber, P., et al. (2014). Normative reference values for lower limb joint range, bone torsion, and alignment in children aged 4–16 years. *Journal of Pediatric Orthopaedics, 23*(1), 15–25.

Munro, A. M., & Malville, J. M. (2011). Ancestors and the Sun: Astronomy, architecture and culture at Chaco Canyon. *Proceedings of the International Astronomical Union, 7*(S278), 255–264.

Nelson, B. A. (1995). Complexity, hierarchy, and scale: A controlled comparison between Chaco Canyon, New Mexico, and La Quemada, Zacatecas. *American Antiquity, 60*(4), 597–618.

Oyebola, D. D. O. (1980). Yoruba traditional bonesetters: The practice of orthopaedics in a primitive setting in Nigeria. *Journal of Trauma, 20*(4), 312–322.

Panda, A. K., & Rout, S. (2015). *Puttur Kattu* (Bandage) – A traditional bone setting practice in South India. *Journal of Ayurveda and Integrative Medicine, 2*(4), 174–178.

Parsons, E. W. C. (1936). *Taos pueblo* [General Series in Anthropology, no. 2]. New York: Johnson Reprint Corp. 1970.

Paul, B. D. (1976). The maya bonesetter as sacred specialist. *Ethnology, 15*(1), 77–81.

Phenice, T. W. (1969). A newly developed visual method of sexing the Os pubis. *American Journal of Physical Anthropology, 30*(2), 297–301.

Pillsbury, B. L. (1978). *Traditional health care in the near east*. Washington, DC: US Agency for International Development.

Plog, S., & Heitman, C. (2010). Hierarchy and social inequality in the American Southwest, A.D. 800–1200. *Proceedings of the National Academy of Sciences of the United States of America, 107*(46), 19619–19626.

Prevezas, N., Antypas, G., Louverdis, D., Konstas, A., Papasontiriou, A., & Sbonias, G. (2009). Proposed guidelines for increasing the reliability and validity of Letournel classification system. *Injury, International Journal of the Care of The Injured, 40*(10), 1098–1103.

Rainey, K. D., & Adams, K. R. (2004). *Plant use by native peoples of the American southwest: Ethnographic documentation* [HTML Title]. Retrieved November 13, 2015, from http://www.crowcanyon.org/plantuses.

Ruatti, S., Guillot, S., Brun, J., Thony, F., Bouzat, P., Payen, J. F., et al. (2015). Which pelvic ring fractures are potentially lethal? *Injury, International Journal of the Care of The Injured, 46*(6), 1059–1063.

Siegmeth, A., Müllner, T., Kukla, C., & Vécsei, V. (2000). [Associated injuries in severe pelvic trauma] translated from German. *Der Unfallchirurg, 103*(7), 572–581.

Simmons, L. W. (1942). *Sun Chief: The autobiography of a Hopi Indian*. New Haven: Yale University Press.

Stefanski, J. L., & Smith, K. J. (2006). The role of nutrition intervention in wound healing. *Home Health Care Management and Practice, 18*(4), 293–99.

Stein, J. R., & McKenna, P. J. (1988). *An archaeological reconnaissance of A Late Bonito Phase Occupation Near Aztec Ruins National Monument, New Mexico*. Santa Fe: National Park Service.

Stimson, L. A. (1899). *A practical treatise on fractures and dislocations*. New York: Lea Brothers and Company.

Subbu, R., & Haddad, F. (2015). Paediatric hip pain: A rare injury. *International Journal of Sports and Exercise Medicine, 1*(3), 1–5.

Tile, M. (1988). Pelvic ring fractures: Should they be fixed? *The Journal of Bone and Joint Surgery, 70-B*(1), 1–12.

Tilley, L., & Cameron, T. (2014). Introducing the index of care: A web-based application supporting archaeological research into health-related care. *International Journal of Paleopathology, 6*(1), 5–9.

Todd, T. W. (1920). Age changes in the pubic bone. I. The male white pubis. *American Journal of Physical Anthropology, 3*, 285–334.

Toll, H. W. (2008). The La Plata, the Totah, and the Chaco: Variations on a theme. In P. F. Reed (Ed.), *Chaco's northern prodigies: Salmon, Aztec, and the Ascendancy of the Middle San Juan Region after AD 1100* (pp. 309–333). Salt Lake City: The University of Utah Press.

Tooker, E. (1962). *An ethnography of the Huron Indians, 1615–1649*. Bulletin, No. 190, Bureau of American Ethnology. Washington, DC: Smithsonian Institution Press.

Turi, C. E., Shipley, P. R., & Murch, S. J. (2014). North American *Artemisia* species from the subgenus *Tridentatae* (Sagebrush): A phytochemical, botanical and pharmacological review. *Phytochemistry, 98*, 9–26.

Vallier, H. A., Cureton, B. A., Schubeck, D., & Wang, X.-F. (2012). Functional outcomes in women after high-energy pelvic ring injury. *Journal of Orthopaedic Trauma, 26*(5), 296–301.

Van Dyke, R. M. (2009). Chaco reloaded: Discursive social memory on the post-Chacoan landscape. *Journal of Social Archaeology, 9*(2), 220–248.

Warren, D. M. (1974). Bono traditional healers. *Rural Africana, 26*(Winter), 25–39.

Waugh, O. C., Byrne, D. G., & Nicholas, M. K. (2014). Internalized Stigma in people living with chronic pain. *The Journal of Pain, 15*(5), 550.e1–e10.

White, T. D., Folkens, P. A., & Black, M. T. (2012). *Human osteology* (3rd ed.). Burlington: Academic Press.

Wilcox, D. R. (1993). The evolution of the Chacoan Polity. In: J. M. Malville, & G. Matlock (Eds.) *The Chimney Rock Archaeological Symposium* (pp. 76–90). General Technical Report, No. RM-227. Fort Collins: U. S. Forest Service.

Wilcox, D. R. (2004). The evolution of the Chacoan polity. In J. M. Malville (Ed.), *The Chimney Rock: The ultimate outlier* (pp. 163–186). Lanham: Lexington Books.

Yamauchi, Y. (1996). Japanese orthopedic surgeons – Survival through the next century. *Journal of Orthopaedic Science, 1*(5), 299–300.

Young, J. W., & Burgess, A. R. (1987). *Radiologic management of pelvic ring fractures*. Baltimore: Urban and Schwarzenberg.

Yount, S. M. (2013). The impact of pelvic floor disorders and pelvic surgery on women's sexual satisfaction and function. *Journal of Midwifery and Women's Health, 58*(5), 538–545.

Chapter 5
Inferring Disability and Care Provision in Late Prehistoric Tennessee

Heather Worne

Introduction

The recent development of the "bioarchaeology of care" (see Tilley, Chap. 2 this volume; Tilley, 2012) provides a methodology and theoretical basis for assessing disability and the provision of care in bioarchaeological contexts. This approach provides a framework for investigating relationships between biological and sociocultural dimensions of physical impairment. The current study presents a case of possible trauma-related disability of a middle-to-older adult female (B271A) from a late prehistoric agricultural community in Tennessee, North America. This individual survived significant traumatic injuries to her pelvis, as well as fractures to her ribs, spine, and facial bones. Her possible disability and likely care are considered within the contexts of both accidental injury and intentional violence. Utilizing the Index of Care (Tilley & Cameron, 2014), her injuries are assessed to determine the immediate and long-term impacts that these may have had on her ability to perform daily activities within her specific social, cultural, and physical context. This chapter also examines the timing of her injuries as well as the type of care she likely received from members of her community.

Biocultural Context of Care

Located in the Middle Cumberland Region (MCR) of north-central Tennessee, the Averbuch site represents a late Mississippian nucleated village (Fig. 5.1). Situated on a broad upland slope on the outer edge of the Central Basin just outside the

---

H. Worne, Ph.D. (✉)
University of Kentucky, Lexington, KY, USA
e-mail: haworn0@uky.edu

© Springer International Publishing Switzerland 2017

L. Tilley, A.A. Schrenk (eds.), *New Developments in the Bioarchaeology of Care*, Bioarchaeology and Social Theory, DOI 10.1007/978-3-319-39901-0_5

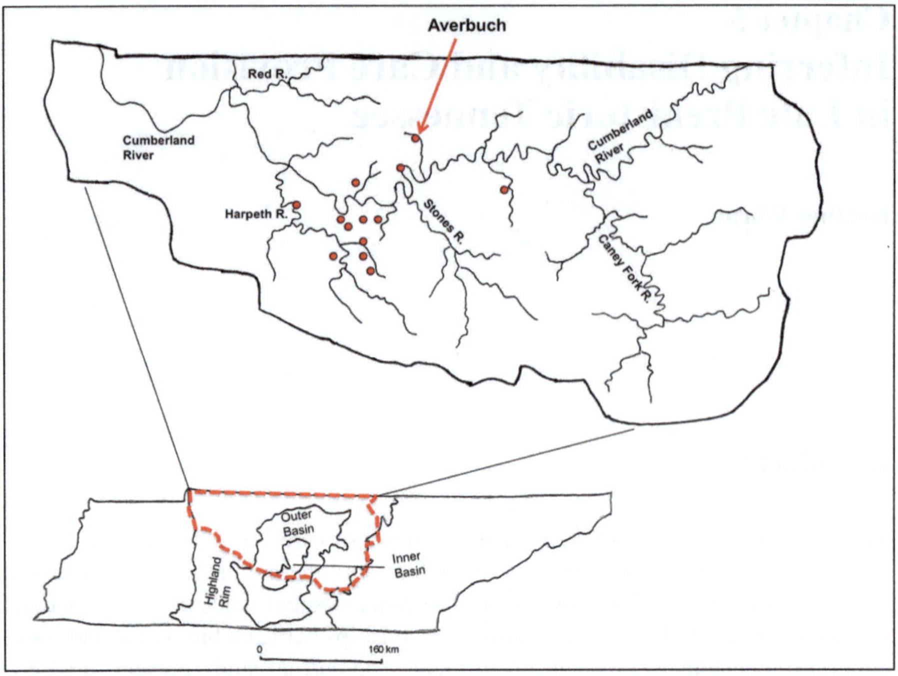

Fig. 5.1 Map of Middle Cumberland Region showing location of Averbuch (after Smith & Moore, 1999, p. 95, Fig. 9.1)

modern day city of Nashville, the site is located on a lesser stream approximately four kilometers to the north of the Cumberland River and two kilometers east of a secondary tributary (Reed, 1984).

Despite its seemingly hinterland location population density at the site was relatively high, with population size estimates averaging between 100 and 200 people living there at any one time (Cobb, Krus, & Steadman, 2015, p. 46). The elevation of the site is 155 m above sea level in an area characterized by rugged, deeply dissected terrain (Miller, 1974). The slopes of the site are prone to erosion, with a particularly steep drop-off to the west. Agricultural potential in the area is relatively good due to the high nutrient content of the soils, and a variety of floral and faunal resources were available within the two adjacent physiographic regions (Highland Rim and Inner Basin). Characterized by a temperate diversified deciduous forest, flora in the area is considered particularly rich and diverse. Groups in the MCR presumably had access to numerous lithic and chert gravel resources from local waterways, with many quarries within walking distance of sites.

The Eastern Salt Basin extends south to the margin between the northern periphery of the Outer Basin and the Highland Rim, providing numerous accessible saline and mineral springs in the region (Smith & Moore, 1996). Salt springs not only provide potential trade goods, but also attract local ungulate populations, providing a concentration of mammals for hunting. Deer was one of the most exploited faunal species in the region. Other faunal mainstays included elk, bear, raccoon, turkey, as well as waterfowl, fish, and mollusks. In addition to maize and other cultigens, people probably also exploited wild berries, nuts, and fruits. There does not appear to be a concentration of power within any one community during the later Mississippian period in the MCR, nor does any group appear to have exclusive control over any particular resource (Moore & Smith, 2009; Smith, 1992). Paleobotanical analyses at the site suggest that, despite the availability of diverse flora in the area, residents at Averbuch focused primarily on a narrow range of plant species (Crites, 1984). Furthermore, isotopic analyses indicate that late prehistoric populations in the region, including Averbuch, had an extreme dietary reliance on maize (Buikstra, William, Emanuel, Leslie, & Nikolaas van der M, 1988).

Recent Bayesian modeling of radiocarbon data indicates that the site was occupied from approximately cal. A.D. 1265–1475 (Cobb et al., 2015, p. 52). A total of 645 burials (887 individuals) were excavated, with the vast majority located in one of three discrete cemeteries (Berryman, 1981). Infants were primarily interred under structure floors. The palisade wall intrudes upon Cemetery 3, suggesting that it was in use prior to the erection of the wall (Berryman, 1981), which was likely built between cal. A.D. 1350 and A.D. 1405 (Cobb et al., 2015, p. 52). Temporal information is not as clear for Cemetery 2. The subject of this chapter, B271A, was buried in the later cemetery (Cemetery 1), which is contained within the fortification walls and was potentially in use between cal. A.D. 1390 and A.D. 1470. Permanent habitation structures excavated at the Averbuch site were square or rectangular, wall-trench or single-post, wattle and daub, and often contained centrally located hearths (Reed & Klippel, 1984). Eleven of the twenty-two domestic structures excavated show evidence for rebuilding. Based on structure floor areas (averaging approximately 28 m^2), domestic structures likely housed an average of five individuals, with some possibly as many as eight (Casselberry, 1974).

Mortuary practices at the Averbuch site (and the wider MCR) usually consisted of rectangular stone box graves accommodating a single extended burial (Brown, 1981; Smith, 1992). Primarily constructed of limestone slabs, stone boxes appear to have been tailored to the size of the interred individual, with the box wider at the head and narrower at the feet. Although typically containing only one individual, graves were often reused, with the original occupants removed or pushed to one end to make room for the newly interred individual (Berryman, 1981; Brown, 1981; Dowd, 2008; Smith, 1992). Based on experiments by Brehm and Evans (1977), it is estimated that a single limestone box grave took approximately 8 h to construct, which suggests the box construction itself was an important aspect of mortuary ritual.

Analyses of mortuary artifacts provide potential insights into the daily lives of individuals at the Averbuch site. There does not appear to be any mortuary distinctions based on social status or rank divisions (Smith, 1992). Only a small proportion of adult burials contain grave goods, most of which are utilitarian in nature and appear to reflect differences in sex or occupation rather than status. The vast majority of nonutilitarian artifacts are buried with infants and children. Exotic goods present in some of the graves likely represent the ability of some individuals or lineages to accumulate wealth during their lifetime. Undecorated (or simply decorated) ceramic vessels associated with domestic household activities are more often buried with female or nonadults (Smith, 1992, p. 273). Small ceramic trowels commonly associated with pottery-making, as well as bone awls possibly used in weaving, are more often located in female burials. Mississippian projectile points likely used for hunting, woodworking tools (i.e., larger ceramic trowels), large plastering trowels (possibly used in house construction), chipped stone, and other mineral artifacts are all primarily associated with male burials.

In order to sustain the rather large sedentary population at Averbuch, all able-bodied adults were likely involved in procuring food and providing protection for those that may not have been able to do so on their own (i.e., the very young or very old, the sick, or part-time craft specialists) (Berryman, 1981; Smith, 1992). Part-time craft or occupational specialists also probably contributed to agricultural production during peak crop seasons (Smith, 1992). The location and size of grain storage vessels in the region suggest that surplus was maintained at the household rather than community level.

Surveys of artifact assemblages from the region indicate that the relatively autonomous villages of the late Mississippian period in the MCR had continual interaction with one another (Smith, 1992). The presence of a variety of nonlocal items throughout the region, (e.g., marine shell, mica, nonlocal chert, quartz, galena, copper, steatite, bison, greenstone) suggests that groups in the MCR, including the community at Averbuch, interacted in the wider Mississippian sphere (Moore & Smith, 2009; Smith, 1992). A number of local products also likely served as export items, such as salt, negative painted vessels, shell gorgets, and mussel shell beads (Smith & Moore, 1999).

Bioarchaeological analyses indicate that residents at the Averbuch site experienced substantial social and biological stress (Berryman, 1984; Eisenberg, 1986, 1991a, 1991b). Life expectancy for the Averbuch skeletal sample is rather low compared to other late prehistoric populations in the region (Berryman, 1981, 1984). Individuals at Averbuch who survived to age 20 had a life expectancy of approximately 32 years (Berryman, 1981; Eisenberg, 1986). Life expectancies at age 20 for other late prehistoric samples in the region range between 31 and 38 years. Relative frequencies of skeletal indicators of stress (i.e., linear enamel hypoplasias, porotic hyperostosis, cribra orbitalia, and tibial periostitis) were rather high compared to other late prehistoric populations in the southeastern and midwestern United States (Eisenberg, 1986, 1991a, 1991b). Relative frequencies of linear enamel hypoplasias for other contemporary sites in the region range from 51 to 90 %, with Averbuch falling towards the upper end of the range at 90 % (Eisenberg, 1986, pp. 165–166). Similarly, the frequency of individuals in the Averbuch sample showing evidence for cribra orbitalia or porotic hyperostosis is 18 %, with other late prehistoric sites in the region ranging from 1.2 to 18 %. Evidence for specific diseases, such as tuberculosis and treponematosis, is present for sites throughout the region, particularly within the Averbuch skeletal sample.

The threat of attack to the Averbuch community apparently warranted the construction of a palisade wall during the mid to late fourteenth century (Cobb et al., 2015). The erection of the wall appears to have been hurried, as the wall passes through graves from an earlier cemetery. Osteological evidence of intergroup conflict has been identified at MCR sites (including Averbuch) in the form of scalping, embedded projectile points, and sharp force trauma (Worne, 2011; Worne, Cobb, Vidoli, & Steadman, 2012). Furthermore, a particularly high proportion of uniformly shaped (round or elliptical) healed cranial depression fractures, showing a sex-specific location on the skull (with wounds more often located on the anterior or superior aspects of the skull in males and on the posterior aspect in females), suggests perhaps the presence of culturally specific interpersonal or intragroup violence. Conflict appears to have escalated in the region over time. This shift follows shortly after region-wide decentralization becomes apparent in the MCR, as groups stopped investing in the construction of earthen mounds and nucleated into smaller, more autonomous palisaded villages and became more defense-oriented (Moore & Smith, 2009; Smith, 1992). Taken as a whole, the osteological evidence from the Averbuch skeletal sample indicates that residents experienced both considerable biological and social stress. Community health was likely adversely affected by multiple synergistic factors, possibly including high population density, the threat of violence, as well as limited access to resources (Berryman, 1981; Eisenberg, 1986; Worne et al., 2012).

There is some evidence suggesting that individuals at the Averbuch site received some amount of care following injury or illness. Several individuals show evidence that they survived bouts of chronic disease (e.g., tuberculosis and treponematosis). Furthermore, at least four victims of scalping (three males and one female) show evidence of infection and/or bone remodeling, indicating that they survived for at least some period of time. However, whether or not the provision of care would have been necessary for these individuals to survive as long as they did has yet to be systematically evaluated. The following case study uses the Index of Care to assess whether care was likely provided for B271A, and what that care may have entailed.

Paleopathology of B271A and Its Implications

B271A, a middle-to-older adult female, was recovered from Cemetery 1 (the later cemetery located within the palisade wall). She was buried in the semi-flexed position, likely due to her placement in a rectangular limestone box grave that was not long enough to accommodate her height. The partial remains of a juvenile were discovered in the burial as well, suggesting that the box was reused for interment of B271A, which was not uncommon at the site. Her remains are relatively well preserved and mostly complete; however, several elements (i.e., ribs, long bones) were fragmentary due to taphonomic processes. Sex estimation was based on morphological characteristics of her skull and pelvis using standard osteological methods of analysis (Buikstra & Ubelaker, 1994). Transition Analysis (Boldsen, George, Lyle, & James, 2002) suggests a maximum likely age of 46.1 years with a 95 % confidence interval of 31.6–67.5 years (Fojas, personal communication 2015).

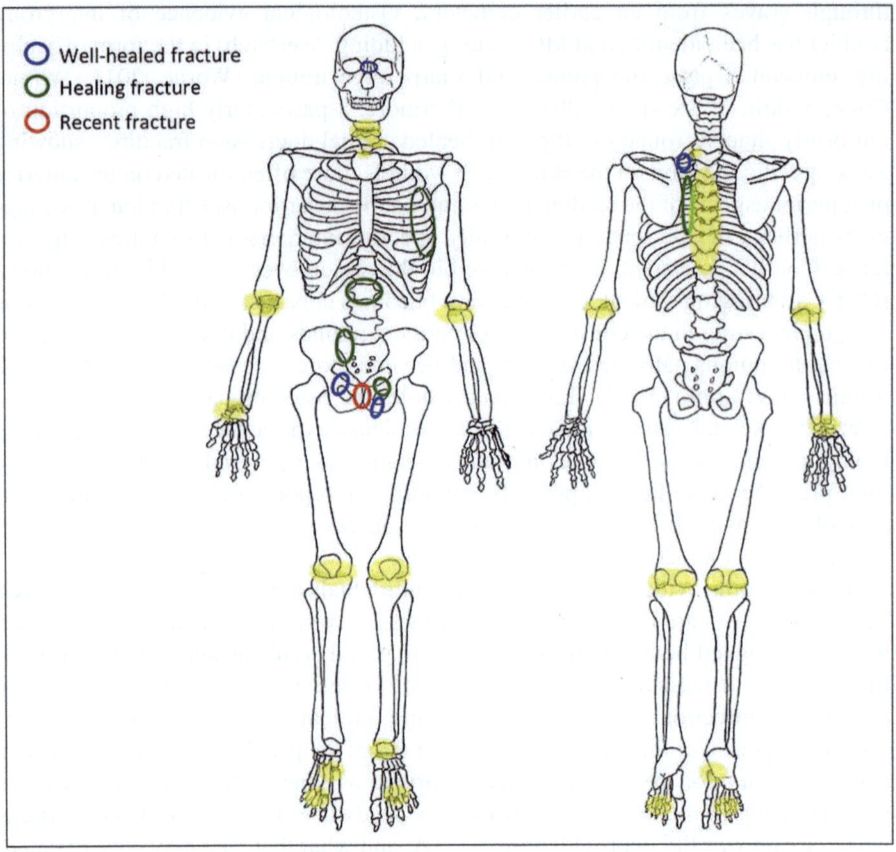

Fig. 5.2 Diagram illustrating relative timing of injuries. Shading and highlighting denote joints affected by osteoarthritis

B271A showed several pathologies, consistent with traumatic injury, in varying stages of healing (Fig. 5.2). Details of her injuries and any other relevant pathologies, as well as potential clinical impacts, are discussed below. It is important to note that the clinical literature generally addresses modern cases from hospital or medical clinic settings. Such reports are based on samples containing a high number of motor vehicle accident victims, and are usually drawn from patient populations where some amount of medical care has already been administered (e.g., analgesics, wounds cleaned, surgery).

The injuries with the most clinical and functional significance for B271A are the multiple fractures of her pelvic ring. There appears to be a well-healed/remodeled callus located on her left ischiopubic ramus just inferior to the pubic body, possibly due to an impact to her groin region, and her right iliopubic ramus has a well-healed fracture with nonunion located near the point where the ilium and pubis meet. There is also a rather large area of woven bone formation on the anterior aspect of the left iliopubic ramus adjacent to the anterior wall of the acetabulum that appears to be a callus. Postmortem breakage to the region makes it impossible to determine the extent of the injury (e.g., complete vs. incomplete fracture; acetabular involvement). The right ala of the sacrum has a compression fracture on the ventral portion of the sacroiliac joint surface at the level of the first sacral vertebra. The fracture line is still visible on the joint surface, with both woven and lamellar bone deposition on the lateral and anterior surfaces. Sacral fractures are associated with neurologic impairment (i.e., damage to the sciatic nerve or L-5 nerve root); however, B271A's injury is located in the alar region (lateral to the sacral foramina), which only results in neurologic deficit in 5.9 % of cases (Denis, David, & Comfort, 1988, p. 71).

The most recent injury involves a compression fracture of the left pubic symphyseal face, causing the dorsal half of the surface to be depressed laterally and angled posteriorly. Minimal woven bone deposition suggests that callus formation is only just beginning. This injury likely resulted in the internal rotation and overlap of the pubic symphyses, which is associated with increased risk of damage to internal abdominal and pelvic organs, bleeding, and death (Bellabarba, Winkelmann, Decker, Bransford, & Krettek, 2009).

While it is difficult to assess the timing of B271A's injuries, it is clear that the pubic symphysis fracture was relatively recent, possibly occurring within a matter of weeks prior to her death. Taking all of her pelvic ring injuries into account, her fractures are consistent with Tile's Type B fractures (Báez-Molgado, Bartelink, Jellema, Spurlock, & Sholts, 2015; Tile, 1988), producing rotational instability of the pelvis. The most recent fracture to her pubic symphysis likely resulted from ipsilateral compression, possibly due to a fall.

Pelvic ring fractures usually cause difficulty standing or walking. Patients generally require a period of bed rest, sometimes lasting weeks or months, depending upon the severity of the injury and stability of the pelvis (Aghababian, 2011; Denis et al., 1988). Physical therapy is often required to regain partial or full mobility (Dutton, 2011). Pelvic bone fractures resulting in damage to internal organs have the potential to cause extensive internal bleeding as well as infection, especially if the peritoneum is compromised (Looser & Crombie, 1976). A review of hospital admissions for pelvic ring fractures found that 29.8 % of individuals with anterior fractures and 83.7 % with posterior fractures suffered retroperitoneal hematoma, with between 28.1 % and 68 % requiring blood transfusion (Looser & Crombie, 1976, p. 639).

Pelvic ring trauma is associated with genitourinary injuries, with frequencies reported between 6.5 % and 30 %. Such injuries include bladder ruptures and urethral damage, which, in females, may result in pelvic organ prolapse, voiding disorders, and urinary incontinence (Bellabarba et al., 2009, pp. 1101–1102). Posttraumatic chronic pain following pelvic ring fracture is common. Gerbershagen et al. (2010, pp. 132–133) found that 67 % of patients with Type B fractures had posttraumatic pelvic pain 52 months after their injury, with 23 % reporting severe pain. They also found a significant correlation between posttraumatic pelvic pain and psychological distress (e.g., anxiety and depression), with 26 % of patients showing signs of clinical depression (Gerbershagen et al., 2010, pp. 134–135). Referring to a previous observation, the above results are taken from research in modern hospital settings. The patients in these samples were likely receiving treatment for pain (e.g., analgesics); without such treatment the number of patients reporting experience of pain would quite possibly have been even higher.

A minimum of two separate injuries caused the fractures observed in B271A's ribs. Her left 2nd rib has a well-healed, remodeled fracture and three unidentified left ribs have healing fractures, all of which are located just distal to the tubercle. Six unidentified and unsided rib fragments have healing fractures located in the anterior half of the rib shafts. All of the healing fractures are consistent with the consolidation stage (see Lovell, 1997, p. 145), with more lamellar bone visible in the posterior fractures. The varying degree of callus formation and remodeling suggests that B271A's rib fractures were sustained as a result of two or more separate traumatic injuries. It is possible that some of the less healed fractures are due to reinjury or continued displacement during healing (Cole, Schroder, & Jacobson, 2009).

Due to the protective location under the shoulder girdle, fractures of the first three ribs are relatively rare. Such injuries are typically caused by high-energy impacts, often resulting in significant chest trauma (Poole & Myers, 1981; Wedel & Galloway, 2014). Because of the amount of force required, and the proximity of the rib to major vessels, upper rib fractures are associated with high mortality (Fermanis, Deane, & Fitzgerald, 1985; Poole & Myers, 1981). Posterior (vertebral end) rib fractures are usually caused by impacts to the posterior aspect of the spine or back of the neck, and are most commonly the result of motor vehicle accidents, falls, or assaults (Wedel & Galloway, 2014). Alternatively, the unidentified left vertebral end rib fractures in B271A could have been caused by indirect forces from lateral compression of the chest cavity, which could also have resulted in the fractures to the anterior portion of the unsided rib fragments. However, the unidentified anterior rib fractures are transverse, which is more consistent with direct blows to the chest (Wedel & Galloway, 2014). Given B271A's age, an underlying condition, such as osteopenia or osteoporosis, may have predisposed her to bone fracture, which could occur from relatively low impact injuries (e.g., falling from standing height, assault, coughing).

Rib fracture can cause significant injury affecting respiratory function (such as flail chest, pneumothorax, hemothorax, pulmonary contusion, and atelectasis or failure to expand lungs), potentially resulting in death (Brickley, 2006; Sirmali et al., 2003). The mortality rates reported for hospital patients with flail chest range from 16 to 33 % (Cole et al., 2009, p. 1552). Fracture of even a single rib can cause acute pain, resulting in loss of workdays and overall reduction in quality of life (Kara, Dikmen, Erdal, Simsir, & Kara, 2003). Such pain can limit the ability to take deep breaths or to cough to clear lungs of mucous, which may lead to respiratory distress as well as increase risk for developing infection (e.g., pneumonia) (Brickley, 2006; Ho, Karmmakar, & Critchley, 2011; Kara et al., 2003; Karmmakar & Ho, 2003). In a study of hospital patients admitted with minor thoracic injuries (not restricted to rib fracture), 53 % reported moderate pain after 2 weeks and 18.2 % still had significant pain after 90 days (Daoust et al. 2013). Another study of hospital patients with traumatic rib fracture found that 22.5 % of individuals had chronic, persistent pain at the injury site after 1 year (Shelat et al., 2012). Among those reporting work-related difficulties, lifting heavy objects was the most frequent cause.

Other pathologies possibly associated with traumatic injury and documented for B271A include a well-healed transverse fracture of the nasal bones and left frontal process of her maxilla, as well as a compression fracture of her second lumbar vertebra resulting in a wedge-shaped central body. The facial fracture is consistent with a lateral impact, possibly due to an assault or a fall (Erdmann et al., 2008; Wedel & Galloway, 2014). Wedge-shaped compression fractures to the vertebral bodies most often occur under compression and flexion resulting in a shortened anterior height (Denis, 1984; Evans, 1982; Ferguson & Allen, 1984) and usually occur during automobile accidents or as a result of falls from considerable height (~3 m) while the spine is flexed. In older individuals (>50 years), these injuries are more commonly caused by skeletal insufficiency (Galloway, Stini, Fox, & Stein, 1990; Wedel & Galloway, 2014).

Several skeletal elements show evidence of osteoarthritis, including multiple ribs, several cervical, thoracic, and lumbar vertebrae, both elbows, the right wrist, both knees as well as foot bones. Two unidentified rib fragments show small (~10 × 20 mm) areas of sclerotic bone deposition on the plural aspect of the shafts, which could indicate past respiratory infection.

Accidental vs. Intentional Trauma?

B271A's multiple rib fractures in varying stages of healing, as well as the facial fracture, are suggestive of assault, possibly resulting from elder abuse or intergroup attack. Given the threat from external groups, raiding violence cannot be ruled out as a possible cause for her injuries. If her fractures are the result of elder abuse, the abuser(s) were also likely responsible for her care and accommodation. In the context of abuse or neglect, her earlier fractures would have rendered her more vulnerable to subsequent injuries (Lachs & Pillemer, 1995; Peh, 1993). Any pre-existing illness or physical impairment would not only hinder her ability to defend herself against physical abuse, but it would also increase her dependence on others for care and support (e.g., assistance walking).

Gowland (2015) has suggested that social marginalization of the elderly could be reflected in the burial record (i.e., uncommon or marginal burials). While burial practices are rather uniform at the Averbuch site (and MCR region), B271A received a relatively less common burial. Most individuals at the site are placed in an extended supine position, in a tailor-made limestone box grave built to accommodate the height of the individual interred. B271A was placed in a box that was too short for her extended body. While the reuse of the grave could suggest that those responsible for her burial were not concerned enough (or did not have the time/energy) to construct a new stone box that would better accommodate her height, there is no evidence to indicate that this practice was restricted to individuals of lower status. It is possible that escalating hostilities in the region affected mortuary practices. For instance, the threat of attack may have hindered the ability of community members to procure the materials (e.g., limestone slabs) required to construct new stone boxes.

The fractures to the pelvis and lumbar vertebra are more consistent with accidental injuries (i.e., falling) (Wedel & Galloway, 2014). If B271A's actual age falls towards the latter end of the estimated range (31.6–67.5 years), it is possible that any of her injuries could have resulted from either normal activities or relatively minor falls due to age-related loss of bone mineral density. Insufficiency fractures, or fractures resulting from stress on abnormal (e.g., osteoporotic) bone, would increase the likelihood of injury recidivism, regardless of the cause (Gubler et al., 1996). Identifying injury recidivism, as opposed to multiple simultaneous injuries, in the skeletal record is problematic, because the chronology is not often clear (Judd, 2002). The amount of time that it takes for a fracture to heal varies considerably based on the bone involved, the severity of the injury, as well as the age or health of the individual (Lovell, 1997).

Discussion

There are many serious and life-threatening complications that could arise from any one of B271A's rib or pelvic fractures; however, most involve the soft tissue and would not leave evidence in her skeletal remains. Given the clinical and functional significance of B271A's injuries, she likely received health-related care in the form of "direct support" immediately following some of her more severe injuries (particularly her pelvic ring fractures), followed by accommodation as her wounds began to heal.

Any of her rib or pelvic ring fractures had the potential to cause damage to internal organs, significant blood loss, infection, as well as immobility. During the acute phase of her injuries, she likely would have needed assistance with several "essential activities of daily living" (see Chap. 2, this volume) such as procuring food and water, cleaning wounds to prevent infection and maintaining overall personal hygiene, dressing herself, standing, and walking. It is not possible to determine the number of distinct incidents resulting in the suite of injuries observed in B271A's remains. Her multiple rib and pelvic fractures would have caused acute pain after her initial injuries, followed by varying periods of chronic pain. The multiple pelvic fractures would likely have resulted in some level of restricted mobility due to discomfort, as well as potential structural constraints. As her injuries accumulated, her pelvis would have become increasingly unstable, which would further limit her ability to walk, as well as render her more susceptible to future injuries. Because the timing of B271A's injuries is unclear, it is not possible to tell the full extent of these impairments. Her limb bones do not show any evidence of prolonged disuse, suggesting that she was not completely incapacitated for any substantial amount of time. It is possible that the most recent injury to her left pubic symphyseal face resulted in significant trauma, potentially contributing to her death.

Given B271A's injuries, she was likely dependent on the assistance of others within her group to perform several "instrumental activities of daily living" (see Chap. 2). In the absence of her injuries, daily life for B271A would likely have involved working in the agricultural fields tending to crops and procuring food for her household. She also may have contributed to the gathering of wild plants for consumption, collecting water from the nearby stream, as well as processing food items (i.e., pounding/grinding maize). Archaeological evidence suggests that females may also have been involved in the production of pottery as well as weaving.

Venturing outside the protection of the palisade wall at the Averbuch site would have been a dangerous endeavor. It is unlikely that B271A would have been able to travel very far, particularly in the rugged terrain surrounding the site, due to her pelvic injuries. She could possibly have used a walking stick for added support. Cosker, Ghanour, Gupta, and Tayton (2005, p. 514) reported that 88 % of elderly patients with pelvic ramus fractures required the use of a walking aid (e.g., walking stick(s), walker, wheelchair) 20 weeks after their injury, compared to only 27 % before their injuries. Sixty-two percent of the same sample was no longer able to walk at least 10 yards. Eighty-six percent reported that they needed "substantial increased support from relatives" (Cosker, Ghanour, Gupta, & Tayton, 2005, p. 515). B271A's fractures would likely result in at least short-term changes to her mobility. Even minor impairments would leave her vulnerable to intergroup attacks and make it more difficult to avoid (or outrun) potential animal threats (e.g., predators, poisonous snakes). She may have been able to take on more work tasks that required less travel and less heavy lifting; for example, preparing meals, caring for older children, and weaving may have been feasible. Intensive labor in the agricultural fields, carrying heavy objects (such as vessels for water), or transporting food would probably have been painful and difficult, if not impossible, without assistance from others.

B271A would probably have required assistance walking down the steep slope to the nearby stream, or she may have needed to enlist the help of others in her household to bring her water for drinking and cooking. An escort may have been needed to support her in the upright position to travel to the water source to bathe. Even if she did not experience long-term changes to her mobility, she would probably still have needed to walk cautiously, or at a reduced speed, due to the instability of her pelvis. While it may have added some burden to others in her family or community, she may have been able to offset any loss of work productivity by taking on other, less arduous duties (such as processing and cooking food, weaving, or making pottery). Even if she did regain full mobility in the long term, her pelvis would likely remain susceptible to future fractures, which would make traversing uneven terrain a potentially dangerous activity.

In an agricultural society that produces surplus, accommodating an individual who is injured or sick may not usually be a significant burden, but several lines of evidence from archaeological and bioarchaeological research indicate that the Averbuch community was undergoing considerable biological and social stress during the period in which B271A lived. The abrupt construction of a palisade wall, as well as skeletal evidence of intergroup conflict, indicates that the threat of violence was quite real. Such threats would probably have restricted travel outside the security of the village walls to acquire food and other resources. The breadth of plant species exploitation was surprisingly narrow despite the resource potential in the region, and skeletal evidence suggests that the population had high frequencies of infectious disease and nutritional deficiencies. Furthermore, if fewer individuals were available to procure food due to violent injury or illness, then the added burden of caring for an extra person for any extended period of time may not have been feasible.

Conclusion

Care provision in an agricultural society would require cooperation and organization, reflecting an emphasis placed on group identity. To care for those who are not able to fully contribute (if at all) suggests that all members of the group (or at least the individual receiving care) are highly regarded and have important contributions to make beyond physical labor. Living in large households often means that many people are responsible for contributing to shared livelihoods. A responsibility to the group likely outweighs individual interests, where individuals contribute, when possible, to benefit the group as a whole.

Anecdotal evidence for the value placed on older women in Mississippian populations can be drawn from the archaeological and ethnohistoric record. Within Mississippian cosmology, the Old-Woman-Who-Never-Dies (other names for her include Earth Mother, Corn Mother, Grandmother, Old Woman) is a seemingly important mythical deity, often portrayed in ceramic effigies as an older woman hunched over showing her prominent spine (Fig. 5.3) (Hammons & Dye, 2012; Sharp, Knight, & Lankford, 2011; Smith & Miller, 2009). Similar characters portrayed in historic Native American mythologies suggest that she represents the mother of humans and plants, giving seeds to humankind for their agricultural crops. Such effigies have been found at sites throughout the Mississippian World, including Averbuch and other MCR sites (Smith & Miller, 2009). Earth Mother was thought to make possible the cycle of life, death, and rebirth (Hammons & Dye,

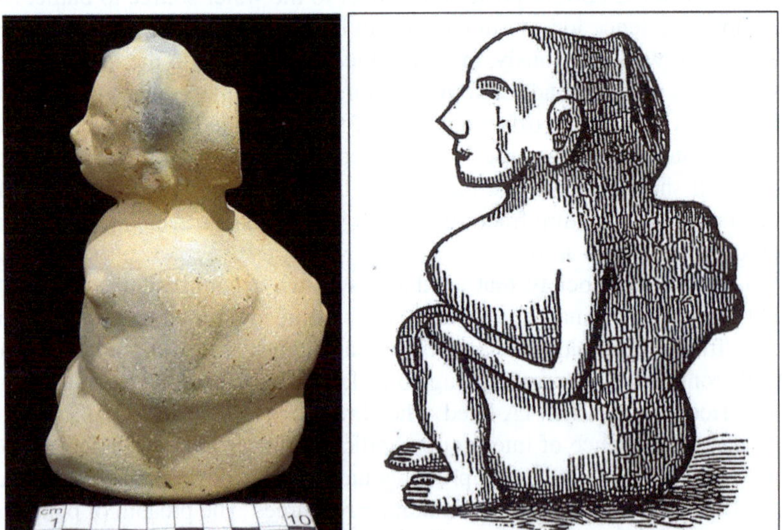

Fig. 5.3 (**a**) Effigy of the Old-Woman-Who-Never-Dies (or Earth Mother) excavated from the Averbuch site; (**b**) Drawing of an Old-Woman-Who-Never-Dies effigy, also from the MCR (Jones, 1876, p. 41, Fig. 4)

2012). Her prominence in Mississippian mythology may reflect the significance or importance of women (or older women) in the community. Perhaps B271A's survival through multiple likely debilitating and potentially life-threatening injuries was due, in part, to the care she received because of her social identity in the community.

Acknowledgements A special thanks to Giovanna Vidoli, Dawnie Steadman, Christina Fojas, Erin Koch, Janet Mansfield, and Hilary Jarvis for their help, as well as Boyce N. Driskell and Jennifer McDonough at the University of Tennessee Archaeological Research Laboratory for granting permission to analyze the skeletal collections. I would also like to thank Lorna Tilley and Alecia A. Schrenk for the invitation to contribute to this volume. This project was supported in part by an NSF grant awarded to D. W. Steadman and C. C. Cobb (BCS-0613173).

References

Aghababian, R. V. (2011). *Essentials of emergency medicine* (2nd ed.). Sudbury, MA: Jones & Bartlett Learning.

Báez-Molgado, S., Bartelink, E. J., Jellema, L. M., Spurlock, L., & Sholts, S. B. (2015). Classification of pelvic ring fractures in skeletonized human remains. *Journal of Forensic Sciences, 60*, S171–S176.

Bellabarba, C., Winkelmann, M., Decker, S., Bransford, R. J., & Krettek, C. (2009). Pelvic ring injuries. In B. B. Browner, J. B. Jupiter, C. Krettek, & P. A. Anderson (Eds.), *Skeletal trauma: Expert consult* (4th ed., pp. 1021–1105). Philadelphia: Elsevier Saunders.

Berryman, H. E. (1981). *The Averbuch skeletal series: A Study of Biological and Social Stress at a Late Mississippian Period Site from Middle Tennessee*, Ph.D. dissertation, Department of Anthropology, The University of Tennessee, Knoxville, Tennessee.

Berryman, H. (1984) The Averbuch skeletal series: A study of biological and social stress at a late Mississippian period site from Middle Tennessee. In W. E. Klippel, & W. M. Bass (Eds.) *Averbuch: A Mississippian manifestation in the Nashville Basin – Observations* (Vol. 1, pp. 5:1–133). Report submitted to the National Park Services, Contract CX 5000-9-5943 between the University of Tennessee and the National Park Service. Copy on file, Department of Anthropology, University of Tennessee, Knoxville, Tennessee.

Boldsen, J. L., George, R. M., Lyle, W. K., & James, W. W. (2002). Transition analysis: A new method for estimating age from skeletons. In R. D. Hoppa & W. V. James (Eds.), *Paleodemography: Age distributions from skeletal samples* (Cambridge studies in biological and evolutionary anthropology, pp. 73–106). Cambridge: Cambridge University Press.

Brehm, H. C., & Evans, E. R. (1977). The preliminary report of an experimental stone box burial. *Tennessee Anthropologist, 2*, 16–23.

Brickley, M. (2006). Rib fractures in the archaeological record: A useful source of sociocultural information? *International Journal of Osteoarchaeology, 16*, 61–75.

Brown, I. W. (1981). A study of stone box graves in eastern North America. *Tenn Anthropol, 6*, 1–26.

Buikstra, J. E., & Ubelaker, D. H. (1994). *Standards for data collection from human skeletal remains*. Fayetteville, Arkansas: Arkansas Archeological Survey.

Buikstra, J. E., William A., Emanuel B., Leslie E., & Nikolaas van der M. (1988). Diet and Health in the Nashville Basin: Human Adaptation and Maize Agriculture in Middle Tennessee. In B. V. Kennedy, & G. M. LeMoine (Eds.) *Diet and Subsistence: Current Archaeological Perspectives* (pp. 243–259). Proceedings of the 19th Annual Chacmool Conference. Archaeological Association of the University of Calgary, Calgary.

Casselberry, S. E. (1974). Further refinement of formulae for determining population from floor area. *World Archaeology, 6*, 117–122.

Cobb, C. R., Krus, A. M., & Steadman, D. W. (2015). Bayesian modeling of the occupation span of the Averbuch site in the Middle Cumberland Drainage, Tennessee. *Southeastern Archaeology, 32*(1), 46–56.

Cole, P. A., Schroder, L. K., & Jacobson, A. R. (2009). Scapula and rib fractures. In B. B. Browner, J. B. Jupiter, C. Krettek, & P. A. Anderson (Eds.), *Skeletal trauma: Expert consult* (4th ed., pp. 1519–1555). Philadelphia: Elsevier Saunders.

Cosker, T. D. A., Ghanour, A., Gupta, S. K., & Tayton, K. J. J. (2005). Pelvic ramus fracture in the elderly: 50 patients studied with MRI. *Acta Orthopaedica, 76*, 513–516.

Crites, G. D. (1984). The Averbuch Skeletal Series: A Study of Biological and Social Stress at a Late Mississippian Period Site from Middle Tennessee. In W. E. Klippel, & W. M. Bass (Eds.) *Averbuch: A Mississippian Manifestation in the Nashville Basin – Observations* (Vol. 1). Report submitted to the National Park Services, Contract CX 5000-9-5943 between the University of Tennessee and the National Park Service. Copy on file, Department of Anthropology, University of Tennessee, Knoxville, Tennessee.

Denis, F. (1984). Spinal instability as defined by the three-column spine concept in acute spinal trauma. *Clinical Orthopaedics and Related Research, 189*, 65–76.

Denis, F., David, S., & Comfort, T. (1988). Sacral fractures: An important problem – Retrospective analysis of 236 cases. *Clinical Orthopaedics and Related Research, 227*, 67–81.

Dowd, J. T. (2008). The Cumberland stone-box burials of middle Tennessee. *Tennessee Archaeology, 3*, 163–180.

Dutton, M. (2011). *Orthopaedics for the physical therapist*. Sudbury, MA: Jones & Bartlett Learning.

Eisenberg, L. E. (1986). *Adaptation in a 'Marginal' Mississippian Population from Middle Tennessee: Biocultural Insights from Paleopathology*, Ph.D. dissertation, Department of Anthropology, New York University, New York.

Eisenberg, L. E. (1991a). Interpreting measures of community health during the late prehistoric period in Middle Tennessee: A Biocultural Approach. In H. Bush, & M. Zvelebil (Eds.) *Health in Past Societies: Biocultural Interpretations of Human Skeletal Remains in Archaeological Contexts* (pp. 115–127). British Archaeological Reports, International Series 567, Tempus Reparatum, Oxford.

Eisenberg, L. E. (1991b). Mississippian cultural terminations in middle Tennessee: What the bio-archaeological evidence can tell us. In M. L. Powell, P. S. Bridges, & A. M. W. Mires (Eds.), *What Mean these bones? Studies in southeastern bioarchaeology* (pp. 70–88). Tuscaloosa, Alabama: University of Alabama Press.

Erdmann, D., Follmar, K. E., DeBruijn, M., Bruno, A. D., Jung, S. H., Edelman, D., et al. (2008). A retrospective analysis of facial fracture etiologies. *Annals of Plastic Surgery, 60*, 398–403.

Evans, D. C. (1982). Biomechanics of spinal injury. In E. R. Gonza & I. J. Harrington (Eds.), *The biomechanics of musculoskeletal injury* (pp. 163–224). Baltimore: Williams and Wilkins.

Ferguson, G., & Allen, B. L. (1984). A mechanistic classification of thoracolumbar spine fractures. *Clinical Orthopaedics and Related Research, 189*, 77–88.

Fermanis, G., Deane, S. A., & Fitzgerald, P. M. (1985). The significance of first and second rib fractures. *Australian and New Zealand Journal of Surgery, 55*, 383–386.

Galloway, A., Stini, R. A., Fox, S. C., & Stein, P. (1990). Stature loss among an older United States population and its relation to bone mineral status. *American Journal of Physical Anthropology, 83*, 467–476.

Gerbershagen, H. J., Dagtekin, O., Isenberg, J., Martens, N., Ozgür, E., Krep, H., et al. (2010). Chronic pain and disability after pelvic and acetabular fractures – Assessment with the Mainz Pain Staging System. *Journal of Trauma, 69*, 128–136.

Gowland, R. L. (2015). Elder abuse: Evaluating the potentials and problems of diagnosis in the archaeological record. *International Journal of Osteoarchaeology*. doi:10.1002/oa.2442.

Gubler, K., Dean, D. O., Maier, R., Davis, R., Koepsell, T., Soderberg, R., et al. (1996). Trauma recidivism in the elderly. *Journal of Trauma-Injury Infection & Critical Care, 41*, 952–956.

Hammons, C., & Dye, D. H. (2012). *Female effigy bottles in the Central Mississippi Valley*. Paper Presented at the 77th Annual Meeting of the Society for American Archaeology, Memphis.

Ho, A. M., Karmmakar, M. K., & Critchley, L. A. (2011). Acute pain management of patients with multiple fractured ribs: A focus on regional techniques. *Current Opinion in Critical Care, 17*, 323–327.

Jones, J. (1876). Explorations of the aboriginal remains of Tennessee. *Smithsonian Contributions to Knowledge, 259*, 1–171.

Judd, M. (2002). Ancient injury recidivism: An example from the Kerma period of Ancient Nubia. *International Journal of Osteoarchaeology, 12*, 89–106.

Kara, M., Dikmen, E., Erdal, H. H., Simsir, I., & Kara, S. A. (2003). Disclosure of unnoticed rib fractures with the use of ultrasonography in minor blunt chest trauma. *European Journal of Cardio-Thoracic Surgery, 24*, 608–613.

Karmmakar, M. K., & Ho, A. M. (2003). Acute pain management of patients with multiple fractured ribs. *The Journal of Trauma-Injury, Infection, and Critical Care, 54*, 615–625.

Lachs, M. S., & Pillemer, K. (1995). Abuse and neglect of elderly persons. *The New England Journal of Medicine, 332*, 437–443.

Looser, K. G., & Crombie, H. D. (1976). Pelvic fractures: An anatomic guide to severity of injury-review of 100 cases. *The American Journal of Surgery, 132*, 638–642.

Lovell, N. C. (1997). Trauma analysis in paleopathology. *Yearbook of Physical Anthropology, 40*, 139–170.

Miller, R. A. (1974) *The geologic history of Tennessee*. Bulletin No. 74. Tennessee Division of Geology, Nashville, Tennessee.

Moore, M. C., & Smith, K. E. (2009). *Archaeological expeditions of the Peabody Museum in Middle Tennessee, 1877–1884*. Research Series No. 16. Tennessee, Division of Archaeology, Nashville, Tennessee.

Peh, W. C. G. (1993). Pelvic insufficiency fractures in the elderly. *Annals of the Academy of Medicine, Singapore, 22*, 818–822.

Poole, G. V., Jr., & Myers, R. T. (1981). Morbidity and mortality rates in major blunt trauma to the upper chest. *Annals of Surgery, 193*, 70–75.

Reed, G. A. (1984). The environmental setting. In W. E. Klippel, & William M. Bass (Eds.) *Averbuch: A Late Mississippian Manifestation in the Nashville Basin* (pp. 1.1–1.10). Department of Anthropology, University of Tennessee, Knoxville. Submitted to the National Park Service, Atlanta.

Reed, G. A., & Klippel, W. E. (1984). Averbuch features and structures. In W. E. Klippel, & William M. Bass (Eds.) *Averbuch: A Late Mississippian Manifestation in the Nashville Basin* (pp. 4.1–4.35). Department of Anthropology, University of Tennessee, Knoxville. Submitted to the National Park Service, Atlanta.

Sharp, R. V., Knight, V. J., Jr., & Lankford, G. E. (2011). Woman in the patterned shawl: Female effigy vessels and figurines from the middle Cumberland River Basin. In G. E. Lankford, F. K. Reilly III, & J. F. Garber (Eds.), *Visualizing the sacred* (pp. 177–198). Austin: University of Texas Press.

Shelat, V. G., Eileen, S., John, L., Teo, L. T., Vijayan, A., & Chiu, M. T. (2012). 2012 Chronic pain and its impact on quality of life following a traumatic rib fracture. *European Journal of Trauma and Emergency Surgery, 38*, 451–455.

Sirmali, M., Turut, H., Topcu, S., Gulhan, E., Yazici, U., Kaya, S., et al. (2003). A comprehensive analysis of traumatic rib fractures: Morbidity, mortality and management. *European Journal of Cardio-Thoracic Surgery, 24*, 133–138.

Smith, K. E. (1992). *The Middle Cumberland Region: Mississippian Archaeology in North Central Tennessee* Ph.D. dissertation, Department of Anthropology, Vanderbilt University, Nashville, Tennessee.

Smith, K. E., & Miller, J. V. (2009). *Speaking with the ancestors: The Mississippian stone statuary of the Tennessee-Cumberland region*. Tuscaloosa: The University of Alabama Press.

Smith, K. E., & Moore M. C. (1996). *On the river and up the creek: Contrasting settlement patterns in the cumberland valley*. Presented paper at the 53rd Annual Meeting of the Southeastern Archaeological Conference, Birmingham, Alabama.

Smith, K. E., & Moore, M. C. (1999). Through many Mississippian hands: late prehistoric exchange in the Middle Cumberland Valley. In E. Peacock, & S. O. Brookes (Eds.) *Raw materials and exchange in the Mid-South* (pp. 95–115). Archaeological Report No. 29, Mississippi Department of Archives and History, Jackson, Mississippi.

Tile, M. (1988). Pelvic ring fractures: Should they be fixed? *Journal of Bone and Joint Surgery [Br], 70B*, 1–12.

Tilley, L. (2012). The bioarchaeology of care. *SAA Archaeological Record: The SAA Archaeological Record: New Directions in Bioarchaeology, Part II, 12*(3), 39–41.

Tilley, L., & Cameron, T. (2014). Introducing the index of care: A web-based application supporting archaeological research into health-related care. *International Journal of Paleopathology, 6*, 5–9.

Wedel, V. L., & Galloway, A. (2014). *Broken bones: Anthropological analysis of blunt force trauma* (2nd ed.). Springfield: Charles C. Thomas.

Worne, H. (2011). *Conflicting spaces: bioarchaeological and geophysical perspectives on warfare in the Middle Cumberland Region of Tennessee* Ph.D. dissertation, Binghamton University, Binghamton.

Worne, H., Cobb, C. R., Vidoli, G. M., & Steadman, D. W. (2012). The space of war: Connecting geophysical landscapes with skeletal evidence of warfare-related trauma. In D. L. Martin, R. P. Harrod, & V. R. Pérez (Eds.), *The bioarchaeology of violence* (pp. 141–159). Gainesville: University Press of Florida.

Chapter 6
Applying the 'Index of Care' to a Person Who Experienced Leprosy in Late Medieval Chichester, England

Charlotte Roberts

In times of stress, pain or of sorrow, the human being will go to any length to find help

(Withers, 1960, p. 1).

Introduction

Definitions, Care Provision and the Epidemiological Transitions

The Oxford English Dictionary defines 'care' as: 'The provision of what is necessary for the health, welfare, maintenance, and protection of someone or something', (medical) 'treatment' as: 'Medical care given to a patient for an illness or injury', and 'compassion' as: 'Sympathetic pity and concern for the sufferings or misfortunes of others'. All these terms are relevant to this paper and are used through its course.

The provision of care and treatment for all people with illness at the point of need in England has always been a subject of debate, with the National Health Service being created in 1958. Today this debate is no more or less intensive as the world's population now lives through the third epidemiological transition, where new infections are emerging and old ones are re-emerging (Harper & Armelagos, 2010). In the first epidemiological transition, a general decline in health was observed at the time our ancestors started to practice agriculture. Establishing settled communities, they encountered new and different health-related hazards in their lives, including population density diseases; they became subject to zoonoses connected to the domestication of animals, and deficiency diseases linked to a less varied and

C. Roberts, B.A., M.A., Ph.D., S.R.N., F.B.A., F.S.A. (✉)
Department of Archaeology, Durham University, County Durham, UK
e-mail: c.a.roberts@durham.ac.uk

© Springer International Publishing Switzerland 2017

L. Tilley, A.A. Schrenk (eds.), *New Developments in the Bioarchaeology of Care*, Bioarchaeology and Social Theory, DOI 10.1007/978-3-319-39901-0_6

unreliable diet than under a hunter-forager regime (e.g. see Cohen & Armelagos, 2013; Cohen & Crane-Kramer, 2007; Roberts & Cox, 2003; Steckel & Rose, 2002). In the nineteenth century, English populations then experienced a further decline in health as they lived and worked in industrialised (usually urban) environments. This second epidemiological transition, occurring from the early modern period to the twentieth century, saw a decline in infections as living conditions improved, and a rise in chronic non-infectious degenerative diseases such as cancer and heart problems as people lived longer; health also became a real concern for governments. For example, in England and Wales today males and females who were born in 2012 will, on average, expect to live until the age of 79.5 and 83.3 years, respectively (Bennett et al., 2015).

As a result of people living longer, the pressures on health care provision in the UK have seen a parallel increase. This has resulted in questions being asked about the quality of care and treatment given in care environments (http://www.theguardian.com/society/2013/feb/06/mid-staffs-hospital-scandal-guide), and the need for more transparent information about hospital care to be provided (http://www.nhs.uk/NHSEngland/AboutNHSservices/NHShospitals/Pages/HospitalsSummary.aspx). Whatever the nature of available care and treatment, while its availability and practice cannot always be proved in the past, it is likely that compassion has been a human trait that has existed in populations throughout time and across the globe.

However, whether care and treatment have always existed in parallel with compassion is an area needing much more research. Even if a person lives in a compassionate community, in some circumstances and for various reasons they may not be cared for (Dettwyler, 1991). For example, while the UK would probably describe itself as a compassionate society, this does not always translate into *actual* compassion; children, the elderly, the poor, the 'disabled' and the sick do not always receive the compassion and care that is warranted (Malmedal et al., 2015; Norman et al., 2012). Indeed, in a study of care and compassion for people with dementia, results showed that there were differences in specific care situations; the level of care that different people experienced varied, with examples of both excellent and poor practices (Crowther et al., 2013). Bioarchaeologists therefore need to be cautious when attempting to infer compassion and care for people purely represented by their skeletal remains; as is seen today, each individual circumstance will differ. The use of a multidisciplinary perspective and engagement with diverse methods of analysis are important.

Bioarchaeological Evidence for Care

Evidence from a range of disciplines indicates that people were cared for in the past and could even have been treated medically and surgically (Porter, 1997). Who was cared for and how is another matter entirely. A person's biological sex, their gender, age, status, and where and when they lived will all affect whether they received care and treatment. However, primary evidence of care and treatment from human remains excavated from archaeological sites is limited to the dentition (Weinberger,

2004): for example, 'fillings' in Medieval carious teeth (Denmark: Møller-Christensen, 1969) and dental prosthetics, such as bridges and false teeth recovered from eighteenth to nineteenth century Christchurch, Spitalfields, London (Molleson & Cox, 1993), and the skeleton: trepanations (see review in Arnottet al., 2003; Jolly & Kurin, Chap. 9 this volume), and amputated body parts and prosthetics, such as the prosthetic toe found with a 21st Dynasty Egyptian mummy (Nerlich et al., 2000). In addition, rarer examples include possible treatment of 'pigeon chest', using compression bandaging of the chest in a high status young woman from late medieval Ripon, North Yorkshire, England (Groves et al., 2003); the application of a linen bandage dressing of sulphur and ivy leaves to a syphilitic skin lesion in a sixteenth-century Italian mummy from Naples, Italy (Fornaciari et al., 1989; Nystrom & Piombini-Mascali, Chap. 10 this volume), and the application of copper plates to infected bones in medieval Sweden, Belgium, and England (Hallback, 1976–1977; Janssens, 1987; Knüsel et al., 1995, respectively). These instances represent direct evidence of interventions to address health problems, but assessing whether a person received mental *and* physical care in any guise, ranging from providing food, water and shelter to attending to personal hygiene, lending a 'helping hand', and even just having a 'shoulder to cry on' or a 'hand to hold', is challenging.

Bioarchaeology is increasingly addressing whether care provision existed (e.g. Tilley & Oxenham, 2011; Tilley, Chap. 2 this volume), and applying modern clinical knowledge to understanding likely disease impact (e.g. Roberts, 2000) and the need for care. Ultimately, for historical periods where medical documentation exists, it becomes increasingly possible to compare and contrast the bioarchaeological and medical historical evidence for care and treatment. Nevertheless, because of the type of evidence available, the often subjective nature of this procedure leaves many questions unanswered, and over-interpretation of the data can be the end result. For example, Lebel et al. (2001) and Lebel & Trinkaus (2002) described antemortem tooth loss in a jaw from a person recovered from the site of Bau de l'Aubesier, Vaucluse, France, who lived in the Middle Pleistocene. The authors interpreted the loss as a debilitating condition, which they said must have needed the person's community to select and manually prepare soft foods, which could have meant extensive use of cooking. This, it was argued, would have enabled the person to survive in their hunter-gatherer group. A challenge to this study came from DeGusta (2002, 2003), who reviewed antemortem loss of teeth in non-human primates and suggested that, because these primates survived loss of teeth and managed well without 'care', the basis of the claim by Lebel was flawed. While DeGusta's work can also be criticised, over-interpretation of data from archaeological human remains to infer care and compassion must be avoided.

However, there have been more convincing examples of studies in the literature that identify likely care scenarios and use multiple lines of evidence to examine these (see chapters in this volume). For example, Hawkey (1998) describes and interprets bone changes consistent with juvenile rheumatoid arthritis in an adult man from Gran Quivira Pueblo, New Mexico, but also documents the progressive effect of the disease by exploring joint mobility range using musculoskeletal marker data. She showed that the entheseal changes in the skeletal remains of this man suggested a dependence on his community as he experienced a disease that began in childhood and which he suffered until his death as an adult. By considering data on this disease's progression in clinical contexts, and estimating the range of joint mobility, it was possible to estimate his potential range of movement at various stages of his life and to infer the extent of his impairment. The entheseal change data also differed when compared to those for other adult males at the site. While Hawkey admits that 'compassion cannot always be determined from the skeletal record alone' she felt on the basis of the evidence that, because the disease appeared to be 'severe', he must have been 'wholly dependent on at least one other member of the group over a long period of time' (1998, p. 326). It should also be noted that there is scope for taking a comparative view of care and compassion, as outlined by Fashing & Nguygen (2011) in their review of compassion and care in other animals.

Concepts of Disease, Levels of Knowledge, the Meaning of Disease and the Importance of Context

Apart from over-interpreting bioarchaeological data, sometimes with little scientific basis, the geographic and temporal contexts of human remains being studied for evidence of care need close consideration. Concepts and attitudes of different cultures towards disease play a large part in how a person may be cared for (e.g. see McElroy & Townsend, 2009) or treated medically and surgically, and medical, surgical, and anatomical knowledge will determine what treatment is possible and attempted.

For example, before human bodies could be legally dissected (first recorded in 1315 in Italy – Porter, 1997, p. 132), practitioners applied anatomical knowledge learnt from animals in treating their patients. Human dissections paved the way for more realistic portrayals of the human body by people such as Vesalius (Belgium, sixteenth century AD) and Leonardo da Vinci (Italy, fifteenth to sixteenth centuries AD). However, a wide range of experiences and outcomes would be expected even for people with the same diseases, past and present. As medical anthropologists who work with populations experiencing ill health in both developed and developing countries indicate, 'disease' can be defined in a range of ways. Disease is usually viewed from a clinical rather than a wider social perspective by clinicians, but what the person actually experiences is 'illness', or the 'interpretation of his or her experience using meanings of notions of causality, provided by the culture to explain misfortune' (McElroy & Townsend, 2009, p. 44). Appreciation of the detailed clinical features and their implications may not be of key importance to the person; it is *their* personal experience that is important to them. A related and relevant term for people with an illness is 'sickness', which is explained as how a person with an illness is 'expected to behave' by their society (McElroy & Townsend, 2009, p. 44).

Anybody studying health and disease, when interpreting their data past or present, should take into account the geographic location, time period, the person affected, the community in which they lived and the agents involved with health care (traditional healer, relatives, surgeon, physician, etc.). What may be classed as a disease in the western sense could be viewed as an illness that, in the eyes of the person experiencing this illness and their community more generally, does not need treatment. These reflections need attention when constructing a 'bioarchaeology of care'. Moreover, even if care provision can be established based on a contextualised study of skeletal remains, the level and type of care may have changed over the course of that person's disease, and of course is dependent on the specific disease experienced (see later with reference to this study).

This introduction and background set the scene for the rest of the chapter. Additionally relevant is the recent publication of the 'Index of Care' (Tilley & Cameron, 2014; Chap. 2 this volume), following on from Tilley & Oxenham (2011), where a more objective method than has been available previously has been outlined for assessing the likely provision of care for people whose skeletons bioarchaeologists study.

The study reported in this chapter is a pilot test of this method on a skeleton with evidence of disease. In this case a skeleton with leprosy was chosen because (1) there can be recognisable bone changes consistent with the infection; (2) in the late medieval period there are many historical data suggesting that most people with leprosy were stigmatised and marginalised, often in leprosy hospitals; and (3) there is a considerable wealth of evidence in this period for 'care' and 'treatment' of those with leprosy (e.g. Demaitre, 2007; Rawcliffe, 2006). Leprosy is a bacterial infectious disease that is caused by *Mycobacterium leprae* or *lepromatosis* and is contracted via the inhalation of exhaled respiratory droplets containing the bacteria (Han et al., 2008; Scollard et al., 2006). It is an infection that affects the skin, peripheral nerves, the mucosa of the upper respiratory tract and the eyes. Today, if it is not treated early with antibiotics, it can lead to damage to the bones of the face, hands, and feet, and other complications (Butlin & Saunderson, 2014). It also has a considerable association with impairment, 'disability', and handicap in the parts of the world where it has been, and is, most frequent (Rodrigues & Lockwood, 2011).

Thus, the aim of this study is to apply the 'Index of Care' to the skeleton of a person who experienced leprosy in late medieval England. In effect, this chapter is set out as a standard scientific paper. As the Index of Care has not yet been widely tested, this pilot study will contribute to the development of further studies that address different time periods and geographic regions and deal with skeletons showing a range of different disease processes.

'Material' and Methods

The skeleton (C148) that is the focus of this study was excavated from the cemetery of St James and St Mary Magdalene, Chichester, Sussex, close to the south coast of England, and around 70 miles south-west of London (Magilton et al., 2008). A late and post-medieval site (twelfth to eighteenth centuries AD) reliant on an agricultural-based economy, this cemetery initially served an urban leprosy

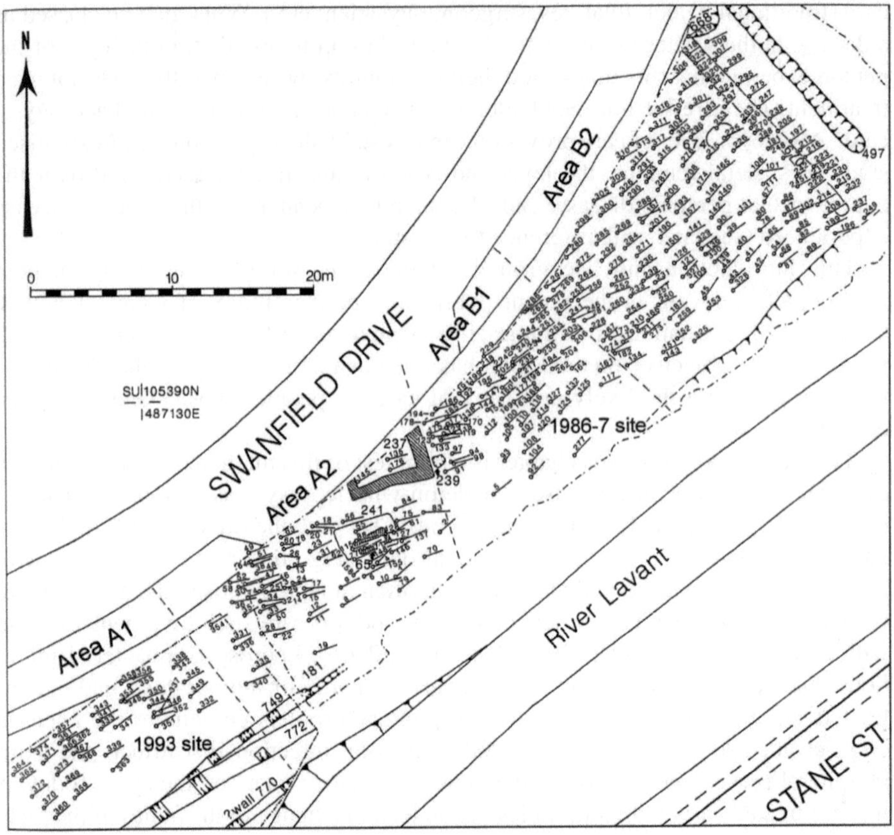

Fig. 6.1 Location of skeleton 148 in the Area A2 part of the cemetery (from Magilton et al., 2008: Fig. 7.9); earlier burials are in Area 1, and later burials in B1 and B2

hospital, which later became a hospital for people with a range of illnesses. The cemetery had different phases, but this skeleton derived from the early part of the cemetery dated to the twelfth to fourteenth centuries AD (Fig. 6.1).

This skeleton had already been analysed as a component of the report on the site (Magilton et al., 2008), and leprosy had already been diagnosed, but original biological data were collected for the purposes of this study. Assessment of the condition of the skeleton C148 was made by compiling an inventory of the bones and observing the nature of bone fragmentation and surface preservation. The sex of the person was estimated through features of the pelvis and skull (described in Brickley, 2004), and age at death was estimated by observing the state of the late fusing epiphyses (basilar suture, sternal end of the clavicle, vertebral epiphyseal rims, heads of the ribs, iliac crest, and sacral segments – Scheuer & Black, 2000: various pages), degenerative changes on the pubic symphysis (Brooks & Suchey, 1990) and the sternal ends of the ribs (İşcan & Loth, 1986); dental attrition was also recorded (Brothwell, 1981). The bones and teeth of the skeleton were assessed for evidence of pathological changes. Lesions caused by bone formation and destruction, and dental destruction (e.g. dental caries, enamel hypoplasia) and accretion (calculus) were recorded, their distribution pattern documented, and differential diagnoses considered (see Roberts & Connell, 2004). Particular consideration was paid to the bone changes of leprosy, as originally described by Møller-Christensen (1961, 1978), with further research considered from Andersen, Manchester, and others (Andersen & Manchester, 1987, 1988, 1992; Andersen et al., 1992; Andersen et al., 1994). The Index of Care steps described by Tilley & Cameron (2014) were followed during analysis and interpretation of the data.

Results: Description, Analysis of Aetiology, and Interpretation

Description

The skeleton was quite well preserved, with intact cortical bone and most of the bones present, including the facial, hand, and foot bones (which are often affected in leprosy). However, some of the bones were fragmented, including, for example, the skull, scapulae, innominate bones, sacrum, and left leg bones. The mandible and maxilla, with their teeth, were particularly well preserved, with only five teeth being lost postmortem (upper left 2nd and 3rd molars, lower right premolars, and lower left first premolar).

The sex of the person was estimated as male (prominent nuchal crest, large mastoid processes, zygomatic arch extending across the external auditory meatus, upright rami and flaring of the right gonial angle, square 'chin'; narrow sciatic notches and sub-pubic angle, and no ventral arc). Age at death was estimated to be between 25 and 35 years. All late fusing epiphyses were fused, the pubic symphyses were estimated to be at stages 3 and 4 (25–35 years), and the sternal rib ends appeared to be 'young'; dental attrition showed an age of between 25 and 35 years.

Pathological changes of the skeleton affected the bones and the dentition. Antemortem tooth loss was noted for the upper right 1st premolar, and the left lower 1st and right lower 3rd molars. Caries was present on the upper right 3rd molar (occlusal); the mesial surfaces of the upper right 1st and 2nd molars; the occlusal and distal surfaces of the lower left 2nd premolar; and the occlusal, distal and buccal surfaces of the lower left 3rd molar. Calculus was present on all teeth present for observation, and the lower canine teeth and upper canine and incisor teeth displayed enamel hypoplastic defects (Fig. 6.2).

Pitting was present on the left side of the superior surface of the greater wing of the sphenoid bone, the sagittal sulcus of the endocranium (also with new bone formation, which was grey in colour), the proximal part of the nasal bones, parts of the ectocranium, the mental protuberance of the mandible, and the anterior part of

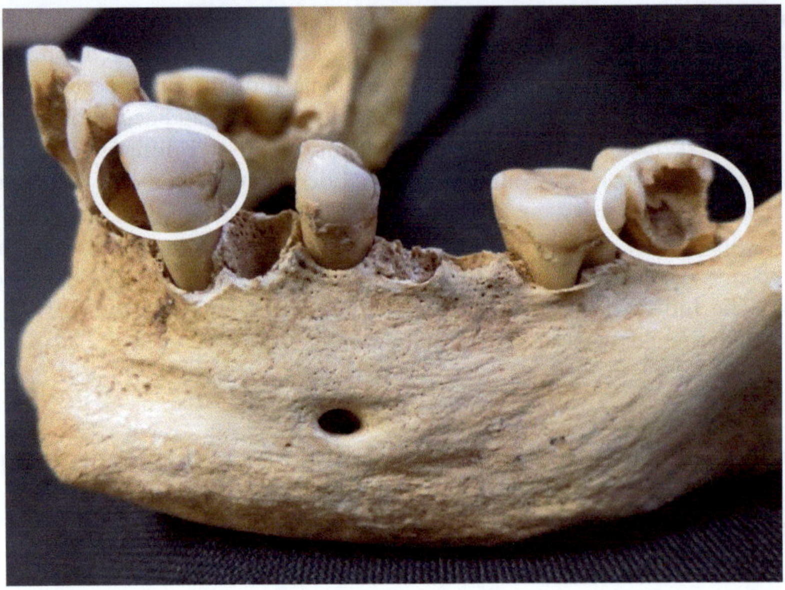

Fig. 6.2 Left side of the lower jaw (*mandible*) showing dental caries of the 3rd molar tooth and an enamel defect on the canine tooth ('groove') - highlighted, along with dental calculus on many teeth

the zygomatic bones; the pitting of the sagittal sulcus was very well remodelled. The anterior nasal spine was resorbed. The 'caucasian' feature of 'silling' (sharp ridges) was present on the base of the nasal cavity (either side of the nasal spine), with some remodelling of the nasal margins close to the absent nasal spine; the rest of the nasal margins superior to the nasal spine that were present for observation were sharp. The tooth roots were exposed to a greater or lesser degree on both the mandible and maxilla and the alveolar margins were in some cases remodelled and rounded, although some margins were clearly damaged postmortem. All the anterior upper teeth, in particular, displayed extensive antemortem exposure of the tooth roots. The nasal surface of the palate had a patch of grey woven bone on the right side, and there was general pitting of the oral surface. The left maxillary sinus contained pitting and well-remodelled new bone (see Figs. 6.3 and 6.4).

Postcranially, five right and four left ribs had well remodelled new lamellar bone formation on their necks, and two unsided rib shafts displayed small patches of woven bone, with one having pitting on its subcostal groove. Five other ribs had degenerative changes on their heads and/or the articular parts of the tubercles (osteophytes and/or porosity [Fig. 6.5]).

The spine was also affected by degenerative changes. Of note, the thoracic and cervical vertebrae had anterior body pitting and new bone formation (C5–7 and T1–4); C5 also had antero-inferior body osteophytes, and T5 also had a large osteophyte on the right side of its inferior body. T6 displayed a corresponding superior right large osteophyte on its body, and also a depression on the inferior body surface.

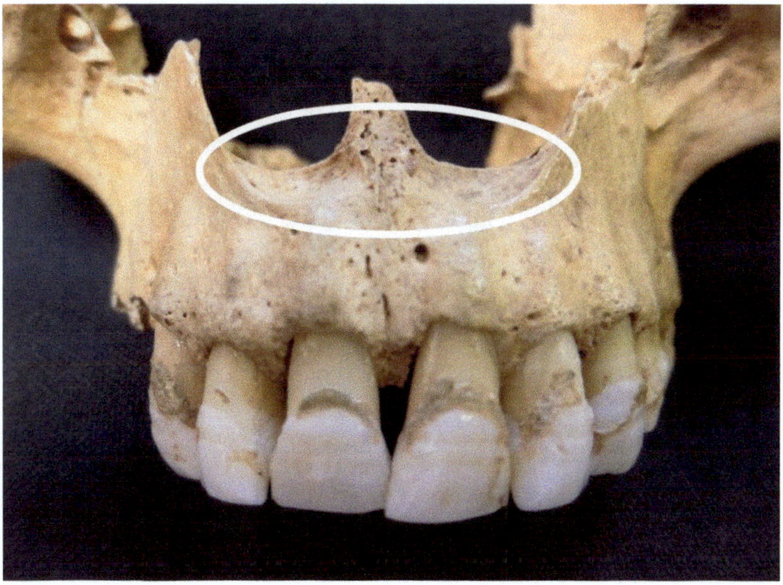

Fig. 6.3 Anterior view of the upper jaw (maxilla) showing recession of alveolar bone around the tooth roots, absorption and remodelling of the inferior nasal aperture area and loss of the anterior nasal spine (highlighted), enamel defects on the incisor teeth, and dental calculus on many teeth

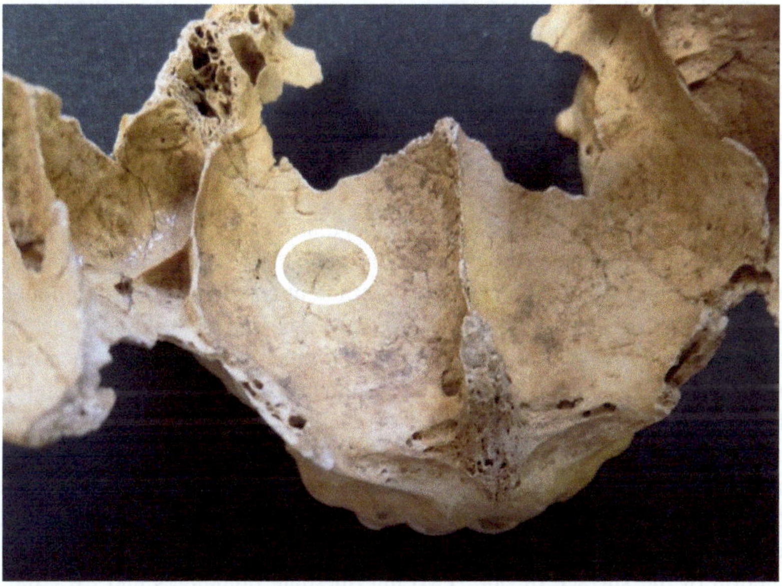

Fig. 6.4 New bone formation on the right nasal surface of the palate (highlighted)

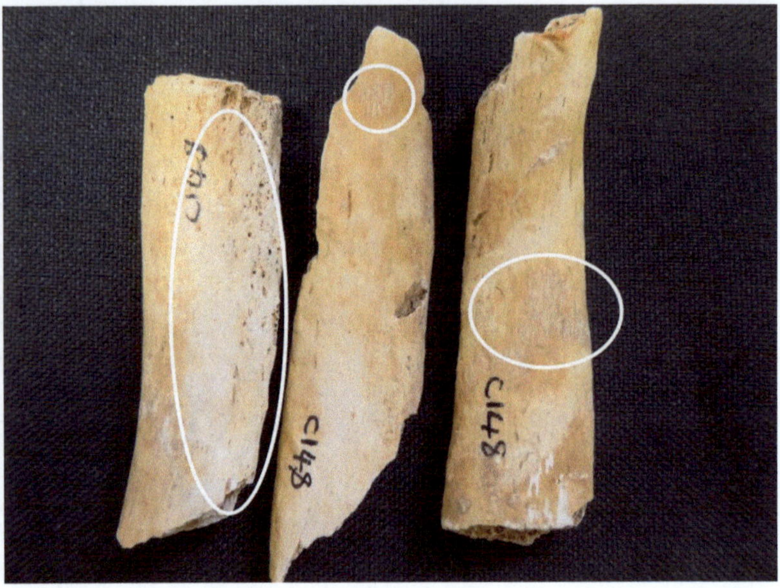

Fig. 6.5 Some of the obvious new bone formation on some of the visceral surfaces of rib shafts (highlighted)

T7–T8 had depressions on their inferior bodies, and a superior body anterior osteophyte on T7. T9 had depressions on both its body surfaces, and a superior anterolateral body osteophyte. T10 had a depression on its inferior body, osteophytes on its transverse processes and on the supero-right body. T11 had depressions on both body surfaces and a right side superior body osteophyte. T12–L3 had depressions on both body surfaces and on L4 superiorly only. The manubrium and body of the sternum had irregular surfaces anteriorly, comprised of well-remodelled new bone formation.

The right humerus displayed a small, irregular, destructive lesion on the capitulum, and the right radius and ulna had marginal osteophytes around their proximal articular surfaces. The left clavicle had a prominent costoclavicular ligament attachment, and pitting of its sternal and clavicular ends. The right-hand bones showed pitting to the anterior shafts of all the metacarpals, and the 2nd metacarpal had a disto-inferior articular marginal osteophyte and surface pitting. The left-hand bones displayed fusion of the proximal and distal hand phalanges of the thumb, and absorption of the distal part of a distal phalanx. There were also absorptive ‘grooves’ on the distal ends of the palmar aspects of five proximal phalanges (two with dorsal shaft pitting) - Fig. 6.6. The pitting was less obvious on three other proximal phalanges, but two had osteophyte formation around their distal articular surfaces, with destruction of the surface of one. Two intermediate phalanges had irregular distal joint surfaces, and one had an absorbed distal end and new bone formation on the proximal end around the joint surface.

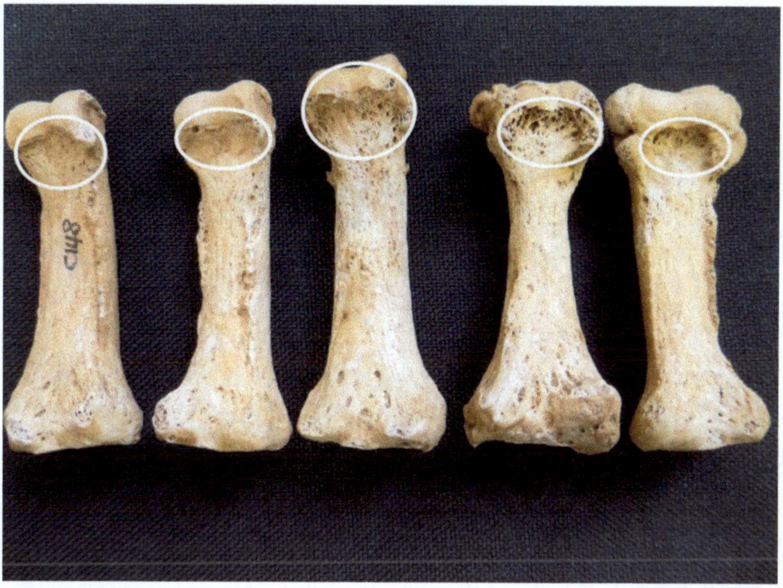

Fig. 6.6 'Absorptive grooves' on the distal (palmar) aspects of the proximal hand phalanges

The left femur, both fibulae and the distal tibiae all had well remodelled new bone formation along their shafts, and the tibiae and fibulae had thickened distal cortices. The fibulae were particularly affected on both sides. On the right side the 1st metatarsal had inferior new bone formation on the shaft, the 5th metatarsal displayed a mid-shaft inferior surface large nutrient foramen and pitting of the shaft, and the calcaneum had pitting to its medial side. On the left side, the calcaneum also had medial surface pitting. The 1st metatarsal was half the length of that of the right side and had a remodelled distal end (Fig. 6.7).

The shaft of the 2nd metatarsal had well remodelled new bone formation, the 3rd metatarsal had new bone formation on the dorsal part of its shaft, and the 4th metatarsal had an enlarged nutrient foramen just below mid-shaft on its medial surface. The 5th metatarsal had a remodelled 'knife edge' shaft with loss and remodelling of its distal quarter, pitting and new bone formation along its shaft, and an enlarged nutrient foramen on the mid-shaft inferior surface. Two intermediate and distal phalanges were fused, and four intermediate phalanges had concentric remodelling (one with loss of the distal end and remodelling).

Diagnosis and Aetiological Interpretation

The dental and skeletal changes indicating pathological processes in the skeleton indicate a number of diagnoses and aetiological interpretations. Dental caries and calculus suggest a diet regularly containing fermentable carbohydrates (starches

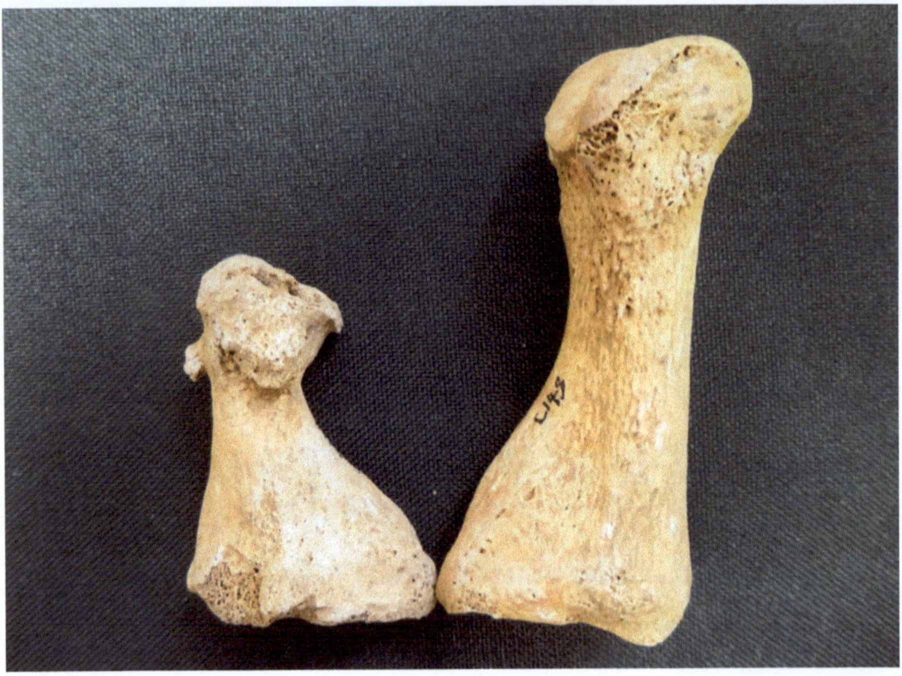

Fig. 6.7 Comparison of the 1st metatarsals showing the difference in length between *left* and *right*, due to bone absorption

and sugars – Hillson, 1996, p. 254), and possibly the milk and dairy product protein casein. Lack of oral hygiene and fluoride in the water may also be contributory factors. Plaque bacteria ferment these constituents of the diet, creating an acidic oral environment and ultimately destruction of the enamel and dentine of teeth. This man experienced antemortem tooth loss, which could have been caused by underlying caries, periapical lesions, or periodontal disease. He had antemortem exposure of many tooth roots, which may be related to periodontal disease, but could also be linked to dental attrition and continuing eruption (Clarke & Hirsch, 1992). The enamel hypoplastic defects suggest a period of 'stress' during development of the teeth, which may be related to a dietary deficiency or childhood disease (Hillson, 1996, p. 177). It is noted that people with leprosy have poorer dental health than those without (e.g. see Reichart et al., 1976).

The pitting observed on many of the bones of the skull suggests either normal variation for the population or an inflammatory process, perhaps as a direct result of infection of the skin (e.g. lupus vulgaris, or tuberculosis of the skin, and the skin lesions of leprosy) or a metabolic disease such as scurvy (Brickley & Ives, 2008, p. 57). The endocranial new bone formation suggests a number of possible diagnoses such as meningitis, skull trauma, anaemia, tuberculosis, scurvy, and rickets (Lewis, 2007, p. 141). The bone changes within the maxillary sinus indicate sinusitis, an inflammatory response to poor air quality, infection, allergens, or any predisposing factor irritating the sinuses. Specific infections such as leprosy can also lead to sinusitis, and have been noted in archaeological skeletons with and without leprosy (Roberts et al., 1998), and in people with leprosy in clinical contexts (Hauhnar et al., 1992). The absorption of the anterior nasal spine and exposure of the anterior tooth roots could be associated with leprosy (Møller-Christensen, 1978), but also with tuberculosis and treponemal disease (Ortner, 2003, p. 69; Hackett, 1976). The pitting and new bone formation of the oral and nasal surfaces of the palate may be caused by inflammation due to infections such as leprosy and treponemal disease, but the pitting could also represent normal variation for the population.

The new bone formation on the ribs suggests inflammation from a pulmonary disease. This could include many conditions, such as chronic bronchitis, tuberculosis, and neoplastic disease (see Roberts et al., 1994). Leprosy is also associated with respiratory infections in general (Kaur et al., 1979).

The spine shows evidence for degeneration in the form of osteophytes and Schmorl's nodes, both associated with increasing age (Reid, 2008, p. 354). Schmorl's nodes are the result of degeneration of the fibrous capsule of the disk and protrusion of the disk's contents into the vertebral body surface. As the nodes here are centrally placed on the vertebrae, this may have led to a painful back (Faccia & Williams, 2008).

There were a wide range of pathological lesions in the hand and foot bones, including inflammatory pitting, degeneration and absorption of articular surfaces, fusion of some bones, remodelling of bone shafts, enlargement of nutrient foramina, and absorptive 'grooves' on proximal hand phalanges. All these changes could be associated with leprosy, but individually they are not in themselves pathognomonic. For example, ulceration of the hands and feet due to sensory nerve damage, contraction of the finger and toe joints due to motor nerve loss, and concentric remodelling caused by autonomic nerve dysfunction, all seen in leprosy, can together be responsible for these changes (Paterson & Job, 1964). Nevertheless, diabetes, treponemal disease, tuberculosis, nervous system disorders leading to paralysis, psoriatic arthritis, infections in general, and frostbite may also cause some of these bone changes.

The tibial and fibular new bone formation has been recognised as a characteristic of leprosy, likely associated with swelling of the legs due to problems with blood and lymph circulation. This perhaps represents 'movement' of the inflammatory changes of the feet in an upwards direction (e.g. see Lewis et al., 1995), or is the result of ulceration, or lesions of the overlying skin (e.g. see Boel & Ortner, 2013), but there are many other conditions that could lead to this bone change (Weston, 2012).

In summary, based on the dental and skeletal changes in this man's skeleton, he appears to have experienced various chronic diseases (i.e. those he experienced during his life and from which he did not die). This interpretation is supported by Wood et al. (1992), who note that a person must suffer a disease for long enough for (chronic) bone changes to occur in their skeleton. The conditions seen in this man's skeleton include dental disease, upper (sinus) and lower (lungs) respiratory disease, spinal degeneration, and an infection, most likely leprosy. The facial bone changes,

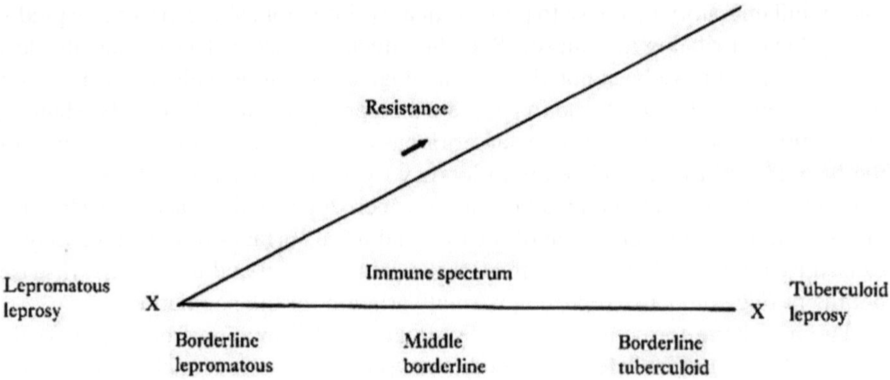

Fig. 6.8 Immune spectrum of leprosy, from low resistance on the *left* (lepromatous leprosy) to high resistance on the *right* (tuberculoid leprosy) – based on Ridley & Jopling (1966) and drawn by Christina Unwin

on which a diagnosis of leprosy usually relies, suggest rhinomaxillary syndrome (Andersen & Manchester, 1992). On the basis of the associated postcranial changes and the context of the skeleton (leprosy hospital cemetery), the changes are therefore most likely due to leprosy.

The type of leprosy this person had was likely the low resistant form (lepromatous leprosy – see Ridley & Jopling, 1966 on the immune spectrum of leprosy (Fig. 6.8)) and it appears that he had it for some time, although it is impossible to say for how long.

The incubation period of leprosy (from infection to expression of the clinical manifestations of the infection) is now thought to be around 5 years (http://www.who.int/mediacentre/factsheets/fs101/en/ accessed July 2015), but different reports suggest periods from a few months to up to 20 years. The first appearance of leprosy is more common in adolescents and adults than in younger people, but this probably reflects the potentially long incubation period. If the incubation period is assumed to have been the same in the past as today (i.e. 5 years), and because this person was aged between 25 and 35 years at death, he could have contracted leprosy during adolescence or his early 20s. Furthermore, the evidence of enamel hypoplasia suggests he was 'stressed' during growth, which may have put him at risk of contracting infectious diseases such as leprosy. Perhaps the presence of enamel hypoplasia indicates a compromised immune system during his growing years and meant that he was more likely to contract the high resistant form of leprosy during that time, eventually progressing to a low resistant form in later life. However, he could also have contracted leprosy later in his adult life, supporting the developmental origins hypothesis (Barker, 1994). Whether initially in adult life he contracted the high or low resistant form is debatable; what is seen here is a person who died with lepromatous leprosy, but the leprosy he experienced may have started as the high resistant form and moved to the other pole of the spectrum (see later for discussion of the immune spectrum of leprosy).

Discussion

Following the application of Step 1 of the Index of Care (*describe, document, diagnose*) described earlier, the discussion of the data of interest recorded from this man's skeleton will follow the remaining Index steps:

- Step 2 (*determine 'disability'*): a consideration of the abnormal lesions seen in the dentition and bones of this man, their potential for functional impacts on his daily life, and the need for 'care'.
- Step 3 (*construct a model of 'care'*): an outline of the care he likely required and with which he was potentially provided.
- Step 4 (*interpretation*): exploration of the implications for this man and his community of the provision and receipt of the care modelled in Step 3.

Step 2: What Can *Be Said About This Man's Experience?*

It is important to first emphasise that it is not possible to say whether this man experienced all of the following challenges as a result of the bone changes observed and, because it is not known when during the man's life these bone changes started, it is not possible to suggest a timeline of events. Essentially, what can be described is a minimalist view of the impact of the infection on his life.

This man had dental caries, which may have been painful and caused problems with eating and a loss of appetite (and weight?). Another factor that could have been associated with a poor appetite may have been loss of his sense of smell and taste due to leprosy related nasal congestion and also, in relation to the former, damage to the olfactory nerve. He had extensive dental calculus, and this may be associated with mouth breathing in leprosy, again as a result of congested nasal passages. He may have experienced chest and sinus pain due to the inflammatory changes he obviously had in his lungs and sinus, and seen represented on his ribs and in one of his sinuses. The sensory loss associated with leprosy most likely led to ulcerations of the feet, and consequently the underlying bone damage; this is less visible in the hand bones, with only one distal phalanx seemingly potentially affected. However, the impact of motor nerve damage was evident in the hand phalanges (fixed flexion of the fingers), suggesting he may have had difficulties with straightening his fingers and using his hands. In addition, if he had problems walking, this may have led to the use of aids for moving around and more 'bed rest', possibly generating pressure sores at points of contact with the underlying surfaces (pressure sores may also be related to loss of skin sensation).

What Cannot *Be Said About This Man's Experience?*

There are a number of features of leprosy that cannot be determined purely from the skeleton. These include whether there actually were skin lesions, facial palsy, or lagophthalmos due to facial nerve damage (inability to close the eyelids fully), blindness or loss of hearing, and his level of back, sinus or chest pain, if he had a hoarse voice (laryngeal involvement in leprosy), or whether he had associated depression, heart problems, fever, inflammation of the lymphatic system, muscle weakness, thinning of eyebrows and eyelashes, the extent of ulceration of the hands, feet, and lower legs, and the level of difficulty he might have had in walking, using his hands, and breathing.

Of course, whether a person develops these changes is variable and determined by many factors, such as at what point on the immune spectrum this person 'falls'. In addition, and very importantly for this particular bioarchaeological study, it is not known whether he was stigmatised by his local community. Although he was indeed buried in a leprosy hospital cemetery, the circumstances of this burial are unknown. While there is an assumption in the published literature that all people in the medieval period were stigmatised and marginalised in leprosy hospitals, this supposition is changing as bioarchaeological and historical data are re-evaluated (Roberts, forthcoming; Rawcliffe, 2006, p. 230; Demaitre, 2007, p. 241).

As seen in many clinical studies, leprosy can cause considerable damage to bones, which can lead to deformity, impairment, and limitations in social participation. Whether this actually happens depends on a range of underlying factors that will be specific to that person, where they live in the world, and in what time period. These include the type of leprosy they have, whether they receive treatment, their age and sex, and their occupation.

While leprosy-associated deformity may not lead to impairment, if it does, then even today people may be stigmatised. In clinical studies, deformity occurred on average 2.9 years after the start of the infection in people with high resistance leprosy (tuberculoid), and 9 years 1 month for people with lepromatous leprosy (Mallac, 1966). This is somewhat counterintuitive, as it would be expected that deformity would occur earlier in the more severe form of leprosy, but possibly the deformity occurred at a later stage in the disease in those with lepromatous leprosy in this study. In another study, 'claw hands', interpreted in this medieval skeleton as 'absorptive grooves' on the proximal hand phalanges, were the most common of the hand deformities (40 % of people). The hands and feet were both affected in 62 % of people (432/700), and 60 % of these had both hands and feet affected. Overall, hand involvement was 1.5 times more common than foot involvement (96.2 % vs. 65.4 %), and this was explained by the fact that hands have a more functional role (Sehgal & Sharma, 1985).

In terms of the effect of hand and foot impairment on function, cutting nails, washing clothes, tying a knot, cutting grass, digging, harvesting, threshing, and milking a cow were the activities most affected in people with leprosy in a Nepalese study group (Van Brakel & Anderson, 1997). People with advanced leprosy and major impairment may also need to rest more (sit, kneel, lie down) or crawl to move between different locations. Crawling, sitting, kneeling, and lying down may lead to damage to the soft tissues of the extremities, knee and elbow joints, buttocks, and the 'sit bones' or ischial tuberosities. These activities may lead to bone changes that have the potential to be recognised in skeletal remains but were not noted in this study.

Step 3: Construction of a Model of Care

Person-centred care that is holistic and all-encompassing is the aim of the Royal College of Nursing in the UK (http://www.rcn.org.uk/development/practice/cpd_online_learning/dignity_in_health_care/person-centred_care). However, there can be a tension about what constitutes 'care' between those practicing nursing, medicine, and surgery, and there has been much discussion of 'cookbook medicine', or clinical stereotyping, versus the 'person-based' approach to caring for and treating an ill person (e.g. Hasnain-Wynia, 2006). It is assumed that this man with leprosy, who was buried in the St James and St Mary Magdalene leprosy hospital cemetery, actually lived within the hospital. However, this cannot be proved, and he may well have lived at home, being buried in the cemetery on his death.

The bone lesions displayed in his skeleton suggest aspects of care that may have been required. He would have needed shelter and sustenance, and that could have come with residence in the leprosy hospital or in a home environment. Because of his potential lack of a sense of taste and smell, and loss of appetite, encouragement with eating and drinking would have been important. Care of ulcers on the hands, feet, and lower legs, and care of other skin lesions related to leprosy, would also have been needed, as would protection of the hands and feet to prevent further damage to sensory deprived appendages. As a consequence of possible impairment in his hands and feet, he may have needed help with everyday tasks and walking, perhaps requiring aids for walking. A holistic approach should also have encompassed psychological support during his life with leprosy, although this is impossible to access through skeletal remains.

What cannot be said for certain is whether his care evolved and changed through time as the disease progressed, although this is highly probable. For example, it is known that people with leprosy today (treated or not) may 'move along' the immune spectrum. While patients can move either way – towards the high or low resistant form – during the course of their illness, the majority of patients today lie in the 'borderline' categories (Bennett et al., 2008; Scollard et al., 2006). Untreated patients have an unstable immunological response and tend to move to the low resistant end of the spectrum (downgrading or decreased cell-mediated immunity), and when patients are treated with chemotherapy they can move towards the high resistant end (improved cell-mediated immunity, termed 'reversal' or 'upgrading' – Bennett et al., 2008). The closer people are to the centre of the spectrum (the borderline forms) the more likely they are to 'move', unlike the polar groups at each end of the spectrum. Some 'movements' are associated with leprosy reactions. 'Reactions' are the sudden onset of acute aggressive inflammation in leprous skin lesions, with specific signs and symptoms (Bryceson & Pfaltzgraff, 1990). Reactions are the body's response to *M. leprae* or its products in the body tissues (Dayal et al., 1990). While their presence does not mean the disease is getting worse, it has been suggested that they are an important factor for permanent 'disabilities' (Fava et al., 2012).

In discussing the course of this medieval man's leprosy, it is very difficult to actually say at what point on the spectrum he would have been at any given time in his life – all we know is that he had bone changes of lepromatous leprosy at the time of his death. As the immune response in leprosy is dynamic, during the normal course of the disease acute clinical reactions can occur in people with untreated *or* treated leprosy (Scollard et al., 2006). As many as 30–50 % of all patients with leprosy today may be affected at least once while they suffer the disease (Kumar, Dogra, & Kaur, 2004). Whether this medieval man experienced these acute reactions is unknown; he may have initially contracted the high resistance form of leprosy, but later in life 'downgraded' to lepromatous leprosy.

Step 4: The Implications for This Man and His Community

It is not known whether this man was a patient in the leprosy hospital in Chichester, or if he was merely buried there when he died. However, the model of care described earlier is only a model, and whether, and what type of, care was given to this man cannot be proved. If it is assumed that he was a patient, does the literature on medieval leprosy hospitals, and specifically on *this* hospital, help us to understand what care and treatment he might have received?

Unfortunately, there is very little information about daily life within individual leprosaria overall (Satchell, 1998), or whether any specific forms of treatment were given; this dearth of information also applies to the hospital of St James and St Mary Magdalene, where there is little documentation that helps us to understand life in the leprosarium. While general ideas can be gleaned about the workings of leprosaria (e.g. see Rawcliffe, 2006), the only specific information of relevance from St James and St Mary Magdalene is that the hospital benefited from gifts, alms, and charity, which all helped it function and provide a place for patients to live (Magilton, 2008, p. 63). Additionally, by the thirteenth century it was tax exempt, and by the fourteenth century Chichester was experiencing famines and the plague. The hospital had an associated garden where food and medicines were grown and there were associated farms, but there is no documentary evidence as to whether this man specifically worked on these farms. How the workings of the hospital impacted the life of this man and shaped his care (if he received care) is unknown.

Nevertheless, he may have received general care, a good diet, positive encouragement from his carers, along with spiritual and psychological help. It is known from descriptions in historical texts that various types of care and treatments were available and practiced, for example bathing, care of ulcers and other skin problems, herbal remedies, and blood-letting and cautery, often reflecting concepts of disease in the medieval mind (see Rawcliffe, 2006, pp. 205–243). One conception of disease was based on the system of the four humours, whereby excess of a humour was believed to cause ill health. For example, the procedure of blood-letting (blood was one of the four humours) was practiced to rid the body of excess humours, alleviating disease – in this case leprosy (Porter, 1997, p. 9).

Specific aspects of this man's care cannot be proven, and what cannot be verified either is whether he was stigmatised by his community and actually segregated by being placed within the hospital. Nevertheless, the context of his burial suggests he could have been a patient and may have received hospital care.

Conclusions

The process of utilising the Index of Care to assess the 'leprosy experience' of this man, buried in a late medieval leprosy hospital cemetery in southern England, has shown what can and cannot be said about one person's 'disease experience' based purely on their skeleton. In doing this it has illustrated the limits to a bioarchaeologist's abilities to shed light on our ancestors' caregiving activities. However, because it is based on a contextualised approach, the Index of Care is a much more objective method for assessing whether care was needed and if it might have been provided than has been employed previously. This is contrary to many previous (subjective) attempts to assess impairment and care provision from archaeological skeletal remains. The Index also takes into account clinical understanding of the disease of interest, which is an essential component of palaeopathology. This approach furthermore enables a detailed 'osteobiography' to be developed, allowing for a much more nuanced appreciation of a person's life with a specific illness and their potential care and treatment.

Global provision of care and treatment today for those experiencing ill health varies in accessibility and quality depending on where a person lives in the world. It should also vary from person to person, even for the same disease. However, pressures on services often lead to the 'cookbook', rather than the 'personalised' medical approach (Malentacchi et al., 2015), because the former is seen as a cheaper and more rapid 'solution' than the latter. Whether these two competing approaches operated in the past is unknown, but discussions of care and treatment in the past *and* the present need to take into account such a possibility. For example, if a person needed a trepanation to treat a head injury, did the surgeon follow a particular process in creating the hole in the skull because this was accepted 'best practice', regardless of the nature of the injury? Likewise, did everybody who had leprosy and who experienced ulcers associated with nerve damage receive treatment for those ulcers and, if so, was that treatment the same regardless of time and place?

All individuals are unique, and past caregiving likely (but not necessarily) reflected a person's individual needs and the cultural milieu in which they lived. In that respect, each person with leprosy today experiences different signs and symptoms, levels of 'disability', attitudes from their communities, types of care given (if any), progress of infection, and rate of recovery. They may also be subjected to drug therapy (antibiotics), which may affect the impact of leprosy on their bodies, including their skeleton. Although it is not always the case, people can adapt well to having an illness and/or 'disability', and bioarchaeologists should never make assumptions about if, and how, a person was cared for in the past. Conversely, it should be remembered that absence of evidence is not evidence of absence. The vagaries of skeletal preservation and skeletal disease manifestation mean there are likely to be many instances where care was given in the past, but for which no physical evidence remains.

Research into caregiving in the past has real potential for providing a deep time perspective on aspects of the disease experience today. Patients visiting their doctors and hospitals in many parts of the world have an inherent level of expectation that they will receive compassion, care, and treatment for their illnesses, although practices, and the quality of these, will vary. Studying the experiences of people with disease centuries ago potentially shows whether such responses featured in their lives. It provides a window on the human condition, on the type of community in which people lived, and on the people who inhabited this community and who gave care. Ultimately, it may show that compassion and caregiving have been around for centuries, and that they should remain a part of people's lives for the very survival of the planet, despite increasing tendencies to narcissism and a lack of concern for the well-being of others (Paris, 2014).

Acknowledgements Jo Buckberry, Biological Anthropology Research Centre, Department of Archaeological Sciences, University of Bradford for enabling access to record the skeleton from Chichester, Lorna Tilley for very insightful comments and suggestions for revising this paper, along with two anonymous reviewers, and Lorna and Alecia for organising the symposium at the Society for American Archaeology Meeting in San Francisco in 2015 at which this case study was presented.

References

Andersen, J. G., & Manchester, K. (1987). Grooving of the proximal phalanx in leprosy: A palaeopathological and radiological study. *Journal of Archaeological Science, 14*, 77–82.

Andersen, J. G., & Manchester, K. (1988). Dorsal tarsal exostoses in leprosy: A palaeopathological and radiological study. *Journal of Archaeological Science, 15*, 51–56.

Andersen, J. G., & Manchester, K. (1992). The rhinomaxillary syndrome in leprosy: A clinical, radiological and palaeopathological study. *International Journal of Osteoarchaeology, 2*, 121–129.

Andersen, J. G., Manchester, K., & Ali, R. S. (1992). Diaphyseal remodelling in leprosy: A radiological and palaeopathological study. *International Journal of Osteoarchaeology, 2*, 211–219.

Andersen, J. G., Manchester, K., & Roberts, C. (1994). Septic bone changes in leprosy: A clinical, radiological and palaeopathological review. *International Journal of Osteoarchaeology, 4*, 21–30.

Arnott, R., Finger, S., & Smith, C. U. M. (Eds.). (2003). *Trepanation. History, discovery, theory*. Lisse: Sweits and Zeitlinger.

Barker, D. J. P. (1994). *Mothers, babies, and disease in later life*. London: BMJ Books.

Bennett, J. E., Li, G., Foreman, K., Best, N., Kontis, V., Pearson, C., et al. (2015). The future of life expectancy and life expectancy inequalities in England and Wales: Bayesian spatiotemporal forecasting. *Lancet, 386*, 163–170. doi:10.1016/S0140-6736(15)60296-3.

Bennett, B. H., Parker, D. L., & Robson, M. (2008). Leprosy: Steps along the journey of eradication. *Public Health Reports, 123*, 198–205.

Boel, L. W. T., & Ortner, D. J. (2013). Skeletal manifestations of skin ulcer in the lower leg. *International Journal of Osteoarchaeology, 23*, 303–309.

Brickley, M. (2004). Determination of sex from archaeological skeletal material and assessment of parturition. In M. Brickley, & J. I. McKinley (Eds.) *Guidelines to the standards for recording human remains* (pp. 23–25). Reading: Institute of Field Archaeologists, Paper 7. Retrieved from http://www.babao.org.uk.

Brickley, M., & Ives, R. (2008). *The bioarchaeology of metabolic bone disease*. London: Academic.

Brooks, S., & Suchey, J. M. (1990). Skeletal age determination based on the os pubis: Comparison of the Ascadi-Nemeskeri and Suchey-Brooks methods. *Human Evolution, 5*, 227–238.

Brothwell, D. (1981). *Digging up bones*. London: British Museum (Natural History).

Bryceson, A., & Pfaltzgraff, R. E. (1990). *Leprosy* (3rd ed.). Edinburgh: Churchill Livingstone.

Butlin, R., & Saunderson, P. (2014). Children with leprosy. *Leprosy Review, 85*, 69–73.

Clarke, N. G., & Hirsch, R. S. (1992). Two critical confounding factors in periodontal epidemiology. *Community Dental Health, 9*, 133–141.

Cohen, M. N., & Armelagos, G. J. (Eds.). (2013). *Paleopathology at the origins of agriculture* (2nd ed.). Gainesville, FL: University Press of Florida.

Cohen, M. N., & Crane-Kramer, G. (Eds.). (2007). *Ancient health. Skeletal indicators of agricultural and economic intensification*. Gainesville, FL: University of Florida Press.

Crowther, J., Wilson, K. C. M., Horton, S., & Lloyd-Williams, M. (2013). 2013 Compassion in healthcare – Lessons from a qualitative study of the end of life care of people with dementia. *Journal of the Royal Society of Medicine, 106*, 492–497.

Dayal, R., Hashmi, N. A., Mathur, P. P., & Prasad, R. (1990). Leprosy in childhood. *Indian Pediatrics, 27*, 170–180.

DeGusta, D. (2002). Comparative skeletal pathology and the case for conspecific care in Middle Pleistocene hominids. *Journal of Archaeological Science, 29*, 1435–1438.

DeGusta, D. (2003). Aubesier 11 is not evidence of Neanderthal conspecific care. *Journal of Human Evolution, 45*(1), 821–830.

Demaitre, L. (2007). *Leprosy in premodern medicine. A malady of the whole body*. Baltimore: Johns Hopkins University Press.

Dettwyler, K. (1991). Can paleopathology provide evidence for compassion. *American Journal of Physical Anthropology, 84*, 375–384.

Faccia, K. J., & Williams, R. C. (2008). Schmorl's nodes: Clinical significance and implications for the bioarchaeological record. *International Journal of Osteoarchaeology, 18*, 28–44.

Fashing, P., & Nguygen, N. (2011). Behavior toward the dying, diseased, or disabled among animals and its relevance to paleopathology. *International Journal ofPaleopathology, 1*, 128–129.

Fava, V., Orlova, M., Cobat, A., Alcaí, A., Mira, M., & Schurr, E. (2012). Genetics of leprosy reactions: An overview. *Memórias do Instituto Oswaldo Cruz, 107*, 132–142.

Fornaciari, G., Castagna, M., Tognetti, A., Tornaboni, D., & Bruno, J. (1989). Syphilis in a renaissance Italian mummy. *Lancet, 2*(8663), 614.

Groves, S. E., Roberts, C. A., Johnstone, C., Hall, R., & Dobney, K. (2003). A high status burial from Ripon Cathedral, North Yorkshire: Differential diagnosis of a chest deformity. *International Journal of Osteoarchaeology, 13*, 358–368.

Hackett, C. J. (1976). *Diagnostic criteria of syphilis, yaws and treponarid (treponematoses) and of some other diseases in dry bone*. New York: Springer.

Hallback, H. (1976–1977). A medieval bone with a copper plate support indicating open surgical treatment. *Ossa 3/4*, 63.

Han, X. Y., Seo, Y. H., Sizer, K. C., Schoberle, T., May, G. S., Li, W., et al. (2008). A new mycobacterium species causing diffuse lepromatous leprosy. *American Journal of Clinical Pathology, 130*, 856–864.

Harper, K., & Armelagos, G. (2010). The changing disease-scape in the third epidemiological transition. *International Journal of Environmental Research and Public Health, 7*, 675–697.

Hasnain-Wynia, R. (2006). Is evidence-based medicine patient-centered and is patient-centered care evidence-based? *Health Services Research, 41*, 1–8.

Hauhnar, C. Z., Mann, S. B., Sharma, V. K., Kaur, S., Mehta, S., & Radotra, B. D. (1992). Maxillary antrum involvement in multibacillary leprosy: A radiologic, sinuscopic, and histologic assessment. *International Journal of Leprosy, 60*, 390–395.

Hawkey, D. (1998). Disability, compassion and the skeletal record: Using musculoskeletal stress markers (MSM) to construct an osteobiography from early New Mexico. *International Journal of Osteoarchaeology, 8*, 326–340.

Hillson, S. (1996). *Dental anthropology*. Cambridge: University Press.

İşcan, M. Y., & Loth, S. R. (1986). Estimation of age and determination of sex from the sternal rib. In K. J. Reichs (Ed.), *Forensic osteology* (pp. 68–89). Springfield, IL: Charles C. Thomas.

Janssens, P. (1987). A copper plate on the upper arm in a burial at the church in Vrasene, Belgium. *Journal of Paleopathology, 1*, 15–18.

Kaur, S., Malik, S. K., Kumar, B., Singh, M. P., & Chakravarty, R. N. (1979). Respiratory system involvement in leprosy. *International Journal of Leprosy, 47*, 18–25.

Knüsel, C., Kemp, R., & Budd, P. (1995). Evidence for remedial medical treatment of a severe knee injury from the Fishergate Gilbertine monastery in the City of York. *Journal of Archaeological Science, 22*, 369–384.

Kumar, B., Dogra, S., & Kaur, I. (2004). Epidemiological characteristics of leprosy reactions. 15 years experience from north India. *International Journal of Leprosy, 72*, 125–133.

Lebel, S., & Trinkaus, E. (2002). Middle Pleistocene remains from the Bau de l'Aubesier. *Journal of Human Evolution, 43*, 659–685.

Lebel, S., Trinkaus, E., Fawe, M., Fernandez, P., Guerin, C., Richter, D., et al. (2001). Comparative morphology and palaeobiology of Middle Pleistocene human remains from the Bau l'Aubesier, Vaucluse, France. *Proceedings of the National Academy of Sciences, 98*, 11097–11102.

Lewis, M. E. (2007). *The bioarchaeology of children. Archaeological and forensic perspectives*. Cambridge: University Press.

Lewis, M. E., Roberts, C. A., & Manchester, K. (1995). Inflammatory bone changes in leprous skeletons from the Medieval Hospital of St. James and St. Mary Magdalene, Chichester, England. *International Journal of Leprosy, 63*(1), 77–85.

Magilton, J. (2008). A history of the hospital. In J. Magilton, F. Lee, & A. Boylston (Eds.), *'Lepers outside the gate': Excavations at the cemetery of the hospital of St James and St Mary Magdalene, Chichester, 1986–87 and 1993* (pp. 57–68). York: Council for British Archaeology.

Magilton, J., Lee, F., & Boylston, A. (2008). *'Lepers outside the gate': Excavations at the cemetery of the hospital of St James and St Mary Magdalene, Chichester, 1986–87 and 1993*. York: Council for British Archaeology.

Malentacchi, F., Mancini, I., Brandslund, I., Vermeersch, P., Schwab, M., Marc, J., et al. (2015). Is laboratory medicine ready for the era of personalized medicine? A survey addressed to laboratory directors of hospitals/academic schools of medicine in Europe. *Drug Metabolism and Personalized Therapy, 30*, 121–128.

Mallac, M. J. (1966). Onset and pattern of deformity in leprosy. *Leprosy Review, 37*, 71–91.

Malmedal, W., Iversen, M. H., & Kilvik, A. (2015). Sexual abuse of older nursing home residents: A literature review. *Nursing Research and Practice, 2015*, 902515. doi:10.1155/2015/902515.

McElroy, A., & Townsend, P. K. (2009). *Medical anthropology in ecological perspective*. Boulder, CO: Westview Press.

Møller-Christensen, V. (1961). *Bone changes in leprosy*. Copenhagen: Munksgaard.

Møller-Christensen, V. (1969). A rosary bead used as tooth filling material in a human mandibular canine tooth. A unique case from the Danish Middle Ages. In *21st International Congress of the History of Medicine, Siena. Atti del Congresso Internazionale di Storia Dela Medicina, Siena (Italia)* (pp. 800–811). Settembre 22–28, 1968.

Møller-Christensen, V. (1978). *Leprosy changes of the skull*. Odense: University Press.

Molleson, T., & Cox, M. (1993). *The Spitalfields project* (The anthropology. The middling sort, Vol. 2). York: Council for British Archaeology Research Report 86.

Nerlich, A. G., Zink, A., Szeimies, U., & Haagedorn, H. G. (2000). Ancient Egyptian prosthesis of the big toe. *Lancet, 356*, 2176–2179.

Norman, R. E., Munkhtsetseg, M., De, R., Butchart, A., Scott, J., & Vos, T. (2012). The long-term health consequences of child physical abuse, emotional abuse, and neglect: A systematic review and meta-analysis. *PLoS Medicine, 9*(11), e1001349.

Ortner, D. J. (2003). *Identification of pathological conditions in human skeletal remains*. London: Academic.

Paris, J. (2014). Modernity and narcissistic personality disorder. *Personality Disorders, 5*, 220–226.

Paterson, D. E., & Job, C. K. (1964). Bone changes and absorption in leprosy. A radiological, pathological and clinical study. In R. G. Cochrane & T. F. Davey (Eds.), *Leprosy in theory and practice* (pp. 425–446). Bristol: John Wright and Sons.

Porter, R. (1997). *The greatest benefit to mankind. A medical history of humanity from antiquity to the present*. London: Fontana Press.

Rawcliffe, C. (2006). *Leprosy in medieval England*. Woodbridge, Suffolk: Boydell and Brewer.

Reichart, P., Ananatasan, T., & Reznik, G. (1976). Gingiva and periodontium in leprosy: a clinical, radiological and microscopical study. *Journal of Periodontology, 47*, 455–460.

Reid, R. (2008). The locomotor system. In D. A. Levison & R. Reid (Eds.), *Muir's textbook of pathology* (14th ed., pp. 330–372). London: Hodder Arnold.

Ridley, D. S., & Jopling, W. H. (1966). Classification of leprosy according to immunity. A five-group system. *International Journal of Leprosy, 34*, 255–273.

Roberts, C. A. (2000). Did they take sugar? The use of skeletal evidence in the study of disability in past populations. In J. Hubert (Ed.), *Madness, disability and social exclusion. The archaeology and anthropology of 'difference'* (pp. 46–59). London: Routledge.

Roberts, C. A. (forthcoming). *Leprosy past and present: dispelling the myths about this infection*. Gainesville, FL: University Press of Florida

Roberts, C. A., & Connell, B. (2004). Guidance on recording palaeopathology. In M. Brickley, & J. I. McKinley (Eds.) *Guidelines to the standards for recording human remains* (pp. 34–39). Reading: Institute of Field Archaeologists. Paper 7. Retrieved from http://www.babao.org.uk.

Roberts, C. A., & Cox, M. (2003). *Health and disease in Britain. From prehistory to the present day*. Stroud: Sutton.

Roberts, C. A., Lewis, M., & Boocock, P. (1998). Infectious disease, sex and gender: The complexity of it all! In A. Grauer & P. Stuart-Macadam (Eds.), *Sex and gender in palaeopathological perspective* (pp. 93–113). Cambridge: University Press.

Roberts, C., Lucy, D., & Manchester, K. (1994). Inflammatory lesions of ribs: An analysis of the terry collection. *American Journal of Physical Anthropology, 94*, 169–182.

Rodrigues, L. C., & Lockwood, D. N. (2011). Leprosy now: Epidemiology, progress, challenges, and research gaps. *Lancet Infectious Diseases, 11*, 464–470.

Satchell, M. (1998). *The emergence of leper-houses in Medieval England 1100–1250*. D.Phil. Thesis, University of Oxford.

Scheuer, L., & Black, S. (2000). *Developmental juvenile osteology*. London: Academic.

Scollard, D. M., Adams, L. B., Gillis, T. P., Krahenbuhl, J. L., Truman, R. W., & Williams, D. L. (2006). The continuing challenge of leprosy. *Clinical Microbiology Reviews, 19*, 338–381.

Sehgal, V. N., & Sharma, P. K. (1985). Pattern of deformities and disabilities in urban leprosy. *Indian Journal of Leprosy, 57*, 183–192.

Steckel, R. H., & Rose, J. C. (Eds.). (2002). *The backbone of history. Health and nutrition in the western hemisphere*. Cambridge: University Press.

Tilley, L., & Cameron, T. (2014). Introducing the Index of Care: A web-based application supporting archaeological research into health-related care. *International Journal of Paleopathology, 6*, 5–9.

Tilley, L., & Oxenham, M. F. (2011). Survival against the odds: Modeling the social implications of care provision to seriously disabled individuals. *International Journal of Paleopathology, 1*, 35–42.

Van Brakel, W. H., & Anderson, A. M. (1997). Impairment and disability in leprosy: In search of the missing link. *Indian Journal of Leprosy, 69*, 361–376.

Weinberger, B. W. (2004). *Introduction to the history of dentistry*. St. Louis: C.V. Mosby Company.

Weston, D. A. (2012). Non-specific infection in paleopathology: Interpreting periosteal reactions. In A. L. Grauer (Ed.), *A companion to paleopathology* (pp. 492–512). Cambridge: University Press.

Withers, R. J. W. (1960). On bone setting. *Ulster Medical Journal, 29*, 1–13.

Wood, J. W., Milner, G. R., Harpending, H. C., & Weiss, K. M. (1992). The osteological paradox. Problems of inferring prehistoric health from skeletal samples. *Current Anthropology, 33*, 343–370.

Chapter 7
Dealing with Difference: Using the Osteobiographies of a Woman with Leprosy and a Woman with Gigantism from Medieval Poland to Identify Practices of Care

Magdalena D. Matczak and Tomasz Kozłowski

This chapter presents the osteobiographies of two women from medieval Poland, together with an analysis of the mortuary treatment they received, as the basis for considering individual experiences of pathology, possible receipt of care, and the influence of social status on both of these. These women, from medieval Poland, would have been visibly different from other members of their community. As a biocultural account of these women's lives, their osteobiographies allow us to address whether their experiences of disease affected how they were treated by society. Both women come from contexts that are representative of society in medieval Poland.

The methodology used in this chapter combines theoretical approaches from osteobiography and the bioarchaeology of care (see Tilley, Chap. 2 this volume) to explore care, healing practices, religious beliefs, emotions, mortuary treatment, and social perceptions of disability and disease in two exceptional case studies from medieval Poland. We also revisit one of the most exceptional discoveries in Polish bioarchaeology – the 'giant woman' – and reinterpret this case in the light of the bioarchaeology of care approach.

Osteobiography

Over the last few years osteobiography has become an established subfield of osteoarchaeology (Robb, 2002; Saul, 1972; Saul & Saul, 1989). As Stodder and Palkovich point out in their recent book, *The Bioarchaeology of Individuals*, osteobiography 'is a uniquely valuable component to the study of prehistory that considers individuals, their

M.D. Matczak, Ph.D. (✉) • T. Kozłowski, Ph.D.
Department of Anthropology, Nicolaus Copernicus University in Toruń, Toruń, Poland
e-mail: magdalenadmatczak@gmail.com

© Springer International Publishing Switzerland 2017

L. Tilley, A.A. Schrenk (eds.), *New Developments in the Bioarchaeology of Care*, Bioarchaeology and Social Theory, DOI 10.1007/978-3-319-39901-0_7

intentions, and their socially contextualized identities as fundamental to understanding the past' (Stodder & Palkovich, 2012a, pp. 2–3). We believe that osteobiography can be an equally powerful contributor to research in the historic context.

There are three approaches to osteobiography in the literature. The first is focused on aspects of life at a population level and is based on evidence from several individuals (Robb, 2002; Saul & Saul, 1989). The second focuses on the life of one individual (e.g., Hawkey, 1998; Knüsel et al., 2010; Robb, 2009; Stodder & Palkovich, 2012b; Tilley & Oxenham, 2011). The third approach restricts the definition of osteobiography to the documentation of osteological material, with data used for demographic analyses, but with no attempt at social interpretation (e.g., Rosado & Vernacchio-Wilson, 2006). In Polish anthropological literature there is a long tradition of producing osteobiographies of this last type (although the term 'osteobiography' has not been used by authors). These osteobiographies typically comprise descriptions of the remains of distinguished and/or powerful historical men and women (e.g., Kozłowski & Drozd, 2009; Reicher, 1933; Rosiński, 1951; Talko-Hryncewicz, 1914).

In this chapter we understand osteobiography as a cultural narrative, based on osteological evidence and cultural context, which tells the story of the personal experience of an individual. Adopting a similar definition, Hawkey (1998) and Tilley and Oxenham (2011) have demonstrated that osteobiography provides a valuable approach for assessing and interpreting individual disability and cultural perceptions of the disabled, and we follow their lead.

Disability During Life and Treatment After Death

The research on disability in archaeology and paleopathology has grown out of the disability studies movement that emerged in the 1980s (see Barnes & Mercer, 2010; Kudlick, 2003). The precise definition of disability is subject to ongoing debate and has evolved in tandem with changes in society's approach to the disabled (Barnes & Mercer, 2010). For instance, the medical model of disability defines disability as a physical or mental deficiency that prevents an individual from fulfilling their social role and results in their dependency on others; this definition has been viewed as contributing to the stigmatization of those with disabilities and their marginalization as members of the society. Conversely, the social model of disability emphasizes disability as a social construction, resulting from the failure of able-bodied people to adjust to the needs of those who are physically challenged. We are not going to discuss definitions of disability in detail here, as this is outside the scope of our study; 'disability,' as defined for bioarchaeology of care purposes, is outlined by Tilley (Chap. 2, this volume), and elaborated by Doat (Chap. 17, this volume). Following we offer a very brief overview of the way archaeologists have approached the issue of definition and explain the definition we are adopting in this chapter.

Over recent decades, many bioarchaeologists and paleopathologists have proposed different interpretations of the term disability. According to Finlay (1999), a universal understanding of the definition of disability does not exist, since disability is a cultural experience. Every society has its own definition of the 'able body' and its opposite: the *dis*abled body (Roberts, 1999). Disability is an experience of lack (Knüsel, 1999), loss, and limitation (Cross, 1999; Roberts, 1999) which results in social exclusion and inequality (Roberts, 1999). Disability is often culturally associated with morality and sin (Hubert, 2000).

The term 'disability' may be a creation of modern Western culture and may not have existed in past societies (Barnes & Mercer, 2010; Horstmanshoff, 2012; Jones, 2012). Furthermore, what is currently referred to as disability may not have been perceived as such in the past. In this study, we use 'disability' as a working term to conceptualize specific physical or mental conditions, inferred from pathological lesions associated with disease, and likely to have disadvantaged the individual's functioning in a way that had an impact on, and was significant in, their everyday lives. Thus, 'disability' is a state of being likely to require some form of care. We emphasize two dimensions of 'disability': the biological and the social, with the social dimension resulting from the individual's biological condition. This two-dimensional approach is especially useful for researchers in reconstructing a past for which historical texts are unavailable, as well as providing a basis for comparison with modern cases of a particular pathology, which may help us to identify both the lived experiences of a person with this pathology in the past and the amount of care necessary for their survival. Archaeological context should then inform us about further possible forms of care, available treatments, and likely social perceptions. The Index of Care, the bioarchaeology of care instrument, attempts to assist in addressing both the biological and social dimensions of disability through constructing an osteobiography of the disabled individual (Tilley & Cameron, 2014) and has been used in this research.

There are two components to investigating the interaction between disability and mortuary evidence in archaeology. The first involves assessment of the pathological condition, while the second consists of assessing the characteristics of the burial itself. Here we would like to elaborate a bit on the implications of mortuary evidence. Several features of burial might indicate disability. The first of these is the 'atypical burial,' such as a burial which contains a body positioned in an abnormal way (for example, placed face down), or interment in an unusual setting (for example, in a bog) (Molleson, 1999; Parker, 2011). The second indicator of potential disability would be the location of the grave in a hospital cemetery or outside the borders of a cemetery (Papadopoulos, 2000). The third indicator consists of items found in a burial that might indicate a certain type of impairment, such as the prosthesis of the big toe found in the grave of an individual from New Kingdom Egypt (Nerlich, Zink, Szeimies, & Hageodorn, 2000).

Some researchers argue that it is sometimes not possible to investigate disability based on mortuary evidence alone. There may be no burial indicators of disability, because the disabled person might have been treated after death in the same way as able-bodied people in their community, regardless of how they were treated during life. Similarly, different mortuary practices may reflect beliefs about the demands of the afterlife, but may not reflect the way the person was perceived nor treatment received when alive (Baker & Bolhofner, 2014). Such variables in postmortem treatment of the disabled (and able-bodied) shows that mortuary evidence is not a reliable indicator for reconstruction of disability, social status, and treatment of the disabled – or that, at least, there may be inherent problems in its use. The obstacles to reconstructing past cultures based on mortuary evidence have been discussed in archaeology since the 1980s, and especially within neomarxist contexts (e.g., Leone, 2005; see Parker, 2011, p. 83). As Mike Parker Pearson (2011, p. 4) writes 'funerary practices serve to create an idealized representation – a 're-presenting' of the individual by others rather than by the man himself.' Mortuary treatment does not passively represent the relationships that existed between people during life but actively creates identity and commemorates the dead.

Context

Following, we present two case studies from medieval Poland: the skeletal remains of a woman with leprosy excavated at Kałdus (known in early medieval times as *Culmen*) (Fig. 7.1; Chudziak, 2010; Kozłowski, 2012), and the skeleton of a woman with gigantism excavated at Ostrów Lednicki Island, which is on Lednica Lake (Szymczyk et al. 1977; Gładykowska-Rzeczycka, Wrzesińska, & Sokół, 2000).

The military, administrative, and religious stronghold on Ostrów Lednicki Island was built in the nineth century (Kurnatowska, 1991). It was an essential part of the Gniezno state (the early Piast state) which later became Poland (Fig. 7.1) and also an important trade center (Tabaka, 2005). Dziekanowice was an agricultural and craft-production settlement located on the Eastern bank of Lednica Lake in front of Ostrów Lednicki Island (Fig. 7.2) and dates to around the mid-eleventh to mid-twelfth century (Wrzesińscy, 1998a, p. 13).

The early Piast state extended its borders and absorbed *Culmen* on the end of the tenth century. Settlement in *Culmen* began at the end of the seventh century, but it only became one of the capitals of Poland in the eleventh century. Both sites are thought to have been capitals – *sedes regni principals* – of the early Piast state, making them two of the most important sites for Polish history and archaeology. In 1038 A.D. the stronghold of Ostrów Lednicki was looted and burnt, and the capital of Poland moved to Kraków (Kurnatowska, 1991). *Culmen* was a castellany from the twelfth to the beginning of the thirteenth century.

The Piast state consolidated in the early Middle Ages, and Christianity was introduced (the official baptism took place in 966 A.D.). In Christianity, burial customs were connected with the belief in and hope for resurrection, emphasizing the specific preservation and placement of the body. This influenced existing burial customs and the then current cremation rite was replaced with inhumation. Graves were orientated from W (head) to E, with all possible variants of this orientation (e.g., NW-SE, SW-NE, NWW-SEE). Skeletons were set in a supine position with arms straight along the body or sometimes placed on the upper legs, on or under the pelvis. Many burials contained grave goods.

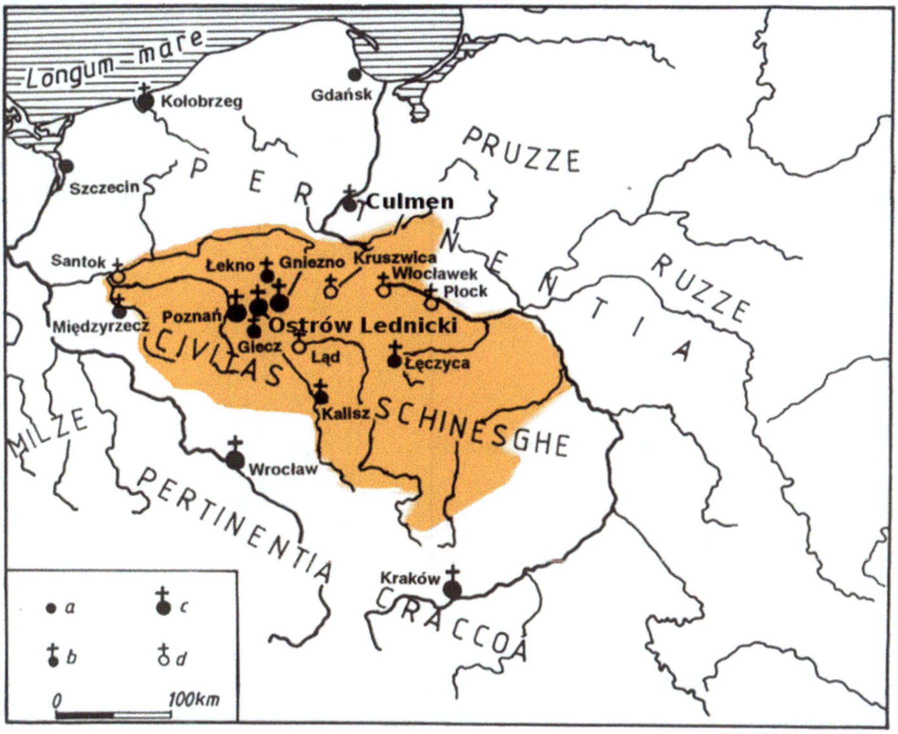

Fig. 7.1 The borders of the Gniezno state (*Civitas Schinesghe*) around 960 A.D. Legend: (**a**) main strongholds, (**b**) sacral buildings, (**c**) sacral buildings in the main strongholds, (**d**) supposed sacral buildings (modified after Chudziak, 2003)

The Woman with Leprosy

Culmen was located in the modern Kałdus village in the Vistula Pomerania in Central-Northern Poland (Chudziak, 2003). Archaeological excavations began in the middle of the nineteenth century and are ongoing (Chudziak, 2010). Archaeologists excavated a strong-hold (Site 3), settlements (Site 2), and cemetery (Sites 1, 2, and 4) in Kałdus (Chudziak, 2003, 2006, 2010). In total, more than 1000 burials were excavated in the cemetery, but the documentation of those excavated in the nineteenth century was destroyed during World Wars I and II.

Paleopathological Description

In 1998, the skeleton of a woman, dated from the twelfth to the beginning of the thirteenth century, was excavated from the grave 101/98, located in cemetery Site 1. Her estimated age at death was 25–30 years old. Skeletal analysis identified

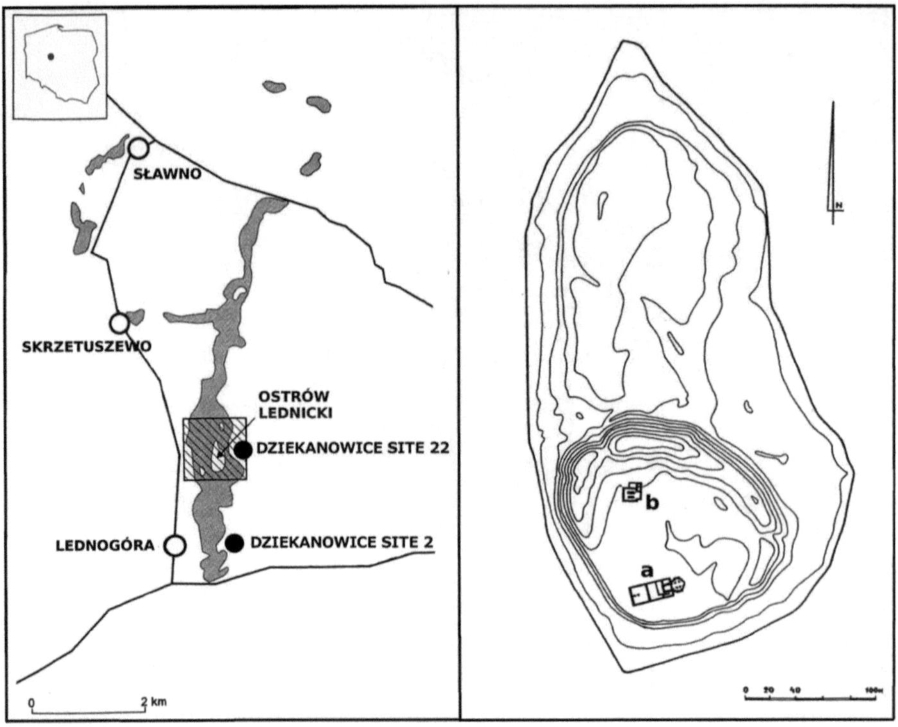

Fig. 7.2 Location of Ostrów Lednicki Island and Dziekanowice sites 2 and 22. The right inset depicts Ostrów Lednicki Island with (**a**) a palace and (**b**) a church (modified after Górecki 1991)

Schmorl's nodes on a number of thoracic vertebrae, morphological deformation of the left tibial shaft, probably caused by healed fractures, and systemic osteoperiostitis on both tibiae and fibulae (Chudziak, Stawska, Weinkauf, & Kozłowski, 2006, p. 374; Kozłowski, 2012, pp. 292–299). X-ray pictures are not clear and the line of fracture is not visible. Only massive periosteal reaction and remodeling are present. Moreover, a congenital fusion of C2 and C3 vertebrae was also identified. Within the roof of the eye sockets there are hypertrophic and porotic changes (*cribra orbitalia*) with little expression (nonactive): a cluster of mostly fine foramina covering a small area ($\leq$1 cm^2), denoted by score 2 according to *Data Collection Codebook* (2006).

The skeleton also presents a complex of typical morphological features resembling those of advanced leprosy. On the skull there is a rounded and receding edge characterizing the anterior nasal aperture with atrophy of the anterior nasal spine, characteristic of *facies leprosa* (clinically known as Bergen syndrome – see Fig. 7.3). The palate is porous, and in the nasal cavity there are signs of chronic inflammation. On the postcranial skeleton, evidence of severe periosteal inflammation, manifesting in slight, discrete patch(es) of reactive bone involving less than one quarter of the long bone surface, denoted by score 3 according to *Data Collection Codebook*

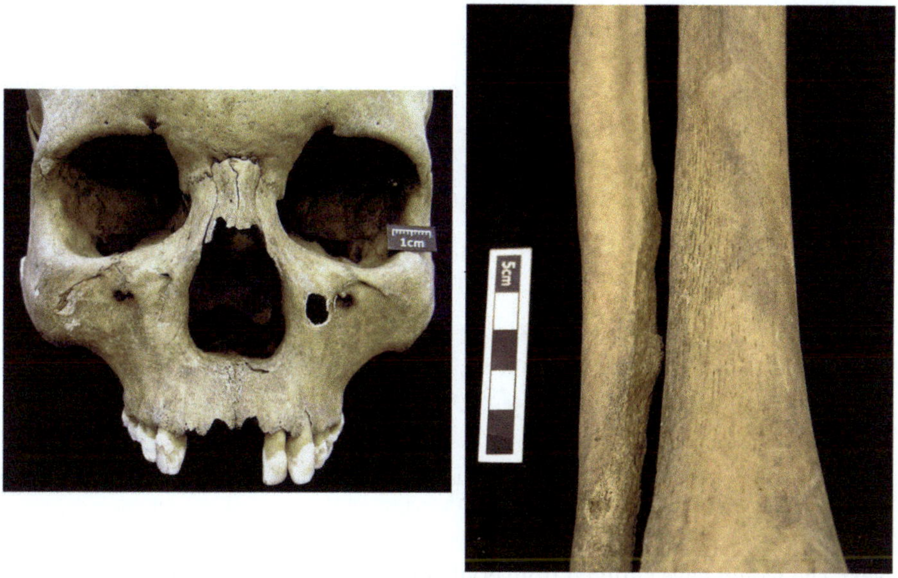

Fig. 7.3 The female from the grave 101/98, Site 1 in Kałdus (Kuyavian-Pomeranian voivodeship). The image on the *left* shows the clear rounded edges of the anterior nasal aperture, resorption of the nasal spine, and atrophy of the frontal surface at the base of nasal cavity (lower edge of anterior nasal aperture) characteristic of *facies leprosa*. The image on the *right* shows signs of periostitis on the surface of right tibial shaft and the surface of the shaft of the right fibula. (Photos by T. Kozłowski)

(2006), is present symmetrically on the bones of the lower limbs. This is particularly true for the tibiae and fibulae (Fig. 7.3). More subtle lesions – markedly accentuated longitudinal striations, denoted by score 2 according to *Data Collection Codebook* (2006) – also occur in other bones, such as the shaft of the humerus and the metatarsal bones. The periosteal inflammation changes are associated with leprosy. Leprosy was confirmed by molecular analysis undertaken by the Department of Molecular Biology at Medical University in Łódź, and based on the nature of pathological lesions we concluded that it was of the form *lepra lepromatosa*.

Estimating Disability and Care

Leprosy is a chronic infection that attacks the nervous system, skin, nasal bones, and postcranial skeleton (Gładykowska-Rzeczycka, 1982; Aufderheide & Rodríguez-Martín, 2006, p. 141). The disease may manifest as either lepromatous or tuberculoid leprosy, dependent on the individual's immune response (Roberts & Manchester, 2010, p. 195). As mentioned earlier, the woman from Kałdus most likely suffered from *lepra lepromatosa* along with the associated clinical symptoms. At the onset of the disease she would have experienced a lack of ability to feel pain.

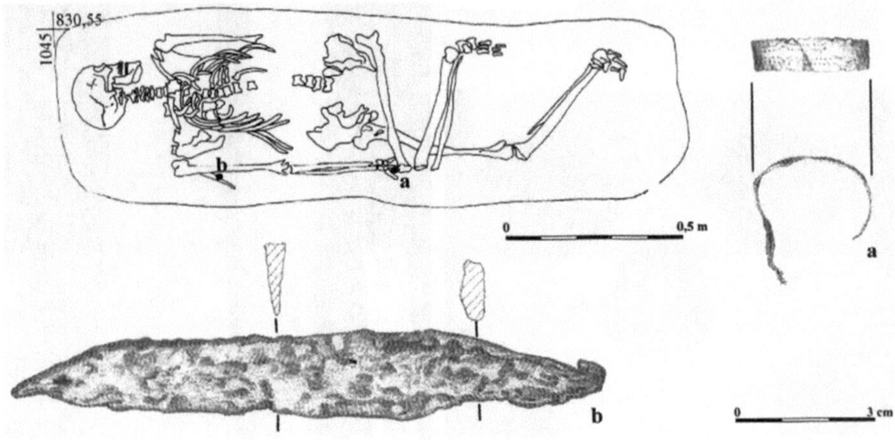

Fig. 7.4 Grave number 101/98, Site 1 in Kałdus (Kuyavian-Pomeranian voivodeship); (**a**) bronze ring; (**b**) iron knife (Chudziak, 2006)

Next, she would have suffered from erythema nodosum, iritis, scleritis, episcleritis, transient fevers, tachycardia, headaches, vomiting, stiffness of the neck, one-sided tremors, muscle pains, and respiratory distress (Longmore, Wilkinson, & Rajagopalan, 2004). Skin nodules, which are characteristic features of *lepra lepromatosa*, would have appeared on her face. Most likely, this woman would have displayed the severe facial changes associated with leonine facies (nodules on the face lead to a resemblance of a lion's forehead).

'As the disease progresses, the peripheral nerves may be enlarged and impaired sensation may occur on the hands, feet and other involved areas. Disabilities may occur as a consequence of this process' (Talhari, Talhari, & Penna, 2015, p. 32). Impaired sensation and loss of fine motor control in leprosy quite commonly leads to secondary injury and infection at the extremities, which may result in the loss of fingers and toes. While the digits of the right upper limb of the woman from *Culmen* are all present, the bones of the left forearm and hand were not found (Fig. 7.4). It is not possible to assess whether their absence is due to burial disturbance, or whether loss of these elements occurred antemortem, but there are no traces suggesting amputation of the left forearm. Even had the woman retained all her digits, it is likely that she experienced difficulties in a range of manual tasks as a consequence of disease impact.

Along with skin nodules, the woman likely would have had other visible changes to her appearance, such as deformation of the nose and hair loss (including eyelashes and eyebrows) (Talhari et al., 2015). Modern clinical studies show that various eye problems, which result in vision difficulties, may be very devastating for an individual with leprosy, since this person uses his or her sight (in place of sensation) to protect anaesthetized limbs from danger (Malik, Morris, & Ffytche, 2011). Before the introduction of multidrug therapy in the 1970s–1980s, ocular complications associated with leprosy occurred in up to 74.2% of patients (Malik et al.,

2011). Even among those who currently benefit from multidrug therapy around 66 % still experience various eye problems such as diminished lid closure, lagophthalmos, ectropion, entropion, trichiasis, episcleritis, scleritis, diminished corneal sensation, mild corneal opacity, acute/chronic iritis, iris atrophy, and synechiae, and around 20–70 % of patients have sight-threatening ocular complications (Malik et al., 2011). Based on such clinical evidence we believe we are justified in suggesting that the woman with leprosy from medieval *Culmen* very likely experienced sight-threatening ocular complications, although because these complications effect soft tissue only we have no 'hard' (i.e., osteological) evidence of this.

Advanced stages of leprosy can result in disability (Ortner & Putschar, 1985; WHO 1988; Roberts & Manchester, 2010, pp. 193–194). In modern Brazil, for example, this occurs in 6 % of cases (Santos et al., 2015). Moreover, 'the lepromatous form has a major impact on the development of disabilities' (Santos et al., 2015, p. 336) associated with loss of function in hands, feet, and eyes, leading to problems such as diminished ability to work, limited social life, and psychological problems. The cranial and postcranial lesions present on the woman's skeleton indicate an advanced stage of leprosy, suggesting that she likely experienced difficulty in aspects of functional capability as a result of her condition. As a result of damage to her hands and possible sight-threatening ocular complications she was probably unable to perform many or all of the daily tasks associated with the role of a typical medieval woman: cultivating vegetables, breeding animals, weaving fabrics, producing ceramics, cooking meals, and raising children. If she developed leprosy early in life, she may have faced difficulties in finding a husband (van Barkel et al., 2012) and, if unmarried, was most likely provided with accommodation and support by relatives. Over the time, the requirements for assistance would have increased as her condition worsened. We are not able to estimate when she may have experienced sight-threatening ocular complications, but it is probable that these were present for several years before death. During the advanced stages of leprosy, particularly if she developed sight-threatening ocular complications, she would have required help in acquiring and preparing food. She may also have required some help with eating, due to difficulties in manipulating utensils or holding food in her hand. Furthermore, if she did develop ocular complications she would have needed somebody to guide her if she wished to venture outside known territory. Help with mobility would have been required, possibly for some months as she recovered from the fracture of her lower limb.

Moreover, the woman had congenital fusion of the C2 and C3 vertebrae. The research shows conflicting results in relation to the potential impacts of this condition; some studies suggest it may affect quality of life (Leivseth, Frobin, & Brinckmann, 2005; Shankar & Kulkarni, 2011), with possible symptoms including limitation of neck movement, myelopathy, or the muscular weakness, atrophy, and neurological sensory loss associated with Klippel-Feil syndrome, whereas other studies have found this condition to be asymptomatic (Leivseth et al., 2005; Shankar & Kulkarni, 2011). Associated symptoms would almost certainly be different for each person, and we would need more data to be confident in speculating about the experience of this woman.

Medical Treatment and Therapies

Care for this woman very probably included therapeutic interventions, and both ethnohistoric and archaeological research identify treatments that may have been practiced in cases of leprosy in medieval Poland. The practices common in nineteenth-century folk culture may have been very similar to those used in medieval times, because folk culture developed in isolation from the culture of major towns and cities (Burszta, 1987) leading to the *longue durée* of some elements of the earlier traditions. Among all of the elements of culture that undergo change, the ones connected with religion and medicine are the most resistant and slow changing (Piątkowski, 2008, pp. 149, 217). Although we cannot know for certain what if any specific treatments this woman received, evidence from Kałdus suggests a range of medical practices that may have been present in the period in which she lived.

For example, ethnographic sources describe the treatment of diseases such as eye problems and gout as 'cut with a sickle,' which metaphorically means killing or ending the particular disease (Kolberg, 1867, p. 95; Kolberg, 1882, pp. 146, 156, 158; Udziela, 1891, p. 118), and it is possible that the subject was treated in this way to alleviate problems with vision and possible pain associated with her various pathologies. In this procedure the patient was seated, and the healer would make gestures over the patient to indicate 'cutting out' the disease and while saying prayers or incantations. A sickle was found in grave 24 at cemetery Site 2 in Kałdus (Haftka, 2007) and could have had double function – for agricultural and for healing purposes. These functions need not have had excluded each other, as the sickle was a multipurpose tool used in cutting plants and in healing depending on need, making its use and functions contextual.

The woman in this study would have experienced weakness and pain when she experienced probable lower limb fracture. The bones of cats were used in folk tradition for healing pain and overcoming weakness (Moszyński, 1967, p. 216), and cat bones (together with some other animal bones) were discovered in pits at the settlement in Kałdus (Makowiecki, 2010) – was this possibly one of the treatments she received? Powder made of belemnites (fossils of an extinct species of cephalopod) was a common remedy for skin ailments, as people believed they had magical powers (Łęga 1961, p. 280); a piece of belemnite was excavated in grave 391/03 at cemetery Site 4, suggesting these may also have been used for medicinal purposes in medieval times (Bojarski et al., 2010, p. 569). The woman in this study likely displayed the nodules symptomatic of lepromatous leprosy – was she offered powder of belemnites as a potential cure? There are many other such remedies recorded, and of course all healing practices were accompanied by prayers and conjurations or enchantments (Łęga 1961).

We do not know what remedies the woman in this study received, but given her context it is virtually a given that she received medical treatments in some form. These treatments would likely have been initiated from the time her symptoms became discernable and could therefore have spanned several months or years.

This woman is an exceptional finding among the remains from Kałdus. There is another possible case of leprosy in *Culmen* (grave 80/98), but due to poor skeletal preservation it is much less certain – molecular confirmation was negative.

Other pathologies identified in the material from Kałdus include anemia, scurvy, tuberculosis (Pott's disease and other locations), periosteal reactions, posttraumatic lesions and fractures, degenerative joint disease, tumors of bones, caries, and abscess (Kozłowski, 2012). In particular, individuals displaying evidence for poliomyelitis, osteomyelitis, rickets, very advanced degenerative lesions of joints that were painful and likely made movement impossible, vertebral disc herniation, hip dysplasia, probably multiple myeloma and amputation could all have suffered considerable limitations in function. In total, there were 40 individuals in *Culmen*, including the woman with leprosy, who likely experienced significant disability (Matczak, 2015). Caregiving was probably a common practice, since so many people are likely to have required care on either a temporary or full-time basis depending on the type and severity of their ailment. Based on our evidence, however, we believe that the subject of this study was one of those who required the most care.

Mortuary Treatment

Despite her very visible disease and associated disability, this woman was buried among others from her community, not relegated to the margins as an 'outcast.' Rather, her grave is located in the Southern-Central part of the cemetery (Chudziak, 2006). She was positioned W–E (the orientation allowing salvation on the Day of Resurrection), supine and with arms by her sides, indicating that she was most probably Christian (Fig. 7.4). Her lower limbs (particularly her left limb) were flexed, which is unusual but may reflect flexure during life that was difficult to redress postmortem. It is possible that the left leg, which at one stage suffered a fracture to the tibia and fibula (although this had healed by time of death), was difficult to straighten since, in comparison to other limbs, it was the most severely affected by periosteal inflammation. Otherwise this grave follows the typical pattern of burial at this site. The woman was interred with grave goods comprising an iron knife and a bronze ring (Chudziak et al., 2006). The location of her grave and the associated grave goods suggest that, despite a disfiguring disease, she received mortuary treatment associated with those of a higher social status.

In the case of this woman the effects of leprosy do not appear to have influenced the way she was treated at death. The reason for this may have been that the woman was the only individual in her community to contract leprosy (leprosy does not appear to have been common in the early Middle Ages in *Culmen*), and therefore while the disease would have marked her out as 'different' from others of her society it was not a source of stigma.

The 'Giant Woman' – A Case Study of Gigantism and Care

The excavation of Ostrów Lednicki cemetery began in the 1930s and revealed a high level of social stratification. In the church of the Ostrów Lednicki stronghold, pre-Romanesque burials of dignitaries dating to the middle the eleventh century were discovered (Górecki 1996, p. 152). In all probability these people were connected with the then prince and later the king of Poland, Bolesław Chrobry (Górecki 1991, 1996). The citizens of the stronghold were buried in the cemetery (Site 1) located near the church. The cemetery burials are dated from the first half of the eleventh century (Górecki 1996). Those who were buried there until the half of the twelfth century could have been connected with the early Piast elite (Górecki 1996). In the second half of the twelfth century the church fell out of use. Burying the people around the ruins of the church continued till the fourteenth century (Wrzesińscy, 1998b, p. 39; Wrzesiński, 2000, p. 236). In total, 2500 burials were excavated at Ostrów Lednicki Island (Wrzesińscy, 2010, p. 92). In contrast, the cemeteries of Dziekanowice (Sites 2 and 22) contained the remains of those who belonged to a lower social rank (Fig. 7.2).

Description of the Female from Grave 23/77

In 1977, the skeleton of a person of exceptional size and stature, most likely female, was recovered from grave 23/77 in the cemetery inside the Ostrów Lednicki stronghold (Szymczyk, Wąsowska, & Ziętek, 1977; Fig. 7.5). Unfortunately, the skeleton, known by researchers as the 'giant woman,' is not complete, because for many years it was used in osteological courses at the Department of Anthropology at Adam Mickiewicz University in Poznań (Gładykowska-Rzeczycka et al., 2000). The grave with the woman's skeleton is dated to between the end of the twelfth and the beginning of the fourteenth century (Wrzesiński, 2000, p. 236).

The subject's estimated age at death was between 25 and 30 years old and her estimated stature was 215.5 cm (c. 7′2″) (Gładykowska-Rzeczycka et al., 2000; Gładykowska-Rzeczycka, Śmiszkiewicz-Skwarska, & Sokół, 1998; Wrzesińscy, 2010). She has been diagnosed as suffering from gigantism during her early years, and from acromegaly in adulthood (Gładykowska-Rzeczycka et al., 2000, p. 272). Aufderheide and Rodríguez-Martín (2006, pp. 326–328) describe characteristic features of gigantism and acromegaly, and the skeleton of the woman from Ostrów Lednicki displays the pathological lesions of both afflictions (Gładykowska-Rzeczycka et al., 1998; Gładykowska-Rzeczycka et al., 2000; Fig. 7.5). The evidence for gigantism in her skeleton includes normally proportioned and structured bones of excessive length (Table 7.1) (compare with Aufderheide & Rodríguez-Martín, 2006, p. 328). The evidence for acromegaly in her skeleton includes an elongated and prognathic mandible, prominence of nasal and facial bones, crowding and malocclusion of the anterior dentition, enlarged vertebrae, and thickened bones in general (Table 7.1) (compare with Aufderheide & Rodríguez-Martín, 2006, p. 328; Bartelink, Willits, & Chelotti, 2014, pp. 39–41).

Aufderheide and Rodríguez-Martín (2006, p. 328) argue that degenerative joint disease is a characteristic feature for both gigantism and acromegaly. Degenerative joint disease in the skeleton of the woman from Ostrów Lednicki was observed in all vertebrae, with Schmorl's nodes on C3–C7, T3–T10 and all lumbar vertebrae,

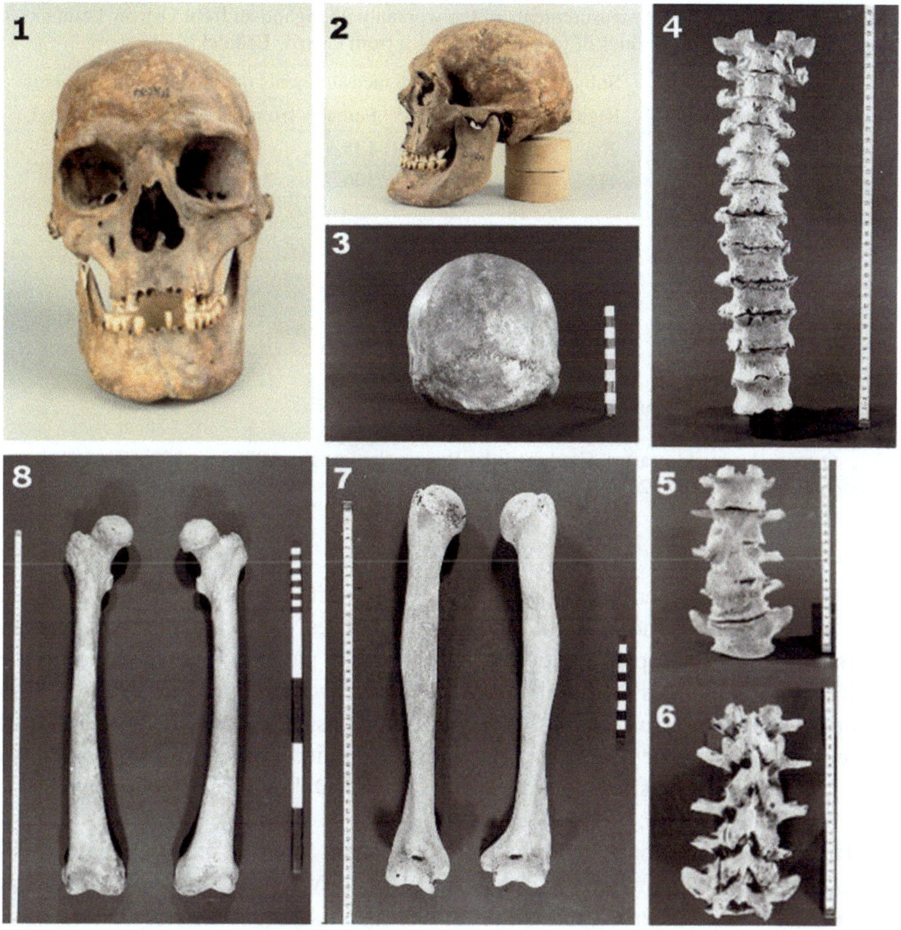

Fig. 7.5 Selected skeletal elements of the woman with gigantism, grave 23/77, Ostrów Lednicki (Greater Poland voivodeship). (*1*) the skull; (*2*) the skull, left view; (*3*) the skull, posterior view; (*4*) thoracic spine – degenerative lesions; (*5*) lumbar spine, anterior view, with syndesmophytes and osteophytes; (*6*) lumbar spine, posterior view, with long costal process; (*7*) left and right humeri; (*8*) left and right femora. Photos by M. Jóźwikowska, *4–8* after Gładykowska-Rzeczycka et al., 2000

and these may have been the result of heavy body weight associated with acromegaly and gigantism. The woman's remains display evidence of healed fractures of the right humerus and left tibia; again, these fractures may have been associated with complications of her pathology, as medical research has found the bones of people with acromegaly, and especially women with acromegaly, to be fragile, because bone mineral density is insufficient to create adequate bone strength (Hong, Kim, Kim, Kim, & Shin, 2016). Other pathologies evident include extensive sclerotization of the left temporal bone and obliterated external auditory canal as a result of

Table 7.1 Values of bones measurements of the woman with gigantism from Ostrów Lednicki in comparison with average values of females and males from Ostrów Lednicki

	Subject		Average measurements of right and left elements		
Location of measurement[a]	Right	Left	Subject	Females from O.L.	Males from O. L.
Length of clavicle	202	203?	202.5	135.5	142.3
Length of humerus	416	416	416	306.3	328.7
Length of radius	–	328	328	226.6	247.5
Length of ulna	364	361	362.5	247.5	268.6
Length of femur	555	548	551.5	416.1	449.5
Cross section of ulna	33	33	33	25.9	26.3
Length of tibia	485	487	486	342.7	367
Length of fibula	478	–	478	334.6	375

[a]measurements are based on Martin & Saller, 1957
The values are in mm
O.L. Ostrów Lednicki. (after Gładykowska-Rzeczycka et al., 1998, p. 152; Gładykowska-Rzeczycka et al., 2000, p. 264)

developmental disorder, partial ossification of the left lateral part of the occipital bone, and sclerotic remodeling of the sphenoid sinuses, dental caries, calculus, dental root abscesses and periodontitis, chondromalacia patellae, and osteomas on the left femur. Small nodes on the ribs indicate that the woman may have suffered from pleurisy. Harris lines on the left and right tibia (possible indicators of periods of malnutrition during development) were also identified (Gładykowska-Rzeczycka et al., 2000; Gładykowska-Rzeczycka, Smoczyński, Dubowik, & Mechlińska, 2001, p. 4; Wrzesińscy, 2010, p. 93).

This woman is the only individual with gigantism found in the Ostrów Lednicki and Dziekanowice cemeteries. The skeleton of a dwarf (Malinowski, 2008) has been recovered, and evidence for skull trauma (from Sites 2 and 22), dental caries, periosteal reactions, congenital pathologies (e.g., spina bifida; Budnik & Ortarzewska, 2010), and trepanation was identified in other remains from these cemeteries (Gładykowska-Rzeczycka, 1981; Wrzesińska, 1998).

Estimating Disability and Care

Acromegaly and gigantism are commonly associated with diabetes, hypertension, headaches, visual deficits, sleep apnea, sweating/oily skin, skin changes, coarse facial features, soft tissue swelling (including the tongue), enlargement of the hands and feet and, in females, menstrual dysfunction (Almalki et al., 2012; Birla, Aggarwal, Sharma, & Tandon, 2014; Dutta et al., 2015; Iuliano & Laws, 2014; Shao & Li, 2013; Wijayaratne et al., 2015). It is probable that the woman from Ostrów Lednicki may have suffered from one or more of these complications, but we cannot be certain because such diseases and ailments do not leave pathological lesions on bones.

Some individuals with gigantism are intellectually impaired and poorly skilled (Gładykowska-Rzeczycka et al., 2000, p. 269), and there is also a relationship between acromegaly and mental disorders. For example, in one study 88 out of 118 acromegalic patients were found to have mental disorders (Bobrov, Starostina, Dreval, & Alexandrova, 2014), and other research has also found that acromegalic patients have increased lifetime rates of affective disorders (Bobrov et al., 2014; Pinto & Safeekh, 2005; Sievers et al., 2009). People with acromegaly may demonstrate lack of initiative and spontaneity, as well as experiencing visual hallucinations and delusions (Pinto & Safeekh, 2005), and are particularly vulnerable to anxiety and dementia (Bobrov et al., 2014). Additionally, women with acromegaly experience psychiatric problems more frequently than men (Anagnostis et al., 2014; Pinto & Safeekh, 2005).

The average height in medieval times in Poland was 154–161 cm for females and 164–172 cm for males (Kozłowski, 2012). The woman with gigantism was around 55–60 cm (22–24 in.) taller than the average female, and due to her exceptional height may well have found it both awkward and uncomfortable to spend long periods inside a typical, small, medieval dwelling; during the winter, when people would have had to spend a lot of time inside their houses, it would have been very claustrophobic for her. (No houses with significantly larger rooms, potentially suitable for accommodating a woman of her stature in comfort, have been found in excavations to date.) At a practical level, it would also have been difficult to find existing furniture, for example a bed or chair, of the right size and strength to meet her needs, meaning that such items would have to be specially constructed.

Physically, other than difficulties associated with her greater-than-normal size and stature, there may have been nothing preventing the woman from Ostrów Lednicki from performing all daily tasks typical for medieval woman (domestic work, weaving, care of children, etc.). She would have encountered limitations while recovering from limb fractures and during likely bouts of pleurisy, however, and if she experienced any of the common complications of acromegaly and gigantism (see earlier) these may also have compromised her ability to undertake work. Minimally, she must have been cared for while recovering from her lower limb fracture, as she would have been unable to walk for this period. If she suffered a hearing deficit due to unilateral auditory atresia people may have had to speak more loudly when talking to her, and she may also have experienced problems in speech development. Nowadays, unilateral auditory atresia is not always medically treated, and people with this ailment can function in society without additional help (Kesser, Krook, & Gray, 2013; Trojanowska et al., 2012).

Willow, elderflower, and narrowleaf plantain (Udziela, 1891, s. 132, 203, 234; Łęga 1961, s. 283; Moszyński, 1967, s. 212–218) were discovered at an archaeological site in Dziekanowice, on the bank of the lake opposite Ostrów Lednicki Island (Makohonienko, 2000; Makohonienko, Wrzesińska, & Wrzesiński, 1998). We can speculate that these plants may have been used in treatment when this woman suffered from pleurisy. More minor likely impacts of her condition (such as headaches, visual problems, possibly symptoms of diabetes, and hypertension) could simply have been treated with rest. If she did have problems with diabetes and/or hypertension, these diseases could have had serious consequences. If such diseases are not medically treated and we assume that in the Middle Ages they were not, diabetes may lead to blindness, to renal failure, insufficiency in blood flow to the legs (ischemia), and heart disease, and hypertension may result in ischemic heart disease, stroke, peripheral vascular disease, heart failure, aortic aneurysms, diffuse atherosclerosis, chronic kidney disease, and pulmonary embolism (Chobanian et al., 2003; www.diabetes.org). Either of these diseases may have led to her death.

Given the correlation between acromegaly and mental disorders, and gigantism and intellectual impairment, it is possible that the woman with gigantism from Ostrów Lednicki suffered from mental or cognitive dysfunction. Of course it is impossible to state whether, or from which, disorder she suffered, and what care – if any – she may have received in response. We know that it is hazardous to speculate about the emotional state of a past individual when we have only her bones to guide us; however, based on modern clinical findings we feel justified in suggesting that the woman with gigantism may have felt any one, or more, of the following at different times, or even concurrently: irritability, anxiety, emotional liability, uncertainty, confusion, sadness, and anger (Anagnostis et al., 2014; Szcześniak, Jawiarczyk-Przybyłowska, & Rymaszewska, 2015). Equally, she may have suffered from depression, sleep disorders, difficulty concentrating, fatigue, high levels of stress, diminished self-esteem, sense of a loss of competence, and loss of control. It is a measure of the severity of possible impact to note that 'the psychological profile of acromegalics does not differ from those with other severe chronic diseases, such as CVD, malignancies, rheumatic diseases and chronic pulmonary obstruction' (Anagnostis et al., 2014, p. 568).

The woman with gigantism may well have needed psychological support, but it is impossible to say if she received it. Her unusual height, which in any society would mark her out as 'different' and may have led to people perceiving her as abnormal in other ways, could have been an obstacle to receiving such care, and being perceived as so very different would likely have an impact on her social life and her relationships with others. A medieval woman was supposed to marry and give birth to children or, alternatively, she might take holy orders and become a nun. We do not know if the woman with gigantism was married, and her treatment after death (see later) seems to exclude her having been a nun. Due to her unusual appearance (and possibly associated emotional problems) she could very possibly have encountered difficulty in finding a husband. If she was indeed unmarried, but at the same time was not part of a religious congregation, she would, in some sense, stand outside the conventional social order – and this would have likely been reflected in the way she was perceived and treated by others in her community.

Mortuary Treatment

The woman with gigantism was buried at a distance of 100–110 cm from the outer wall of the ruins of the former church (Wrzesiński, 2000). The church was in use until mid of the twelfth century (Wrzesiński, 2000, p. 235). At the time of the burial of the woman with gigantism (the end of the twelfth – beginning of the fourteenth century) the church was no longer in use. Her burial was located in the area of the former cemetery reserved for the elite (Górecki 1996, p. 153; Wrzesiński, 2000). She was the only individual of those buried around the church (and its later ruins) with her head orientated to the East and with no grave goods present (Fig. 7.6). Her skeleton sloped at an angle, which might indicate either that the surface of the grave was not flat or that she had been placed on material that had since decomposed. Her skeleton was lying on the left side, with her left hand close to her skull. The right upper limb was bent at the elbow. The left lower limb was bent at the knee to an angle of just less than 110° (Gładykowska-Rzeczycka et al., 2000, p. 239; Wrzesiński, 2000).

It is hard to interpret the anomalous burial orientation of the 'giant woman.' Possibly it was connected with an older pagan ritual, as an eastern orientation of graves was quite popular in early medieval Poland (although it was less popular than the western orientation, and disappeared in the thirteenth century – Miśkiewicz, 1969). Burial close to the ruins of the church indicates that the woman with gigantism was probably Christian. If she was buried at this location (i.e., the site of the elite cemetery) at the end of the twelfth century she may have come from a higher social class, as at this time memory of elite burial practices would be still vivid and these practices might still endure. However, her grave is potentially dated to any time between the end of the twelfth and the beginning of the fourteenth century. It cannot be assumed that earlier customs relating to elite burial were observed during the thirteenth and into the fourteenth century, and therefore we cannot safely draw any firm conclusion about the social class to which the woman with gigantism belonged.

This woman's remains did not receive a standard burial, which suggests she was perceived as 'different' in death (Gładykowska-Rzeczycka et al., 2000, p. 272), whatever her social status in life. Her body was placed in very unusual way and apparently without attention to detail; very different to the typical disposition of the dead, which was supine, with arms and hands extended along the body or hands placed on the pelvis. Indeed, the unusual burial orientation, disposal of the body without care, and lack of grave goods may indicate that this woman belonged to a lower social stratum. During her lifetime, as well, she may have been subject to different treatment by her community because of her physical abnormalities and/or possible psychological or cognitive problems. However, her survival to middle adulthood, together with the evidence indicating she likely received health-related care – minimally nursing during bouts of respiratory disease and recovery from fracture – suggests that she was not rejected by her society.

Discussion

We have chosen the osteobiographies of these two women to present a wider view of aspects of life in medieval society, including care, emotion, social perception, status of the diseased and the disabled, and the meaning of burial ritual. Our osteobiographical approach has allowed us to tell the stories of two particular individuals and their lives.

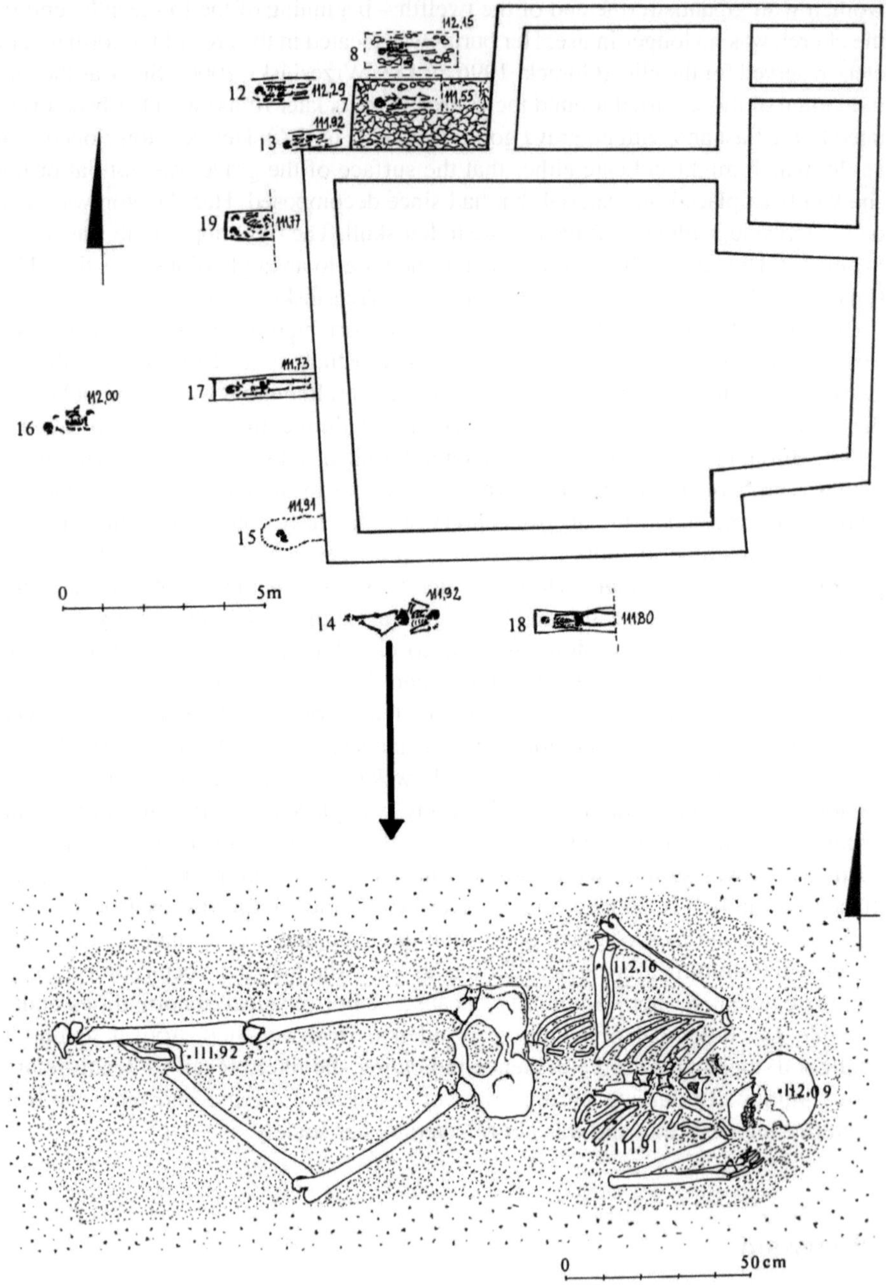

Fig. 7.6 The *top* part of the image shows the plan of the ruins of the church and cemetery at Ostrów Lednicki. The *arrow* indicates disposition and burial orientation of the 'giant woman' from grave 23/77 (modified after Górecki 1996)

Two Types of Care

The bioarchaeology of care methodology can help us to focus on two kinds of care: health-related care received during life, and 'care' after death. In the first case, examining likely disability impact helps us to assess care provision to an individual during his or her life. In the second case, analyzing the type of burial provided may help us to understand social attitudes toward the individual at time of their funeral. The first type of care is achieved by analogy with modern clinical cases, ethnography, and historical texts. This study showed us that the woman with leprosy was cared for. People probably provided her with food, accommodation, clothing, therapies, and guidance when she wanted to walk outside the home. In the case of the woman with gigantism, care was provided to her during recovery from limb fractures and experiences of pleurisy – both pathologies with physical consequences. Yet it is very hard (if not impossible) to assess whether any care was provided to this same woman in the event that she experienced mental health issues – which it is likely she did.

Consideration of the second type of care – 'care' in relation to the mortuary treatment afforded an individual – is based on archaeological evidence. This might be called 'care after death.' Burial custom is a lens of three forms of such care. The first form occurs when the people care for the memory of the dead, commemorating the deceased. Therefore, we argue that the woman with leprosy from Kałdus was commemorated as a community member with quite a high social status in her society with 'care after death.' The woman from Ostrów Lednicki was commemorated in a different way to others in her society, evidenced in the different orientation of her body and in the disposal of her body without care. Possibly her unusual height and probable mental difficulties had an impact on the way she was commemorated.

The second form of 'care after death' is realized in the care shown in providing a proper burial to ensure the successful passage of the individual into the afterlife. The woman from Kałdus was buried according to all Christian rules to ensure her place in the afterlife. Interpreting the significance of the burial of the woman with gigantism is hard, since she was interred close to the ruins of the church, which might indicate that she was Christian. On the other hand, she was the only person buried with her head to the east, which might indicate a pagan element of ritual. Maybe the community sought to emphasize the difference of this woman by orientating her body to the east. Maybe people thought that God caused her to be abnormally tall as a punishment for her pagan attitude.

The third form of 'care after death' is, in fact, directed toward the living and refers to measures taken in burying the dead to ensure that the dead will not cause any harm to those left behind. In medieval times people feared some of the dead, especially those of the dead who, for various reasons, were perceived as vampires. Vampires were thought to bring death and harm to society, and communities developed elaborate burial customs and antivampire practices to protect themselves; such behaviors have been extensively discussed in the literature (e.g., Betsinger & Scott, 2014; Matczak, 2014, 2015). In our case studies, we did not identify any practices that could indicate an attempt to protect the living against vampires. As already discussed, the grave of the woman from Kałdus conformed to the norms of the time. The grave of the woman with gigantism is unusual, but it does not display characteristics associated with the burial treatment of vampires. In a strict sense, it is also hard to classify it as an 'atypical' grave from Polish medieval times. Atypical graves are characterized by much more explicit features, such as prone positioning of the body, placement of the body on its side, curled (fetal) positioning of the body, stones directly placed on the body, removal of body parts, double graves, or chamber graves (Matczak, 2014, 2015). The grave of the woman with gigantism does not conform to any of these recognized atypical treatments and is therefore problematic. However, while the grave is not atypical in the formal sense, the burial treatment of the woman with gigantism suggests lack of attention to detail that may, perhaps, indicate a lack of affection or respect felt for her, at least at the moment of her funeral. Although she may not have been completely rejected by her society, perhaps neither was she considered a full member of it. Possibly she had a form of liminal status, which saw her understood not as good, or bad, but as different.

As the earlier discussion illustrates, in some circumstances it is possible to use skeletal and mortuary evidence reflexively to inform analysis of various forms of care, and in certain cases, indeed, these forms of evidence are so closely entwined as to be inseparable. As we mentioned at the beginning of this chapter, burial ritual is a complex topic, which has different meanings according to the archaeological context and approach of the researcher. In the light of traditional approaches to mortuary evidence, care taken to ensure proper burial might tell us many things about an individual – such as their social status, social acceptance of their disease experience, whether they evoked fear or compassion. However, if we follow this line of thinking we are likely to encounter the same obstacle we discussed in the section 'Disability during life and treatment after death.' If funerary practices create an idealized representation (Parker, 2011), then this representation creates idealized conception of care. Careful placement of the body in the grave and a proper grave according to the social rules may not directly represent care of the individual when he or she was alive. That is why pathological assessment of physical evidence in remains is the most reliable way to assess care in the past.

Care and Disability

As we mentioned earlier, interpretation of care is intimately associated with assessing disability. According to Tilley and Oxenham (2011), disability can be either temporary (e.g., fracture followed by a period of recovery) or long term, and both can be associated with care. In this sense, both women examined here – one with leprosy and one with gigantism – were disabled. In contrast to Tilley and Oxenham (2011), we would rather define disability only as a long-lasting condition, which worsens over time and results in an inability to perform daily tasks. We acknowledge that compound fractures may cause complications that might lead to long-lasting disability, as is indicated in contemporary clinical studies (e.g., Marks, 2011). However, we do not consider a simple fracture that was healed as a temporary disability.

The study reported in this chapter is based on osteological and ethnographic materials and on contemporary clinical studies, which we use to construct the perception of disability. For instance, ethnographic texts (Kolberg, 1867, 1882; Łęga 1961; Moszyński, 1967; Udziela, 1891) indicate that people considered fractures to be different to what they considered 'impairments' and 'handicaps,' which were usually congenital disabilities. Normal fracture healing takes up to 12 weeks, which is circa 3 months (Brown, *How to Speed Fracture Healing*, www.betterbones.com). This is a comparatively short time in comparison to some of the conditions associated with disease or illness (e.g., leprosy, anemia, and tuberculosis last for years). A person with a fracture of one upper limb could still perform daily tasks with the other upper limb. A person with only one upper limb could have functioned and even participated in a fight (Jones, 2012). If a person had fractured leg she or he could still have temporarily performed daily tasks using their hands. There were still plenty of such tasks for both women and men in medieval society. For instance, women still could have nursed children, cultivated vegetables, weaved fabrics, produced ceramics, and cooked. The men would still have been able to skin, tan, and produce tools. People with different and severe physical conditions were a larger proportion of the society in the past than nowadays because of high levels of warfare, risky daily jobs (e.g., hunting), and lack of advanced medicine. Moreover, Knüsel (1999) argues that whether impairment was perceived as taking from the value of the individual concerned, or not affecting estimation of their value, was dependent on contextual factors: for example, lifeways demands on the individual, their social status, and the way the impairment was acquired. As we can see, the term 'disability' is ambiguous, contextual, and depends upon different factors. For these reasons, we do not think that the woman with gigantism suffering from a fracture (that was healed) was temporarily physically disabled. The question as to whether the woman with gigantism was intellectually or psychologically disabled remains open, because we do not have enough data to ascertain this.

Text Sources

The interpretation of care based on evidence from historical times would be much richer if it were supplemented with textual sources. Some of the Polish historians have approached the topic of health and disease through medieval sources of information, but such studies may not be fully reliable because their authors have not examined the chronicles and other document sources to establish which elements genuinely correspond to Polish history and culture, and which are shared as *topoi* between many other European texts. There is a need for detailed and heuristic research on this problem, with an approach that takes a comparative perspective in relation to other European texts. The current state of historical studies on past health and disease does not allow bioarchaeologists to approach the topic of caregiving using historical sources. This is very unfortunate, because we believe that such texts could contribute significant information to our studies. We argue that using textual sources without proper heuristic analysis would be superficial and would result in treating such sources in an instrumental way.

Conclusions

Our study uses osteobiography and the bioarchaeology of care methodology with an aim to investigate disability and care of the disabled in medieval times. We presented the life history of two individuals within the context of their societies from a comparative perspective. We conclude that the woman from Kałdus was disabled, but she was cared for by her society rather than excluded from it. The various forms of care she received included provision of food, accommodation, clothing, therapies, and guidance outside of the house. Care was likely provided to the woman for a considerable time, possibly from the first visible symptoms of leprosy until her death, and such care could have lasted for several years. Her burial also indicates that care was taken to provide proper burial according to the prevailing cultural ideology, highlighting her social status and ensuring her afterlife.

The other individual – the woman with gigantism – displayed no skeletal evidence of physical disability, and the question of whether she was intellectually or psychologically disabled remains open. She was temporarily injured (fractures) and incapacitated (pleurisy), and care was provided for her at that time. This indicates that care could have been provided not only to those who were long-term physically disabled, but also to the ill and those with traumatic injury. The placement of her body in the grave is unusual. In medieval society, it was probably her unusual height and (possible) problems with mental health that had an impact on the social perception of her as being 'different.'

Mortuary evidence can significantly add to research on past caregiving, as we have demonstrated in our study. Typical and atypical burials give new insights into our perception of the ill, the disabled, and the society in which their possible care occurred. Mortuary evidence is an essential part of research into care and disability, and should be accepted as an integral part of the bioarchaeology of care methodology. We have also identified the importance of undertaking an heuristic analysis of disability, disease, and health-related care practices in Polish history, and we hope that, in the future, it will be possible to conduct an interdisciplinary research project that will meet this need.

Acknowledgements We would like to thank Lorna Tilley and Alecia A. Schrenk for the invitation to contribute to this volume and their stimulating comments that helped to elaborate on many issues that are described in this chapter. We thank to anonymous reviewers for their comments, which contributed to the shape of this text, Harsha Vardhan Simhadri for consultation and criticism, and Jacek Wrzesiński for consultation and giving us access to the photographs of the woman with gigantism. This work was supported by the National Science Centre from Poland under grant UMO-2014/13/N/HS3/04602.

References

Almalki, M. H., Chesover, A. D., Johnson, M. D., Wilkins, G. E., Maguire, J. A., & Ur, E. (2012). Characterization of management and outcomes of patients with acromegaly in Vancouver over 30 years. *Clinical and Investigative Medicine, 35*(1), 27–33.

Anagnostis, P., Efstathiadou, Z. A., Charizopoulou, M., Selalmatzidou, D., Karathanasi, E., Poulasouchidou, M., et al. (2014). Psychological profile and quality of life in patients with acromegaly in Greece. Is there any difference with other chronic diseases? *Endocrine, 47*, 564–571.

Aufderheide, A. C., & Rodríguez-Martín, C. (2006). *The Cambridge encyclopedia of human paleopathology*. Cambridge: Cambridge University Press.

Baker, B. J., & Bolhofner, K. L. (2014). Biological and social implications of a medieval burial from Cyprus for understanding the leprosy in the past. *International Journal of Paleopathology, 4*, 17–24.

Barnes, C., & Mercer, G. (2010). *Exploring disability. A sociological introduction*. Cambridge: Polity Press.

Bartelink, E. J., Willits, N. A., & Chelotti, K. L. (2014). A probable case of acromegaly from the Windmiller culture of prehistoric Central California. *International Journal of Paleopathology, 4*, 37–46.

Betsinger, T. K., & Scott, A. B. (2014). Governing from the grave: Vampire burials and social order in post-medieval Poland. *Cambridge Archaeological Journal, 24*(3), 467–476.

Birla, S., Aggarwal, S., Sharma, A., & Tandon, N. (2014). Rare association of acromegaly with left atrial myxoma in Carney's complex due to novel PRKAR1A mutation. *Endocrinology, Diabetes & Metabolism Case Reports, 2014*, 140023. doi:10.1530/EDM-14-0023.

Bobrov, A., Starostina, E., Dreval, A., & Alexandrova M. (2014). Psychopathology in patients with acromegaly. *The Journal of the European Psychiatric Association* 29.

Bojarski, J., Chudziak, W., Drozd, A., Koperkiewicz, A., Kozłowski, T., & Stawska, V. (2010). Katalog źródeł. In W. Chudziak (Ed.), Wczesnośredniowieczne cmentarzysko szkieletowe w Kałdusie (stanowisko 4) (Mons Sancti Laurentii 5, pp. 437–603). Toruń: Wydawnictwo Naukowe UMK.

Brown, S. E. *"How to speed fracture healing"(PDF). Center for better bones*. Retrieved December 27, 2015, from www.betterbones.com.

Budnik, A., & Ortarzewska, K. (2010). Spina bifida occulta a asymetria fluktuująca w średniowiecznej populacji z mikroregionu Ostrowa Lednickiego. In T. Kozłowski & A. Drozd (Eds.), *Biokulturowe uwarunkowania stanu zdrowia populacji ludzkich w okresie średniowiecza* (pp. 17–22). Wrocław: Wydawnictwo DN.

Burszta, J. (1987). Kultura ludowa. In Z. Staszczak (Ed.), *Słownik etnologiczny. Terminy ogólne* (pp. 195–198). Warszawa, Poznań: Państwowe Wydawnictwo Naukowe.

Chobanian, A. V., Bakris, G. L., Black, H. R., Cushman, W. C., Green, L. A., Izzo, J. L., Jr., et al. (2003). Seventh report of the Joint National Committee on Prevention, Detection, Evaluation, and Treatment of High Blood Pressure. *Hypertension, 42*(6), 1206–1252.

Chudziak, W. (2003). *Wczesnośredniowieczna przestrzeń sakralna in Culmine na Pomorzu Nadwiślańskim* (Mons Sancti Laurentii 1). Toruń: Wydawnictwo Uniwersytetu Mikołaja Kopernika.

Chudziak, W. (Ed.). (2006). *Wczesnośredniowieczne cmentarzysko szkieletowe w Kałdusie (stanowisko 1)* (Mons Sancti Laurentii 3). Toruń: Wydawnictwo Naukowe UMK.

Chudziak, W. (Ed.). (2010). *Wczesnośredniowieczne cmentarzysko szkieletowe w Kałdusie (stanowisko 4)* (Mons Sancti Laurentii 5). Toruń: Wydawnictwo Naukowe UMK.

Chudziak, W., Stawska, V., Weinkauf, J., & Kozłowski, T. (2006). Katalog. Część II. Badania Instytutu Archeologii i Etnologii UMK w Toruniu w latach 1997–1999. In W. Chudziak (Ed.), *Wczesnośredniowieczne cmentarzysko szkieletowe w Kałdusie (stanowisko 1)* (Mons Sancti Laurentii 3, pp. 345–388). Toruń: Wydawnictwo Naukowe UMK.

Cross, M. (1999). Accessing the inaccessible: Disability and archaeology. *Archaeological Review from Cambridge, 15*(2), 7–30.

Data Collection Codebook (2006). R. H. Steckel, C. S. Larsen, P. W. Sciulli, & P. L. Walker (Eds.). The global history of health project. Retrieved August 13, 2015, from http://global.sbs.ohio-state.edu/docs/Codebook-12-12-05.pdf.

Dutta, P., Hajela, A., Pathak, A., Bhansali, A., Radotra, B. D., Vashishta, R. K., et al. (2015). Clinical profile and outcome of patients with acromegaly according to the 2014 consensus guidelines: Impact of a multi-disciplinary team. *Neurology India, 63*(3), 360–368.

Finlay, N. (1999). Disability and Archaeology. *Archaeological Review from Cambridge, 15*(2), 1–6.

Gładykowska-Rzeczycka, J. J. (1981). A short review of paleopathological research in Poland. *HOMO, 32*, 125–130.

Gładykowska-Rzeczycka, J. J. (1982). Schorzenia swoiste ludności z dawnych cmentarzysk Polski. *Przegląd Antropologiczny, 48*, 39–55.

Gładykowska-Rzeczycka, J. J., Śmiszkiewicz-Skwarska, A., & Sokół, A. (1998). A Giant from Ostrów Lednicki (XII-XIIIc), Dist. Lednogóra, Poland. *The Mankind Quarterly, 39*(2), 147–172.

Gładykowska-Rzeczycka, J. J., Smoczyński, M., Dubowik, M., & Mechlińska, J. (2001). Rare developmental disorder of the sound-conducting system of the skeleton from an early medieval cemetery in Poland. Endoscoping and CT findings. *The Mankind Quarterly, 42*(1), 3–16.

Gładykowska-Rzeczycka, J. J., Wrzesińska, A., & Sokół, A. (2000). Morfologiczne i radiologiczne badanie szkieletu olbrzymki z wczesnośredniowiecznego cmentarzyska na Ostrowiu Lednickim. *Studia Lednickie, 6*, 239–276.

Górecki, J. (1991). Preromańskie pochówki panujących dostojników w tzw. II kościele na Ostrowie Lednickim. *Studia Lednickie, 2*, 117–132.

Górecki, J. (1996). Nekropola tzw. II kościoła na Ostrowie Lednickim. *Studia Lednickie, 4*, 137–156.

Haftka, A. (2007). *Wczesnośredniowieczne cmentarzysko szkieletowe w Kałdusie. Stanowisko 2*, M.A. thesis, Nicolaus Copernicus University in Toruń.

Hawkey, D. (1998). Disability, compassion and the skeletal record: using musculoskeletal stress markers (MSM) to construct an osteobiography from Early New Mexico. *International Journal of Osteoarchaeology, 8*, 326–340.

Hong, A. R., Kim, J. H., Kim, S. W., Kim, S. Y., & Shin, C. S. (2016). Trabecular bone score as a skeletal fragility index in acromegaly patients. *Osteoporosis International, 27*(3), 1123–1129.

Horstmanshoff, M. (2012). Disability and rehabilitation in the Graeco-Roman world. In R. Breitwieser (Ed.) *Behinderungen und Beeinträchtigungen/disability and impairment in antiquity. BAR International Series. Studies in Early Medicine 2* (pp. 1–9). Oxford: British Archaeological Reports.

Hubert, J. (2000). Introduction: The complexity of boundedness and exclusion. In J. Hubert (Ed.), *Madness, disability and social exclusion. The archaeology and anthropology of "difference"* (pp. 1–8). London: Routledge.

Iuliano, S. L., & Laws, E. R., Jr. (2014). Recognizing the clinical manifestations of acromegaly: Case studies. *Journal of the American Association of Nurse Practitioners, 26*(3), 136–142. doi:10.1002/2327-6924.12076.

Jones, T. E. (2012). "A lame man can ride… a deaf man can kill… a dead man is of no use to anyone". When was a deformity not a disability in Early Medieval Europe? In R. Breitwieser (Ed.) *Behinderungen und Beeinträchtigungen/disability and impairment in antiquity. BAR International Series. Studies in Early Medicine 2* (pp. 131–135). Oxford: British Archaeological Reports.

Kesser, B. W., Krook, K., & Gray, L. C. (2013). Impact of unilateral conductive hearing loss due to aural atresia on academic performance in children. *The Laryngoscope, 123*(9), 2270–2275.

Knüsel, C. J. (1999). Ortopaedic disability: Some hard evidence. *Archaeological Review from Cambridge, 15*(2), 31–53.

Knüsel Ch, J., Batt, C. M., Cook, G., Montgomery, J., Müldner, G., Ogden, A. R., et al. (2010). The identity of St Bees Lady, Cumbria: An osteobiographical approach. *Medieval Archaeology, 54*, 271–311.

Kolberg, O. (1867). *Dzieła Wszystkie* 1, Kujawy, Warszawa.

Kolberg, O. (1882). *Dzieła Wszystkie* 15, Wielkie Księstwo Poznańskie.

Kozłowski, T. (2012). *Stan biologiczny i warunki życia ludności in Culmine na Pomorzu Nadwiślańskim (X-XIII wiek): studium antropologiczne* (Mons Sancti Laurentii 7). Wydawnictwo Naukowe UMK: Toruń.

Kozłowski, T., & Drozd, A. (2009). Ludzkie szczątki kostne z krypty północnej w prezbiterium kościoła katedralnego w Kwidzynie w świetle badań antropologicznych i paleopatologicznych. In M. Grupa & T. Kozłowski (Eds.), *Katedra w Kwidzynie—tajemnica krypt* (pp. 43–67). Kwidzyń: Kwidzyńskie Centrum Kultury.

Kudlick, J. C. (2003). Disability history: Why we need another "other". *The American Historical Review, 108*(3), 763–793.

Kurnatowska, Z. (1991). Z badań nad przemianami organizacji terytorialnej w państwie pierwszych Piastów. *Studia Lednickie, 2*, 11–22.

Łęga, W. (1961). *Ziemia chełmińska*. Wrocław: Polskie Towarzystwo Ludoznawcze.

Leivseth, G., Frobin, W., & Brinckmann, P. (2005). Congenital cervical block vertebrae are associated with caudally adjacent discs. *Clinical Biomechanics, 20*, 669–674.

Leone, M. P. (2005). *The archaeology of liberty in an american capital: Excavations in Annapolis*. Berkeley: University of California Press.

Longmore, M., Wilkinson, I. B., & Rajagopalan, S. R. (2004). *Oxford handbook of clinical medicine*. Oxford: Oxford University Press.

Makohonienko, M. (2000). Analiza palinologiczna zawartości ziemi z misy brązowej z wczesnośredniowiecznego cmentarzyska w Dziekanowicach, stanowisko 22. *Studia Lednickie, 6*, 207–212.

Makohonienko, M., Wrzesińska, A., & Wrzesiński, J. (1998). Analiza palinologiczna wypełniska jam grobowych. *Studia Lednickie, 5*, 95–102.

Makowiecki, D. (2010). *Wczesnośredniowieczna gospodarka zwierzętami i socjotopografia in Cumine na Pomorzu Nadwiślańskim*. Toruń: Wydawnictwo UMK.

Malik, A. N., Morris, R. W., & Ffytche, T. J. (2011). The prevalence of ocular complications in leprosy patients seen in the United Kingdom over a period of 21 years. *Eye, 25*(6), 740–745.

Malinowski, A. (2008). Medyczno-antropologiczne aspekty Lednickiego Parku Krajobrazowego i Muzeum Pierwszych Piastów na Lednicy. *Homines Hominibus, 1*(4), 25–32.

Marks, R. (2011). Physical activity and hip fracture disability: A review. *Journal of Aging Research, 2011*, 741918. doi:10.4061/2011/741918.

Martin, R., & Saller, S. (1957). *Lerbuch für Anthropologie*. Stuttgart: Gustav Fischer.

Matczak, M. D. (2014). Tak zwane pochówki antywampiryczne a zagadnienie zmian patologicznych. Próba reinterpretacji. In W. Dzieduszycki, & J. Wrzesiński (Eds.) *Królowie i biskupi, rycerze i chłopi – identyfikacja zmarłych. Funeralia Lednickie* 16 (pp. 437–457). Poznań: SNAP.

Matczak, M. D. (2015). *The Ill, the disabled in early medieval Culmine. The archaeological and anthropological perspective,* PhD dissertation, Adam Mickiewicz University (in Polish).

Miśkiewicz, M. (1969). Wczesnośredniowieczny obrządek pogrzebowy na płaskich cmentarzyskach szkieletowych w Polsce. *Materiały Wczesnośredniowieczne, 6*, 241–301.

Molleson, T. (1999). Archaeological evidence of attitudes to disability in the past. *Archaeological Review from Cambridge, 15*(2), 69–77.

Moszyński, K. (1967). *Kultura ludowa Słowian* (Vol. 2(1)). Warszawa: Książka i Wiedza.

Nerlich, A. G., Zink, A., Szeimies, U., & Hageodorn, H. G. (2000). Ancient Egyptian Prothesis of the big Toe. *The Lancet, 356*(9248), 2176–2179.

Ortner, D. J., & Putschar, W. G. J. (1985). *Identification of pathological conditions in human skeletal remains*. Washington: Smithsonian Institution Press.

Papadopoulos, J. K. (2000). Skeletons in wells: Towards an archaeology of social exclusion in the ancient Greek word. In J. Hubert (Ed.), *Madness, disability and social exclusion. The archaeology and anthropology of 'Difference'* (pp. 96–118). London: Routledge.
Parker, P. M. (2011). *The archaeology of death and burial*. Stroud: Sutton Publishing Limited.
Piątkowski, W. (2008). *Lecznictwo niemedyczne w Polsce. Tradycja i współczesność. Analiza zjawiska z perspektywy socjologii zdrowia i choroby*. Lublin: Wydawnictwo UMCS.
Pinto, M., & Safeekh, T. M. (2005). Psychotic symptoms in acromegaly. *Indian Journal of Psychiatry, 47*(1), 58–59.
Reicher, M. (1933). Niektóre cechy anatomiczne szczątków królewskich z Bazyliki Wileńskiej. *Pamiętnik XIV Zjazdu Lekarzy i Przyrodników Polskich w Poznaniu 11-15 IX 1933*, 1, 391–393.
Robb, J. (2002). Time and biography: Osteobiography of the Italian neolithic lifespan. In Y. Hamilakis, M. Pluciennik, & S. Tarlow (Eds.), *Thinking through the body: Archaeologies of corporeality* (pp. 153–171). New York: Kluwer Academic/Plenum.
Robb, J. (2009). Towards a critical Ötziography: Inventing prehistoric bodies. In H. Lambert & M. McDonald (Eds.), *Social bodies* (pp. 100–127). New York: Berghahn Books.
Roberts, C. A. (1999). Disability in the skeletal record: assumptions, problems and some examples. *Archaeological Review from Cambridge, 15*(2), 79–97.
Roberts, C. A., & Manchester, K. (2010). *The archaeology of disease*. Stroud: The History Press.
Rosado, M. A., & Vernacchio-Wilson, J. (2006). Paleopathology and osteobiography of the people of Peñuelas, Chile's semiarid north. *Memórias do Instituto Oswaldo Cruz, 101*(Suppl. II), 85–95.
Rosiński, B. (1951). O szczątkach kostnych rodziców Fryderyka Chopina. *Przegląd Antropologiczny, 17*, 303–319.
Santos, V. S., Santos de Matos, A. M., Alves de Oliviera, L. S., Dolce de Lemos, L. M., Gurgel, R. Q., Reis, F. P., et al. (2015). Clinical variables associated with disability in leprosy cases in Northeast Brazil. *The Journal of Infection in Developing Countries, 9*(3), 232–238.
Saul, F. P. (1972). *The human skeletal remains of Altar de Sacrificios: An osteobiographic analysis* (Vol. 63(2)). Papers of the Peabody Museum of Archaeology and Ethnology. Cambridge, MA, Peabody Museum of Archaeology and Ethnology, Harvard University.
Saul, F. P., & Saul, J. M. (1989). Osteobiography: A Maya example. In M. Y. Iscan & K. A. R. Kennedy (Eds.), *Reconstruction of life from the skeleton* (pp. 287–301). New York: Alan R. Liss.
Shankar, V. V., & Kulkarni, R. R. (2011). Block vertebra: Fusion of axis with the third cervical vertebra – A case report. *International Journal of Anatomical Variations, 4*, 15–16.
Shao, S., & Li, X. (2013). Clinical features and analysis in 1385 Chinese patients with pituitary adenomas. *Journal of Neurosurgical Sciences, 57*(3), 267–275.
Sievers, C., Dimopoulou, C., Pfister, H., Lieb, R., Steffin, B., Roemmler, J., et al. (2009). Prevalence of mental disorders in acromegaly: A cross-sectional study in 81 acromegalic patients. *Clinical Endocrinology, 71*(5), 691–701.
Stodder, A. L. W., & Palkovich, A. M. (2012a). Osteobiography and bioarchaeology. In A. L. W. Stodder & A. M. Palkovich (Eds.), *The bioarchaeology of individuals* (pp. 1–8). Gainesville: University Press of Florida.
Stodder, A. L. W., & Palkovich, A. M. (2012b). *The bioarchaeology of individuals*. Gainesville: University Press of Florida.
Szcześniak, D., Jawiarczyk-Przybyłowska, A., & Rymaszewska, J. (2015). The quality of life and psychological, social and cognitive functioning of patients with acromegaly. *Advances in Clinical and Experimental Medicine, 24*(1), 167–172.
Szymczyk, B., Wąsowska, E., & Ziętek, A. (1977). Przypadek gigantyzmu we wczesnośredniowiecznym materiale szkieletowym z Ostrowa Lednickiego. *Przegląd Antropologiczny, 43*(2), 334.
Tabaka, A. (2005). Domniemane miejsce targowe na Ostrowie Lednickim. *Studia Lednickie, 8*, 131–144.

Talhari, C., Talhari, S., & Penna, G. O. (2015). Clinical aspects of leprosy. *Clinics in Dermatology, 33*, 26–37.

Talko-Hryncewicz J. (1914). Odtworzenie kilku typów postaci historycznych spoczywających na Wawelu. *Rozprawy Wydziału Matematyczno-Przyrodniczego PAU, seria 3, dział B, 54*, 105–139.

Tilley, L., & Cameron, T. (2014). Introducing the Index of Care: A web-based application supporting archaeological research into health-related care. *International Journal of Paleopathology, 6*, 5–9.

Tilley, L., & Oxenham, M. F. (2011). Survival against the odds: Modeling the social implications of care provision to seriously disabled individuals. *International Journal of Paleopathology, 1*, 35–42.

Trojanowska, A., Drop, A., Trojanowski, P., Rosińska-Bogusiewicz, K., Klatka, J., & Bobek-Billewicz, B. (2012). External and middle ear diseases: Radiological diagnosis based on clinical signs and symptoms. *Insights Imaging, 3*(1), 33–48.

Udziela, M. (1891). *Medycyna i przesądy lecznicze ludu polskiego/Przyczynek do etnografii polskiej.* Wisła 7. Warszawa: Księgarnia M. Arcta.

van Barkel, W. H., Sihombing, B., Djarir, H., Beise, K., Kusumawardhani, L., Yulihane, R., et al. (2012). Disability in people affected by leprosy: The role of impairment, activity, social participation, stigma and discrimination. *Go Health Action, 5*, 18394.

WHO. (1988). *Expert committee on leprosy, sixth report.* World Health Organization Technical Report Series. 789.

Wijayaratne, D. R., Arambewela, M. H., Dalugama, C., Wijesundera, D., Somasundaram, N., & Katulanda, P. (2015). Acromegaly presenting with low insulin-like growth factor-1 levels and diabetes: A case report. *Journal of Medical Case Reports, 9*(1), 241. doi:10.1186/s13256-015-0736-z.

Wrzesińscy, A. J. (1998a). Próba interpretacji struktury społecznej ludności na cmentarzysku. Doniesienie wstępne. *Studia Lednickie, 5*, 13–27.

Wrzesińscy, A. J. (1998b). Odtworzenie stanu i dynamiki biologicznej ludności pochowanej na cmentarzysku wczesnośredniowiecznym Dziekanowice, stanowisko 22. *Studia Lednickie, 5*, 29–40.

Wrzesińscy, A. J. (2010). Wyjątkowe kobiety–choroby w przeszłości. Wybrane przykłady. *Nowiny Lekarskie, 2*, 89–97.

Wrzesińska, A. (1998). Charakterystyka urazów czaszki z cmentarzyska. *Studia Lednickie, 5*, 53–64.

Wrzesiński, J. (2000). Odkrycie i stratygrafia w rejonie grobu 23/77 na Ostrowie Lednickim. *Studia Lednickie, 6*, 231–237.

Websites

www.diabetes.org – American Diabetes Association

Talhari, C., Talhari, S., & Penna, G. O. (2015). Clinical aspects of leprosy. *Clinics in Dermatology, 33*, 26–37.

Tatko-Hryniewicz, J. (1914). [illegible]

Tilley, L., & Cameron, T. (2014). Introducing the Index of Care: A web-based application supporting archaeological research into health-related care. *International Journal of Paleopathology, 6*, 5–9.

Tilley, L., & Oxenham, M. F. (2011). Survival against the odds: Modeling the social implications of care provision to seriously disabled individuals. *International Journal of Paleopathology, 1*, 35–42.

[illegible]

Chapter 8
A Post-mortem Evaluation of the Degree of Mobility in an Individual with Severe Kyphoscoliosis Using Direct Digital Radiography (DR) and Multi-Detector Computed Tomography (MDCT)

Gerald Conlogue, Mark Viner, Ronald Beckett, Jelena Bekvalac, Ramon Gonzalez, Melinda Sharkey, Kenneth Kramer, and Brenda Koverman

Introduction

Generally most anthropological imaging studies of skeletal and/or mummified remains have two primary objectives: to acquire optimal images and to reach a diagnosis. The first may be only limited to plane radiographs or endoscopic images. However, if the remains are in a stable condition and additional

G. Conlogue, M.H.S., R.T.(R.)(M.R.)(C.T.) (✉)
Diagnostic Imaging Program, Quinnipiac University, Hamden, CT, USA

Bioanthropology Research Institute, Quinnipiac University, Hamden, CT, USA
e-mail: Gerald.Conlogue@quinnipiac.edu

M. Viner, F.C.R., M.Sc., H.D.C.R., M.C.S.F.S., S.R.R.
Barts and London School of Medicine and Dentistry, Queen Mary University of London, London, UK

Cranfield University Forensic Institute, Swindon, UK

R. Beckett, Ph.D.
Bioanthropology Research Institute, Quinnipiac University, Hamden, CT, USA

J. Bekvalac, B.A. Hons., M.Sc., F.S.A.
Centre for Human Bioarchaeology, Museum of London, London, UK

R. Gonzalez, M.D.
Diagnostic Imaging Program, Quinnipiac University, Hamden, CT, USA

M. Sharkey, M.D.
Yale University School of Medicine, New Haven, CT, USA

K. Kramer, M.D.
Connecticut Orthopaedic Specialists, Hamden, CT, USA

B. Koverman, M.B.A., M.S., O.T.R/.L.
Rush University Medical Center, Chicago, IL, USA

© Springer International Publishing Switzerland 2017

L. Tilley, A.A. Schrenk (eds.), *New Developments in the Bioarchaeology of Care*, Bioarchaeology and Social Theory, DOI 10.1007/978-3-319-39901-0_8

information deemed necessary, multi-detector computed tomography (MDCT) may be included in the study. Once acceptable images have been acquired, the next step in the process is to arrive at a diagnosis by consensus. The pool of individuals reviewing the images would include not only radiologists and anthropologists, but also orthopaedists, pathologists and other medical specialists whose expertise can generate a more accurate diagnosis. Although there may sometimes be more than one possible conclusion, the approach is to arrive at a diagnosis that is generally agreed upon by consensus.

This is usually where the process stops and the team moves onto the next project. However, Tilley and Cameron (2014) have encouraged moving the process further in the case of individuals who demonstrate severe pathological conditions by endeavouring to determine the nature and extent of care that might have been required. Their web-based method permits a four-step analysis to assess all the factors that contribute to the status of the individual and the possible care required. Application of the bioarchaeology of care concept is thoroughly addressed in Chap. 2 of this volume.

In this case study, the Index of Care was applied to the skeletal remains of an adult male individual with severe kyphoscoliosis from the crypt at St Bride's Church, Fleet Street, London, England.

Materials and Methods

The Site and Its History

The male individual had been interred in a lead coffin in the crypts at St Bride's Church, Fleet Street, London, England, during the eighteenth century (Georgian period), and would have been a man of wealth. In association with the skeletal remains were remnants of what may have been parts of a supportive harness. The present church represents the eighth Christian place of worship on the site, which has been occupied since the Roman occupation of Londinium. The sixth church that stood on the site was one of many consumed by flames during The Great Fire of London in 1666. It was rebuilt by Sir Christopher Wren, beginning in 1672 and completed in 1703, with a distinctive *wedding cake* steeple and the inclusion of the crypt spaces that were subsequently used as places of interment for wealthier individuals.

Burials in the crypt stopped in 1854, following a cholera epidemic in London. A series of Acts of Parliament in the 1850s, intended to regulate burials, culminated in the 1852 Metropolitan Burial Act; this Act closed places of burial that were often in an appalling condition, and encouraged burials in cemeteries outside the City. On 29th December 1940, during WWII and the *Blitz* on London, an incendiary bomb hit the church and all but the steeple and outer wall were destroyed. In 1952, prior to reconstruction, a mandatory architectural survey, which included the excavation of the crypts and a medieval charnel house, was directed by Professor William

Francis Grimes, a noted medieval archaeologist. Grimes would later become the director of the Institute of Archaeology at the University of London and director of the Museum of London.

Although few details of the original excavation relating to the processes and recording of the coffins and remains have survived, Scheuer and Black (1995) collated a variety of sources of documentary information related to the remains found in the crypts. Nearly 300 wooden coffins, with middle lead shells and associated metallic coffin plates with inscribed biographical information, were recovered from the vault spaces in the crypt. Skeletal remains and associated coffin plates were removed from the coffins and placed into Army surplus metal munitions boxes. Unfortunately, insufficient boxes were available and, as noted by Scheuer and Black, in many instances more than one skeleton was placed in the same box. Individuals that were not skeletonized were reburied in an area just outside the church.

The munitions boxes were moved from the crypts and fortunately, due to *Section 25* of the *Burial Act of 1857*, records exist for the *Licenses for Removal of Human Remains* that document possession of the remains. On 30th April 1953, Dr. Keith Simpson and Professor Wood Jones of the Royal College of Surgeons, London, transported the remains to the Faculty of Anthropology at Cambridge. On 18th October 1956, Dr. I. Steel of the London Hospital transferred the skeletons from the Army surplus boxes into 'specially commissioned white plastic containers' (Scheuer & Black (MacLaughlin), 1995). It appears that if more than one skeleton was contained in the munitions box Dr. Steel attempted to separate each individual and associated coffin plate, and then place them into their own plastic container. Unfortunately, the plastic containers were not an ideal means for storing the skeletal remains, causing damage to the bones by creating a warm and damp environment that encouraged mold growth, as well as the oxidation of lead coffin plates.

In 1989, Scheuer and Black received a 3 year grant from the Leverhulme Trust to conduct an anthropological study of the 227 identified individuals, and Dr. J.E. Bowman participated as a research assistant. During this period, all of the skeletal remains were transferred from the plastic containers into the cardboard boxes in which they are presently stored, with separate boxes for the cranial and postcranial elements. Between 2008 and 2009 J Bekvalac, from the Centre for Human Bioarchaeology (CHB) at the Museum of London (MOL), conducted an osteological analysis of the same individuals and entered the data onto the Wellcome Osteological Research Database (WORD). All the data were recorded to standard osteological methods and are accessible through the CHB in Microsoft *Excel* format. Funding for the recording was provided by the CHB and the City of London Archaeological Trust (CoLAT).

The Radiographic Study

Between 2010 and 2013, on four occasions, a temporary radiographic facility was established in the crypt at the church using portable direct digital radiographic (DDRM) system (Conlogue et al., 2011). All X-ray exposures were taken with a Sedecal SP-HF 4.0 kW X-ray source set at 60 kV-peak (kVp), 3.2 mA-seconds (mAs) at 100 cm source-to-image receptor distance (SID), acquired with a Cannon Lanmix CXDI-50C imaging plate and processed with 'foot' algorithm to maximize bony detail. In all, the skeletal remains of 227 individuals were either partially or completely radiographed, and these radiographs are available for research on request.

One of the individuals, SB79-105, manifested a case of severe kyphoscoliosis. The associated coffin plate was badly corroded, making it difficult to read. The name that could be discerned was Samuel Lord, but the dates were not legible. In October 2013, the skeletal remains were transported to St. Bartholomew's Hospital (Barts) for a multi-detector computed tomography (MDCT) scan. All scans were accomplished with a Siemens Definition DS scanner acquired at 0.6 mm slice thickness, 64 slices per revolution, using 100 kV and 30 mA (mA).

Bioarchaeology of Care

Step 1A: Description of the Remains

The skeletal remains, recovered from a lead lined coffin in the crypt at St Bride's Church, Fleet Street, London, were of a completely skeletonized male, and assessed for sex estimation based upon the morphological features of the skull and pelvis, following Ferembach, Schwidetzky, and Stoukal (1980), Brothwell (1981), and Bass (1995). The associated coffin plate identified the individual as Samuel Lord; however, due to the extensive corrosion on the plate, no other information could be deciphered relating to the age at death or date of death. Accessing parish records for the church through the London Metropolitan Archive (LMA) there is a reference to a Samuel Lord, and using this information a time period date range for the individual was estimated between the 1790s and 1830s.

Attempts to estimate the age of the individual was markedly hindered by antemortem tooth loss and by pathological processes affecting the sternal rib ends and pelvis. Therefore the standard age estimate methods used in the WORD database, based on the indicators of tooth wear, following the criteria of Brothwell (1981), sternal rib ends, pubic symphysis and auricular surface following Iscan, Loth, and Wright (1984, 1985), Brooks and Suchey (1990) and Lovejoy, Meindl, Pryzbeck, and Mensforth (1985) were not possible to apply. However, an estimate of age for the individual was based upon the maturation of the bones, obliteration of the epiphyseal lines and fusion of the sternal end of the clavicle, and his age at the time of death was estimated to be between mid- to late 30s.

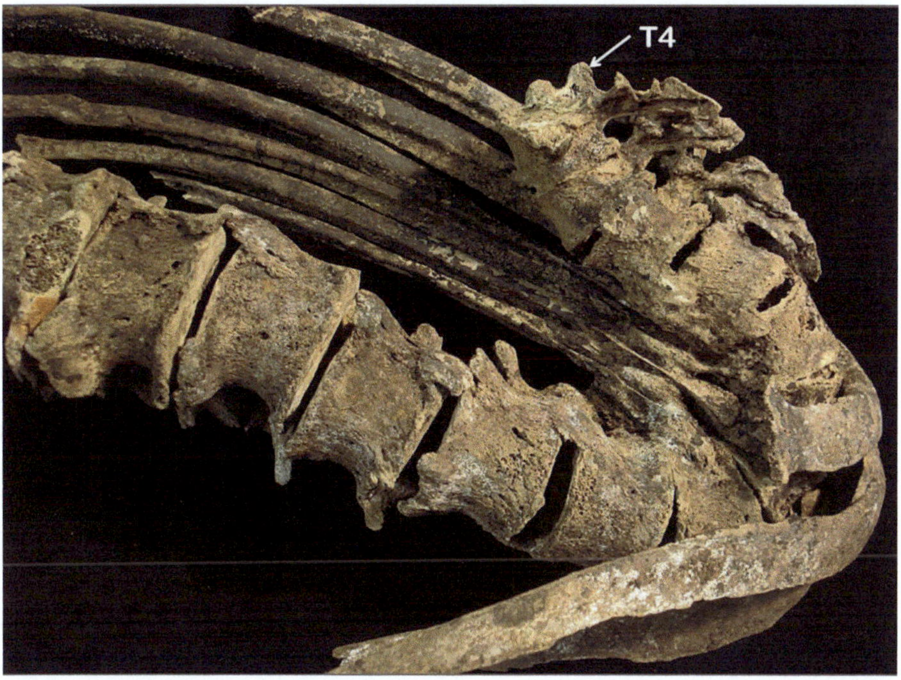

Fig. 8.1 A photograph of the section of fused section of spine. The fourth thoracic vertebrae (T4) is indicated for orientation

There was a suite of congenital and pathological processes observed in the macroscopic analysis of the individual. There was asymmetry of the skull seen in the facial bones and alteration in shape of the cranium, notably in the base, and variance in the mandible, with the left side longer than the right. This left side variation was observed in the cranial shape and with atresia of the left auditory meatus. The most visible and extreme skeletal alteration was the severe kyphoscoliosis of the spine with deformation of the associated ribs (Aufderheide & Rodríguez-Martín, 1998; Ortner, 2003).

The gross curvature affected the thoracic and lumbar vertebrae from Thoracic (T) 4 to lumbar (L) 1 (Fig. 8.1). The cervical (C) vertebrae were also affected and had hypoplastic defects of the spinous processes of C3–C6, with C3 and C4 having scooped features of the apex of the bifid spinous processes. The spinous processes of C5 and C6 had the most pronounced hypoplastic defects, with the processes being simply thin, tapered, bony projections. When the cervical vertebrae were articulated there was a slight anterior curvature going towards the left side. The most pronounced changes in the vertebrae were in the thoracic vertebrae; the first three thoracic vertebrae were not fused and were able to articulate normally, but were affected in their development, with mild unilateral multiple hemimetameres hypoplasia producing lateral wedging of the left side (Barnes, 1994). This alteration also produced changes in the facets on the left side. The inferior vertebral body of

T3 was wedged and had a deep concavity on the right side, with osteophytic lipping more pronounced on the left side of the centrum that was either fused (then broken post-mortem) or almost at the point of fusion at the time of death.

From thoracic T4 to L1 the vertebrae were grossly contorted in being twisted, curved and fused, with associated fusion and contortion of the ribs. When looking at the affected vertebrae as one solid formation, it was possible to see that T4 and T5 faced anteriorly in their normal anatomical position. The gross distortion began with the following thoracic vertebrae (T6–T9) gradually becoming more twisted and distorted towards the left aspect, until T10 was virtually at a posterior aspect in its rotation out of the normal alignment, the inner part of the curve at its severest point occurring at T9 and T10. T11–L1 vertebrae were twisted and turned at an almost 90° angle towards the right side.

The vertebrae all appeared to have developed individual centrums, and fusion occurred between the thoracic vertebrae and alternated between the sides of the affected centrum. The spinous processes were at points completely distorted in their form and fused, but there were apophyseal joint articulations. The lumbar vertebrae, of which there were six, with L6 being completely sacralized, were not fused to one another, but were affected developmentally with multiple unilateral hypoplasia of the hemimetameres of the left side producing lateral wedging. There was distortion to the articular facets to accommodate the severe curvature of the thoracic vertebrae, and also osteophytic lipping at the sides of the vertebral bodies, with syndesmophytes producing bony bridges on the right side and grosser lipping on the left aspect of L4–L5. Eburnation of the joint surface was observed in the inferior left facet of L5 and corresponding superior left facet of L6.

The ribs were affected by the gross curvature of the vertebrae, with fusion of some of the ribs in the mid-thoracic area, and there was marked alteration to the shape and formation of the ribs, with the right side having a very sharp angle to the heads and the left being broad and flattened. The mid-thoracic ribs were contorted with fusion and were compressed together, causing some to have a tapered appearance. The eighth right rib, close to the sternum, had a healed fracture with good remodelled callus formation.

There was bilateral ankylosis of the sacroiliac joints, and the sacrum was contorted towards the right side with a slight anterior protrusion to the juncture between L6 and S1. The acetabulae did not appear to have been adversely affected, with no gross indication of any hip dysplasia problems. The depth of the acetabulae appeared to be normal, as did the formation of the femoral heads and the articulation between the acetabulae and femora. The femora had pronounced medio-lateral flattening in the proximal 1/3, giving them the appearance of being bowed and curved. The tibiae had an 'S' shape curve midshaft causing bowing and pronounced concavity on the lateral aspect. The fibulae were correspondingly curved and flattened in a way that matched the concavity of the tibiae. The flattened fibulae shafts were expanded, producing a very sharp edge to the anterior margin, and were almost 'boomerang' in appearance. The changes observed in the leg bones represent changes most often attributable to the effects of residual rickets and vitamin D deficiency during youth, and in this case might also be related to, and/or exacerbated by, the biomechanical alteration resulting from the [mal]alignment of the spine. Interestingly, all of the long bones (upper and lower) were robust in appearance and did not give the indica-

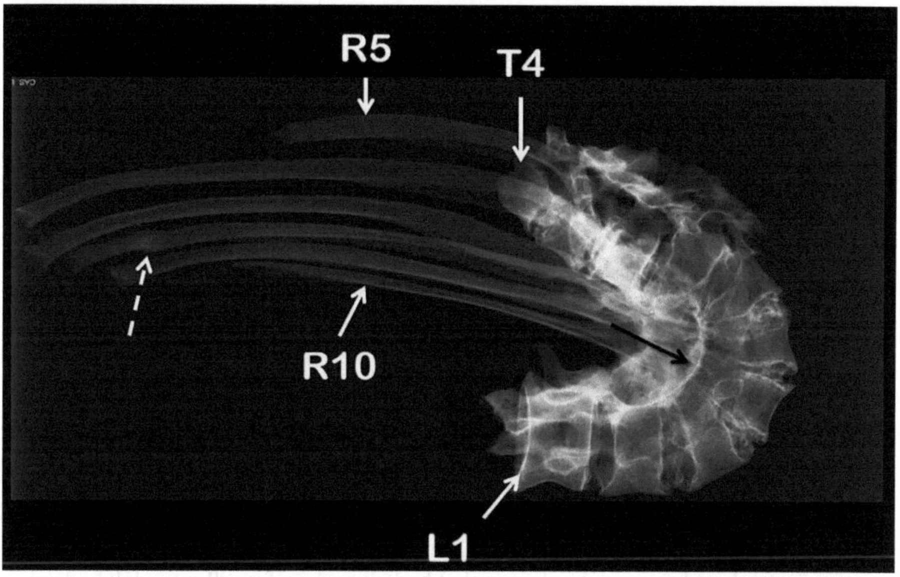

Fig. 8.2 A radiograph of the deformed region of the thoracic spine demonstrating a unilateral bar on the concavity (*black arrow*). The image also reveals the fused regions from the fourth thoracic (T4) to the first lumber (L1) vertebrae and the right fifth (R5) to the tenth (R10) ribs. Note the healing fracture on the distal eighth rib (*dashed arrow*)

tion of being atrophied from lack of use. Also interestingly, and perhaps surprisingly, there was no indication on the bones of lesions indicative of any infectious processes. This is particularly so in relation to the visceral surface of the ribs, where it would be considered more likely to see some inflammatory response because of the pulmonary restrictions typically associated with an increased vulnerability to respiratory infections. The distortion of the vertebrae and ribs would have caused an abnormal shape to the thoracic cavity and compromised the normal functioning of the lungs causing pulmonary restrictions and disorders.

Knüsel and Bowman (1996) examined the skeleton and reached a diagnosis of possible neurofibromatosis. Spinal deformity is one of the most common orthopaedic manifestations of the disease (Tsirikos, Saifuddin, & Noordeen, 2005).

Step 1B: Differential Diagnosis

Radiographs of the deformed region of the spine revealed a unilateral bar on the concavity (Fig. 8.2), differentiating the condition as congenital kyphoscoliosis and not the idiopathic form. Since the non-idiopathic type of spinal deformity is consistent with neurofibromatosis, the radiographs support the Knüsel and Bowman diagnosis. A more complete description of the radiographic findings is presented later in this chapter.

Step 1C: Document the Cultural, Social, Economic and Environmental Context

London is a place that is forever changing and the eighteenth and nineteenth century was a significant time of change. SB79-105 lived during the Georgian period (1714–1830), which '...was an extraordinary period in the city's history' shaped by four defining events: 'Restoration, Plague, Fire, Revolution' (Inglis, 2013, p. 1). This was the era of the Industrial Revolution, which saw transformations in London's physical and social appearance, as well as an increase in its population. People were leaving the land to work in the cities, and this saw a shift in population that had dramatic consequences for the general standard of living conditions. In eighteenth century England '... the striking characteristic of that society was the vast and profound influence exercised by its capital, the metropolis of London, a concentration of population which set against its hinterland had no parallel or precedent in European history' (Cunningham & French, 1990, p. 5). There was a building boom that increased the demand for tradesmen and merchants and saw the creation of a new London, and this period also saw the advent of new inventions and developments in mechanisation changing the nature of jobs. London was a landscape that had altered profoundly; '... [i]t had solidified first into brick and then to stucco, as the outlying marshes and green fields were slowly eaten up by speculative builders...', and by 1831 the population of the city was over 1.5 million (Inglis, 2013, p. 10) (Fig. 8.3).

As London expanded, connecting suburbs around the city created a diverse landscape with a mixed populace and individuals of differing social status (White, 2013). Pollution increased as a by-product of the processes of manufacturing, the growing populace created ever larger quantities of waste, and with an increase in the number of coal fires in homes, coal imports rose (Inglis, 2013). A study by Bernofsky (2010) investigated respiratory health in the past, looking at sinusitis and rib periostitis as potential indicators for poor air quality and respiratory disorders. It produced interesting results, ascertaining that there were patterns over time with a prevalence rate of 30.6 % for sinusitis and 29.7 % for rib periostitis in the Post Medieval individuals, but also indicating that the causes of respiratory disease were complex.

London was becoming an urban environment with new building developments and improved thoroughfares, but in many areas there were still large sections of old London with poor housing, filthy streets, unhygienic and unsanitary conditions in which the masses lived and worked, and areas in the vicinity of the church were no exception (White, 2013). Fleet Street was the main route connecting the City of London and the City of Westminster; the Fleet River, which ran close to the church, had once been crowded with river traffic but gradually became filled with rubbish from residents up stream and with foul waste from a number of trades, including those of the butchers. It was eventually covered over in 1736, having become '... a mere sluggish and plague breeding sewer' once more (Inglis, 2013, p. 29).

This combination produced unhealthy environmental conditions that were rife with a host of infectious diseases, and led the well-being of the majority of the population to be negatively impacted over time. The Bills of Mortality recorded

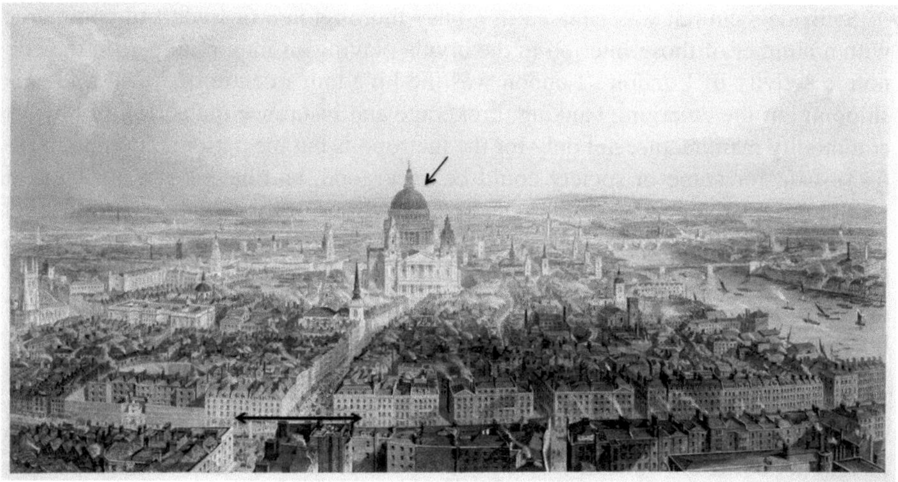

Fig. 8.3 Panorama view of the City of London, circa 1832–1846 showing St Paul's (*single headed arrow*) in the background and Farringdon Road (*double headed arrow*, foreground), the main road cutting across the bottom, where the Lower Churchyard of St Bride's was located. ©Museum of London

deaths for the parishes, and are an interesting source of information for gaining a sense of the types of diseases affecting the population and of the numbers that succumbed to these. Although not necessarily an exact and absolute record of the numbers, they provide an indication of the diseases present and an insight into their prevalence. Accessing the parish records for St Bride's it was apparent that diseases such as consumption and phthisis (tuberculosis) were common during this time period and often the most frequent cause of death. Analysis of skeletal remains from a number of post medieval collections (Brickley & Miles, 1999; Henderson, Miles, Walker, & with Brian Connell & Robin Wroe-Brown, 2013; Miles, Powers, Wroe-Brown, & with Don Walker, 2008; Molleson, Cox, M. with Waldron H. A, & Whittaker, 1993) has also shown that the rate of specific infections such as tuberculosis and syphilis increased, as did the metabolic disorders rickets and scurvy, particularly exacerbated for the poorer members of society. These lower status individuals would have experienced close quarter living, poor nutrition and general living conditions that deprived them of access to the necessities for a life of economic and social quality. Those of higher status, however, were not exempt from such diseases, although their social status provided advantageous living conditions. Individuals interred in the crypts at St Bride's, although of a better social status, were still exposed and susceptible to disease, but their superior living conditions, including fewer occupants in a household and access to good food stuffs, were a buffer against the threats posed by the city environment. Despite this, many of these individuals, predominantly males, would have worked in the city and would have encountered its health hazards in the process.

St Bride's church was situated in a busy thoroughfare of trade and commerce, with a number of those interred in the crypts playing an important part in the economic activity of London. 'London was the kingdom's centre of world trade and shipping, of the emerging banking, brokerage and insurance industries, of finished commodity manufacture not only for the metropolis but the nation…'(White, 2013, p. 3). Life for some in society could be very good, and having the attributes of wealth provided a good quality home in the environs of the city or on its outskirts, with more open spaces and cleaner air. On a number of occasions the church burial records for those interred in the crypt provides address details, with some individuals recorded as living not far from the church, in the heart of the cosmopolitan morass of London, and others living on the outskirts in greener areas such as Peckham and Parsons Green, which although today are part of the ever sprawling London were not in the eighteenth century. Unfortunately, with the limited information relating to Samuel Lord, it was not possible to ascertain his address and gain insight about the environs of where he lived in London. In view of his burial location it can be presumed that his living conditions were of a better standard than those of the poorer workforce members, who would have been confined to multiple-occupancy rooms in crowded households.

The demographic profile of those interred in the crypt, taking in to account the inherent bias of the sample, was an 'older age at death' profile similar to that of Christ Church Spitalfields (Molleson et al., 1993), a contemporary burial population. In comparison, individuals analysed from burials of a similar period, but from lower status backgrounds, have a different demographic profile (Brickley & Miles, 1999; Henderson et al., 2013; Miles & Conheeney, 1990). The diseases observed in the crypt individuals were primarily those associated with age and with a lifestyle providing the means for access to medical and dental care.

Step 1D: Mortuary Practices

The poorer parishioners were buried in the Lower Churchyard on Farringdon Street, where excavations in an area of the cemetery carried out in 1990 found that the coffins were stacked to accommodate more burials, and that these coffins, based on the traces of wood found, were of the cheaper sort (Miles & Conheeney, 1990). In contrast, the crypt burials were reserved for persons of means who could afford the higher cost of interment within the church, and these individuals were interred in triple shell coffins, with a lead inner coffin, associated funereal ornamentation, and inner and outer coffin plates.

Unfortunately, the records for excavations undertaken in the 1950s (when the coffins were first discovered in the crypts) are not all present and did not always record the type of information that would be pertinent and beneficial to fully appreciating the mortuary practices in the crypt spaces at St Bride's. As such, the mortuary practices for the individuals buried at St Bride's can only be inferred in a general way, based upon data from contemporary crypt burials, such as those at Christ

Church Spitalfields, which have been excavated more recently (Reeve & Adams, 1993). From the information available it appears there were a series of differently named vaults in the crypt spaces that may have had differing costs associated with them. The coffins were placed in the vaults, possibly stacked and, based on biographical information and parish data, families were interred together. Accounts from the 1950s excavation indicate that the preservation of the remains varied, with some individuals still quite well preserved (with remaining soft tissue) and who were subsequently reburied in an area just outside the church; the accounts note in relation to some individuals that they were clothed. None of the funereal ornamentation was retained, other than the coffin plates, and so it is not possible to compare funereal furnishings to get an idea of individual variety in selection. Such information can be found by reference to undertaker trade books, and it can be an aid in considering the social wealth and standing of the individuals.

It was interesting to observe that craniotomies had been performed on a small number of the individuals who dated to before the Anatomy Act 1832. This Act was passed by parliament in the United Kingdom in response to the illegal trade in corpses that had provided bodies for dissection and the teaching of anatomy. The context and integrity of the skeletal remains of the individuals with craniotomies from St Bride's are indicative of post-mortem investigation, carried out to better understand and ascertain the causes of death. These medical explorations occurred at a time of a burgeoning interest in science and a period of Enlightenment or Age of Reason that had a radical impact on thinking and social outlook. The Age of Enlightenment was the major philosophical movement of seventeenth and eighteenth century Western Europe, which sought to bring about a reformation of society through establishing the primacy of science, reason and the role of the individual. Many of the individuals buried at St Bride's would have lived during the period of the Enlightenment and were potentially influenced by it, and this may explain decisions to allow the post-mortem examination of deceased family members to verify cause of death. This was by no means a normal mortuary practice of the time as religious mores dictated that the integrity of the body was paramount, and this scientific medical intervention would have been deemed repugnant by the majority of the populace.

The next stage of this bioarchaeology of care analysis assesses whether SB79-105 experienced disability likely to have required care. It does this in two steps, first reviewing the clinical characteristics of the pathology identified in this individual's remains, and then considering the range of possible consequences of these for his ability to function successfully within the society of the day.

Step 2A: Clinical Characteristics

Plane radiographs and MDCT scans were used to document the pathologic conditions of the skeleton. An agenesis of the left external auditory canal was noted, however, both semicircular canals were present. The spine exhibited a severe kyphosis, with fused and rotated vertebral bodies T4-L1. In addition, right ribs 5–10

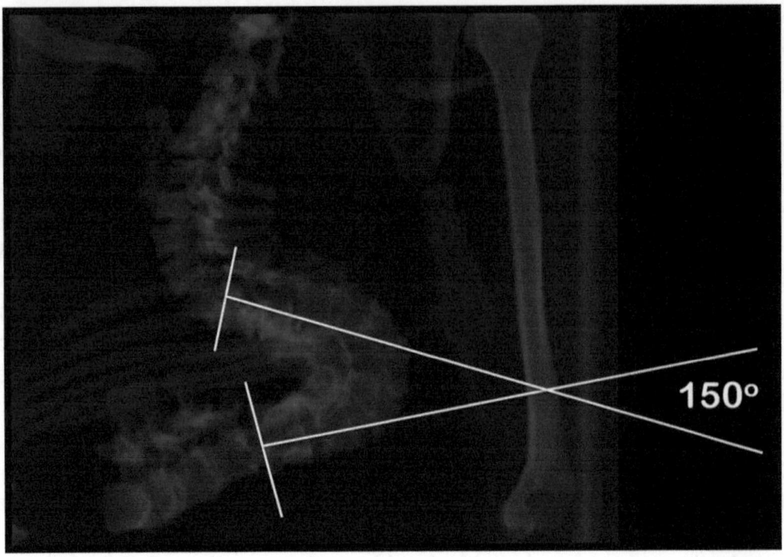

Fig. 8.4 The radiograph of the spine, employing the Cobb Method to measure the curvature of the spine

were fused at the vertebral articulations (Fig. 8.2). Using the Cobb Method (1948), the curvature of the spine measured 150° (Fig. 8.4) and, with the associated fusion of the ribs, would have resulted in impaired thoracic development leading to pulmonary hypoplasia.

The appendicular skeleton, although abnormalities were noted, was generally robust. The humeri were both well mineralized, with normal cortical thickness. Slight bowing was noted on the left humerus. Asymmetry was seen in the forearms, with the right radius and ulna appearing more robust. However, on the anterior-posterior (AP) projection, 15° anteromedial bowing of the proximal third of both ulnae was seen (Fig. 8.5).

Other than bilateral ankylosis of the sacroiliac joints, the pelvis appeared normal. Although the femora were both well mineralized with normal cortices, the trabeculae within each femoral neck were unorganized, suggesting a lack of the normal biomechanical forces. The decreased angulation of the femoral necks also implied a rachitic appearance. Using the Keats Method (1966), the angle of the right femoral neck measured 110° and the left 112°, while the normal male femoral neck angle should be 128° (Fig. 8.6). On the lateral projection of the femora a posterior angulation was noted bilaterally, with the right femur angled approximately 20° and the left 10° (Fig. 8.7). The AP projection of the lower legs demonstrated bilateral severe diaphyseal lateral bowing of the tibiae (Fig. 8.8a) with transverse linear radiopacities suggestive of Harris' arrest line on the distal metaphyses (Fig. 8.8b). Lateral projections of the tibiae revealed posterior angulation measuring 13° on the right and 16° on the left (Fig. 8.9). The fibulae, on the AP projection, were not as bowed, but appeared to be thinner than normal. However, the distal two-thirds appeared flattened on the lateral projection (Fig. 8.10).

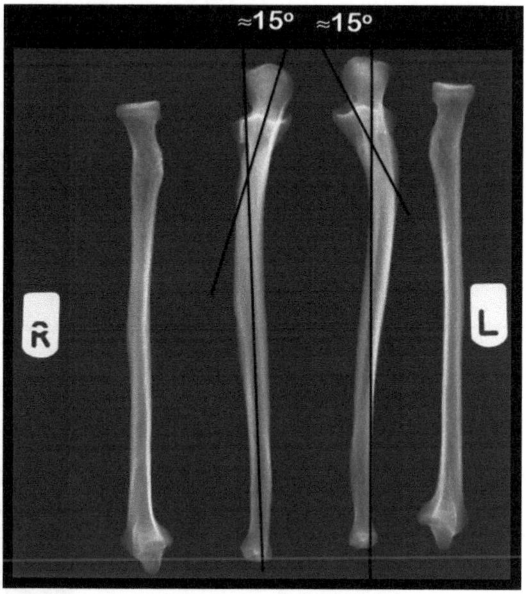

Fig. 8.5 AP projection of the bones of the forearm revealing an approximate 15° anteromedial bowing bilaterally of the proximal third of both ulnae

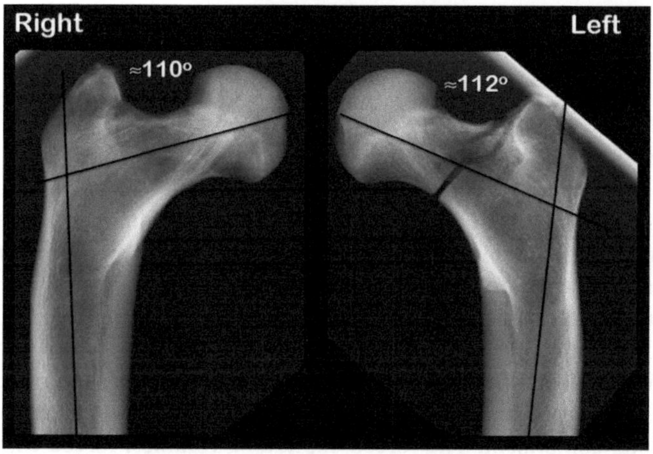

Fig. 8.6 AP radiograph of the right and left femoral heads indicated the calculated angles of the femoral necks. Noted the post-mortem intertrochanteric fracture of the left femoral neck

In addition to orthopaedic impairments, severe scoliosis, as represented in this case, would have presented clinically as a severe restrictive pulmonary process. Restrictive lung diseases are classified as disorders that decrease all lung capacities, including the total lung capacity (TLC) and the vital capacity (VC). Reductions in lung capacities reduce pulmonary reserves, leading to an inability to increase ventilation when the individual is challenged with an increased metabolic demand (McCance, Huether, Brashers, & Rote, 2010). When the metabolic demand increases

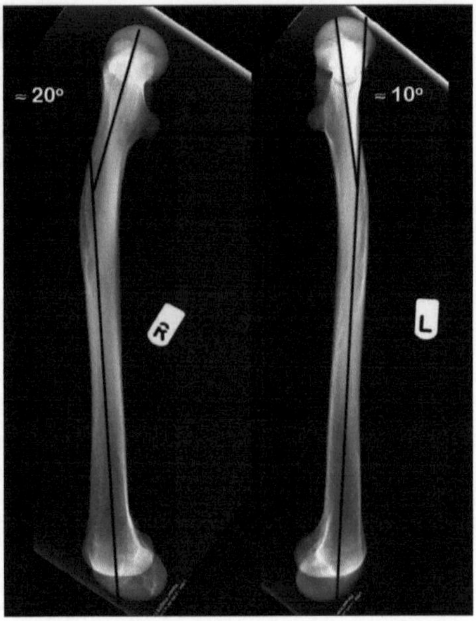

Fig. 8.7 Lateral radiographs of both femora demonstrating the posterior angulation

from increased workload, the pulmonary system increases the depth and rate of ventilation in an attempt to attain more oxygen (O_2) and to eliminate excess carbon dioxide (CO_2). However, in individuals with restrictive pulmonary disease attempts at increasing ventilation exacerbate the poor oxygenation status, and impose physiologic stress on the cardiovascular and other body systems.

Another clinical characteristic associated with severe restrictive lung disease is a marked reduction in normal pulmonary defense mechanisms. The sub-normal TLC and VC would reduce the individual's ability to move air in and out of the lungs efficiently, due to mechanical inability of the pulmonary musculature and limitation of the skeletal component. The forced expiratory volumes, forced expiratory flow rates and Peak Flow rates would all be reduced (DiBari et al., 2004). The inability to take a deep breath, coupled with the inability to move air through the conducting airways effectively, would have compromised this individual's pulmonary defenses and his ability to produce an effective cough. Mucociliary clearance would have been markedly impaired. Considering the air pollution as described earlier in this paper, this reduction in pulmonary defenses would result in a high susceptibility to frequent and recurrent pulmonary infections.

Finally, there is the potential for the development of Cor Pulmonale (right sided-heart enlargement) resulting from increased pulmonary vascular resistance on the affected side. It is very likely that a shift in the mediastinal contents (including the heart) would have placed an increased workload on the heart.

a

b

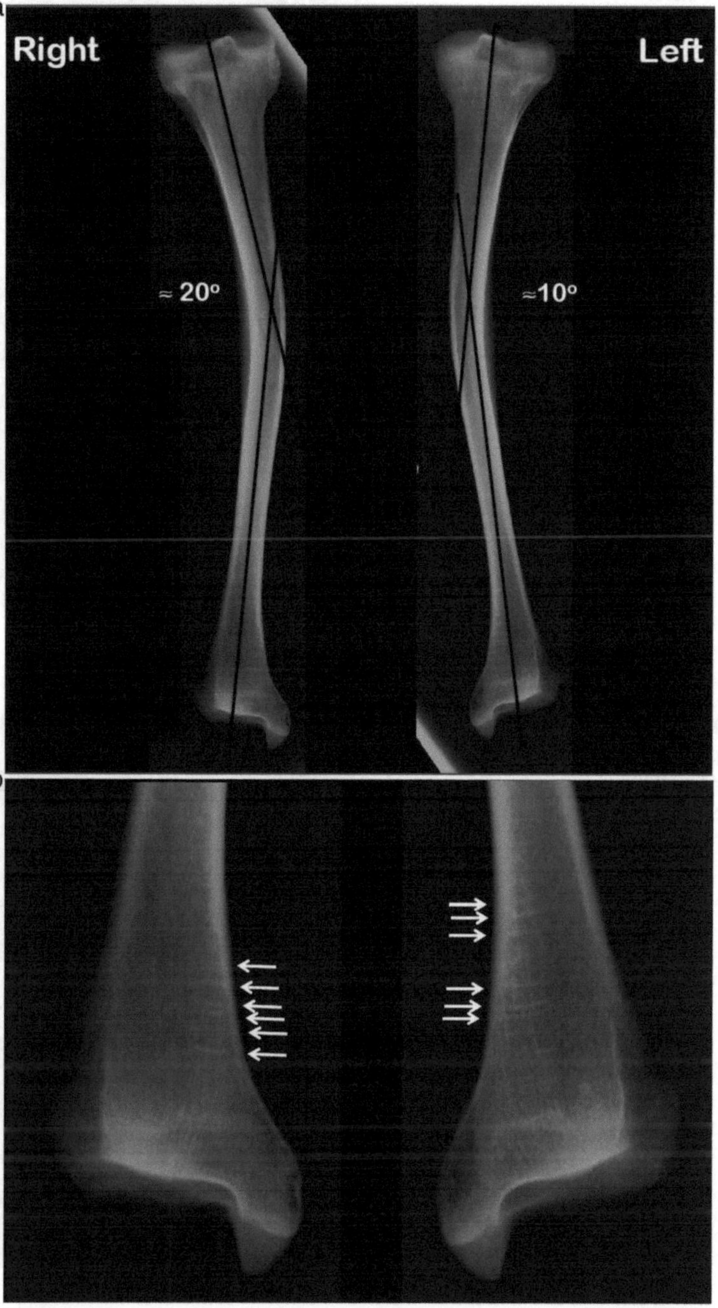

Fig. 8.8 (**a**) AP radiographs of the tibiae revealing lateral angulation of approximately 20° on the right and 10° on the left. (**b**). AP radiograph of both tibiae displaying multiple transverse linear radiopacities suggestive of Harris' *arrest lines*, several indicated by *arrows*, on the medial aspect bilaterally

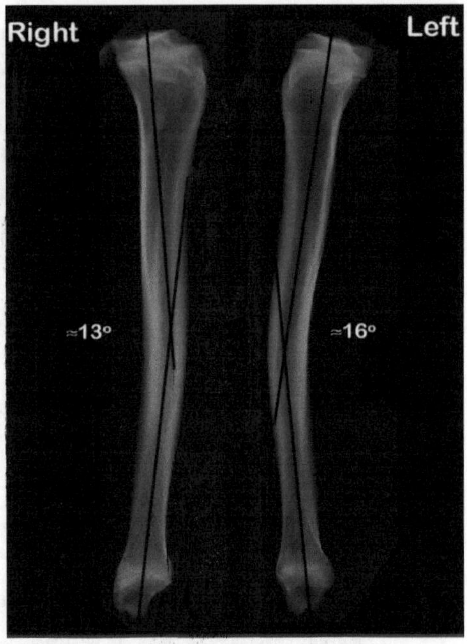

Fig. 8.9 Lateral radiographs of both tibiae indicating posterior angulation of approximately 16° on the left side and 13° on the right

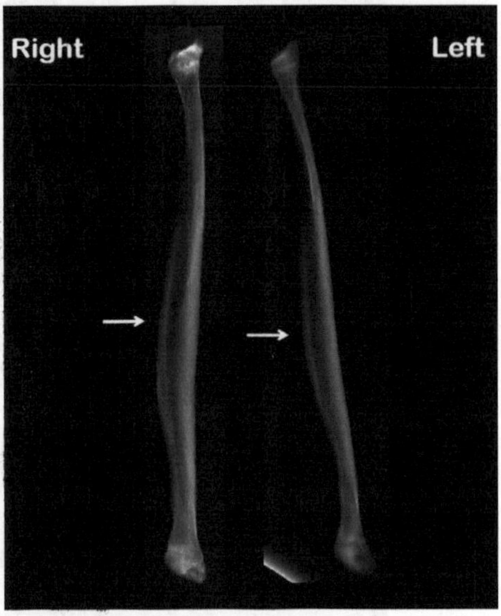

Fig. 8.10 Lateral radiographs of both fibulae revealing flattening of the distal two-thirds

Step 2B: Functional Consequences

It is difficult to make an objective analysis of this individual's functional abilities or the value he placed on self-reliance, however, it is possible to consider certain requirements identified as basic activities of daily living (BADL), which include the need to dress, bathe, obtain and prepare food, etc. It would appear that the BADLs involving lower body functions, for example, getting shoes on and off, washing feet and lower legs, and possibly toileting, would have been the most difficult activities for this individual. However, it may have been possible for this individual to perform BADLs in a seated or supine position, taking breaks to compensate for the impact of the cardiac and pulmonary limitations described. The left lateral curvature would result in the individual having some difficulty in reaching his right foot. Arm length would also be a factor in toileting, affecting his ability to reach all areas for hygiene purposes. However, grooming and eating would not appear to have been a problem.

The mechanical ability to carry loads, lift objects or manoeuvre around challenging environments would be markedly reduced, due to an unstable centre of gravity associated with the physical presentation in this case. Further, a lack of balance would predispose this individual to falls and potential associated injuries.

Pulmonary and Cardiac Functional Impairment

Based on primarily his pulmonary impairment, it is concluded that this individual would certainly have had poor pulmonary reserves in terms of increasing ventilation and altering oxygenation status when challenged with an increased workload. Given the degree of scoliosis and the resultant restrictive pulmonary disease, this individual would have been unable to respond to even a marginal increase in workload, making him symptomatically short of breath, expressed as an impaired exercise capacity (EC). Performance of instrumental activities of daily living (IADLs) such as walking up an incline or up a street, walking up stairs, or lifting/carrying would have presented marked challenges because of limited lung capacity. Indeed, this individual would have encountered difficulties in undertaking any activity that required more than minimal physical strength or effort, given the restrictions to physiological work imposed by severe limitations to cardiac and pulmonary function. The reduced pulmonary defenses would have increased his susceptibility to pulmonary infections. The restriction of pulmonary blood flow may have created and increased pulmonary vascular resistance, followed by the development of Cor Pulmonale, although this is speculative. And it is certain that, with advancing age, he would likely have required increasing assistance with some or all of his ADLs.

While we cannot, in good conscience, identify those specific ADLs that he was able to conduct nor those that he needed assistance with, we can be confident that he faced impediments to lifting and carrying loads, and perhaps to climbing stairs, associated with the physiologic limitations imposed by his restrictive pulmonary disease. What is less sure is his need for assistance in other activities. The human characteristics of motivation and determination are highly variable and, sadly, not recorded in bones or tissues that remain for us to examine. Considering the functional consequences imposed on this individual, he may have been highly functional or not. This uncertainty is based on his mechanical challenges, his pulmonary (and cardiac) limitations, his determination/motivation, his available support system, the nature of those support systems (enabling or encouraging) and the physical environment in which he was challenged to interact.

In sum, as we examine the available information, it is clear that on the balance of probability this individual required and received both direct care and accommodations. As we consider a 'model of care', and given the physical and physiological constraints imposed upon this individual, it is clear that this individual required direct support to varying degrees throughout his life, although we cannot establish the precise extent of support needed at any given time. Considering the associated cold, damp and poor air quality conditions, the individual would have certainly suffered from repeated bouts of condition-related pulmonary infections requiring direct support in relation to BADLs, including feeding, water, bedding and hygiene, as well as receiving any available interventions such as manipulation, positioning, nursing or therapeutic methods. When free of active infectious processes, this individual would have needed assistance with many IADLs, while his BADLs may have been supported through various accommodations. The individual may not have required many dedicated caregivers, other than when afflicted with an active disease process. Likely one or two individuals looked after this subject throughout his life, with other professionals of the times intervening as the need arose.

Discussion

This man is a most interesting individual, and one who faced great challenges to survive with such a severe deformity into adulthood. With the severity of his kyphoscoliosis and associated impairments, it can be conjectured that he must have had to overcome a variety of problems in dealing with everyday tasks of life that those of us not similarly affected take for granted. It is also important to factor in the period in which he lived and how he would have been perceived by society. Having a disability at this time was seen to affect your role as a citizen and compromised the ability to participate in the labour market (Borsay, 2004), although if this individual belonged to a higher social class his social status could potentially have mitigated some of the problems typically encountered. His interment in the crypt at St Bride's provides an indication of his social status, as to afford to be buried in such a place suggests that he was a man of means. It is not possible for us to fully know how active he was within his social group, but his ability to interact and play an active role would no doubt have relied upon the care and support of those around him.

Georgian London was a time when there was 'a great emphasis placed on the body's appearance and the aesthetic concept, instead of bodily function…with the pursuit of ideal beauty' (Turner, 2012). The perception of those with disabilities was inherently gendered and associated with the poor, with 'cripples' and 'the lame' a common sight in large cities such as London (Turner, 2012). In society at that time being a male would have been advantageous; disabled men were more visible in the eighteenth and nineteenth century than females (Turner, 2012), not surprisingly, when one considers the place of women in a male dominated society. People with disabilities were vulnerable and at an increased risk of poverty (Borsay, 2004), so again, SB79-105's interment in the St Bride's crypt is confirmation that he was not a poor man. It may well have been that he was seen as a cripple by others, but while being disabled, and having to deal with all this entailed in terms of performing activities in daily life, his social standing would have been a buffer against hardship. There would have been no need for him to use his disability or deformity as a means of 'display' to scrape a living to survive.

His social status would also have had a part to play in the type and degree of access to care that he had in life. The presence of the remains of what look like leather and hessian straps may well indicate that he had some sort of corrective and support brace as an aid to support his upper body. If they are the remnants of such a device, it provides an indication that he had access to medical care and an apparatus not available to those of a poorer status. In the time period in which we believe he lived, such a support brace would have been made as a bespoke item for him. The braces of the eighteenth and nineteenth century would in their function and construction have resembled those of later dates, with the exception of the materials used (Bick, 1948). A number of surgeons before and during the eighteenth century investigated the treatment of spinal deformities, and produced a variety of apparatuses and methods for attempting to prevent and cure these (Bick, 1948). In 1885, E. Fischer produced a monograph on the treatment of scoliosis over a 400 year period, with detailed descriptions and illustrations (Bick, 1948). With what is remaining of the possible straps it is not possible to ascertain precisely what the support brace may have looked like, but from examples of such devices (Bick, 1948) the construction would have involved provision of a supportive frame for back and front (possibly with a collar for neck support) that would be strapped to the upper body.

It would, of course, have been an advantage to have known with confidence the name of SB79-105 and the exact dates of his birth and death, as this information would have provided greater certainty for accessing documentary sources for research. Unfortunately, the corroded condition of the coffin plate did not enable this, but these problems aside, it is still possible to use the Index of Care to analyse this man's experience. For the essence of what we hoped to achieve was not solely focused on his 'formal' biography, but was an attempt to understand him in a more holistic manner in relation to his impairments and care requirements. It is difficult for us today to fully appreciate the perceptions of disability in the past and the experiences of those with disabilities (Turner, 2012). It is impossible for us to know every detail of how this man adapted to his situation, coped with the inevitable obstacles he encountered, and generally made his way through society. However, the Index assisted us in carrying out a systematic appraisal of this man's experience of health and disease, his social and economic environment, as well as the clinical characteristics and the functional impacts of his impairment. It provided a framework to consider what all these factors suggest about the care he may have needed and a basis for thinking about the nature of the medical (and social) assistance that may have been at his disposal. We stopped our analysis at this point, but given that he survived into his mid- to late 30s, in a future study it would be interesting to reflect upon the trajectory of his care in his transition from childhood to adulthood. In addition, the needs associated with this man's condition and his care would have had a continuing effect upon the daily lives of those around him – and possibly a future study might also include consideration of his family and friends, who would have taken on different roles in his care and in their social interactions with him, as part of the greater story.

It is a privilege to have had the opportunity to learn from this individual. We have attempted to understand – and appreciate – the life this man faced with severe disability within the constructs of the social era in which he lived. Ultimately, we were able to consider how he lived with the severe impairments that would have profoundly challenged his physical health and had a major impact on his functional abilities, causing detriment to his general well-being and generating the need for care.

References

Aufderheide, A. C., & Rodríguez-Martín, C. (1998). *The Cambridge encyclopedia of human paleopathology*. Cambridge: Cambridge University Press.

Barnes, E. (1994). *Developmental defects of the axial skeleton in paleopathology*. Boulder, CO: University Press of Colorado.

Bass, W.M. (1987). *Human osteology. A laboratory and field manual*, 3rd edition. USA: Missouri Archaeological Society, Inc.

Bernofsky, K. S. (2010). *Respiratory health in the past: A bioarchaeological study of chronic maxillary sinusitis and rib periostitis from the Iron Age to the Post Medieval Period in Southern England*. Doctoral thesis, Durham University.

Bick, E. M. (1948). *Source book of orthopaedics* (2nd ed.). Baltimore: The Williams and Wilkins Company.

Borsay, A. (2004). *Disability and social policy in Britain since 1750. A history of exclusion*. Basingstoke: Palgrave Macmillan.

Brickley, M., & Miles, A. (1999). *The cross bones burial ground, Redcross Way Southwark London*. Archaeological Excavations (1991–1998) for the London Underground Limited Jubilee Line Extension Project. Museum of London Archaeology Service, Monograph 3

Brooks, S. T., & Suchey, J. M. (1990). Skeletal age determination based on the os pubis: A comparison of the Ascadi-Nemeskeri and Suchey-Brooks methods. *Human Evolution, 5*, 227–238.

Brothwell, D. R. (1981). *Digging up bones* (3rd ed.). London: BM (NH) and OUP.

Cobb, J. R. (1948). *American Academy of Orthopaedic Surgery, 5*, 261–275.

Conlogue, G., Viner, M., Farmer, M., Gulliver, D., Bekvalac, J., & Eggleton, K. (2011). *Tales from the Crypt: Preliminary findings of a Digital Radiographic Study of Skeletal Remains Under St*

Bride's Church in London, England. 38th Annual North American Paleopathology Association Meeting. Minneapolis, Minnesota.

Cunningham, A., & French, R. (1990). *The medical enlightenment of the 18th century*. Cambridge: Cambridge Press.

DiBari, M., Melisenda, C., Matteuzzi, D., Zacchei, S., Pozzi, C., Bellia, V., et al. (2004). Thoracic kyphosis and ventilatory dysfunction in unselected older persons: An epidemiological study in Dicomano, Italy. *Journal of the American Geriatrics Society, 52*(6), 909–915.

Ferembach, D., Schwidetzky, I., & Stoukal, M. (1980). Recommendations for age and sex diagnoses of skeletons. *Journal of Human Evolution, 9*, 517–549.

Fischer, F. E. (1885). *Geschite und Behandling der seitlichen Rukratsverkrummung (skoliose)*. Strassburg.

Henderson, M., Miles, A., & Walker, D., with Brian Connell and Robin Wroe-Brown. (2013). *'He being dead yet speaketh' Excavations at three post-medieval burial grounds in Tower Hamlets, east London, 2004–2010*. Museum of London Archaeology, Monograph 64.

Inglis, L. (2013). *Georgian London into the streets*. Penguin Books.

Iscan, M. Y., Loth, S. R., & Wright, R. K. (1984). Age estimation from the rib by phase analysis: White males. *Journal of Forensic Sciences, 29*, 1094–1104.

Iscan, M. Y., Loth, S. R., & Wright, R. K. (1985). Age estimation from the rib by phase analysis: White females. *Journal of Forensic Sciences, 30*, 853–863.

Keats, T. E., et al. (1966). *Radiology, 87*, 904.

Knüsel, C. J., & Bowman, J. E. (1996). A possible case of neurofibromatosis in an archaeological skeleton. *International Journal of Osteoarchaeology, 6*, 202–210.

Lovejoy, C. O., Meindl, R. S., Pryzbeck, T. R., & Mensforth, R. P. (1985). Chronological metamorphosis of the auricular surface of the ilium: A new method for the determination of adult skeletal age at death. *American Journal of Physical Anthropology, 68*, 15–28.

McCance, K. L., Huether, S. E., Brashers, V. L., & Rote, N. S. (2010). *Pathophysiology, the biologic basis for disease in adults and humans* (6th ed., pp. 310–311). Mosby/Elsevier. ISBN: 978-0-323-06584-9.

Miles, A., & Conheeney, J. (1990). *A Post-medieval population from London: Excavations in the St Bride's Lower Churchyard* (pp. 75–82). MoLAS Studies Series. Farringdon Street City of London, EC4.

Miles, A., Powers, N., Wroe-Brown, R., with Don Walker. (2008). *St Marylebone church and burial ground in the 18th to 19th centuries: Excavations at St Marylebone school, 1992 and 2004–2006*. Museum of London Archaeology Service, Monograph 46.

Molleson, T., & Cox, M. with Waldron H. A., and Whittaker, D. K. (1993). *The Spitalfields Project*. The anthropology: The Middling Sort (vol. 2). CBA Research Report 86, Council for British Archaeology.

Ortner, D. J. (2003). *Identification of pathological conditions in human skeletal remains* (2nd ed.). London: Academic.

Reeve, J., & Adams, M. (1993). *The Spitalfields Project*. The archaeology: Across the Styx (vol. 1). CBA Research Report 85, Council for British Archaeology.

Scheuer, J. L., & Bowman, J. E. (1995). Correlation of documentary and skeletal evidence in the St. Bride's crypt population. In S. R. Saunders & A. Herring (Eds.), *Grave reflections: Portraying the past through cemetery studies* (pp. 49–70). Toronto: Canadian Scholar's Press.

Tilley, L., & Cameron, T. (2014). Introducing the Index of Care: A web-based application supporting archaeological research into health-related care. *International Journal of Paleopathology, 6*, 5–9.

Tsirikos, A., Saifuddin, A., & Noordeen, M. H. (2005). Spinal deformity in neurofibromatosis type-1: Diagnosis and treatment. *European Spine Journal, 14*(5), 427–439.

Turner, D. M. (2012). *Disability in eighteenth-century England: Imaging physical impairment*. Routledge studies in modern British history; 8.

White, J. (2013). *London in the 18th century a great and monstrous thing*. Vintage Books.

Chapter 9
Surviving Trepanation: Approaching the Relationship of Violence and the Care of "War Wounds" Through a Case Study from Prehistoric Peru

Sarah Jolly and Danielle Kurin

Introduction: Trepanation as Care

Trepanation, or the surgical removal of part of the cranium, has long fascinated scholars, collectors, medical practitioners, and the interested public alike, as a surprisingly universal form of prehistoric surgery, one that existed in the premodern medical world without modern forms of anesthesia, antibiotics, or painkillers. While ethnopharmacology has identified indigenous forms of perioperative treatments, present-day observers of trepanned skulls may still cringe at the thought of undergoing surgery without a modern medical infrastructure, although people often survived prehistoric trepanations, as evidenced by skeletal healing (Weber & Czarnetzki, 2001; Andrushko & Verano, 2008; Erdal & Erdal, 2011). These low mortality rates speak to a complex system of care and medical knowledge attained by prehistoric practitioners. Yet scholars are still trying to understand how and why this skillset was achieved. Bioarchaeological analyses, in particular, can help to comprehensively reconstruct the experience of trepanation to better understand the development of these prehistoric "operating rooms."

Worldwide, trepanation is generally performed using one of four techniques: (1) scraping, or the repeated abrasion of the ectocranial surface; (2) circular grooving, or the creation of a circular furrow and bone plug; (3) boring and drilling, or the

S. Jolly, M.A. (✉)
Department of Anthropology, University of Pittsburgh, Pittsburgh, PA, USA
e-mail: sarahannejolly@gmail.com

D. Kurin, Ph.D.
Department of Anthropology, University of California, Santa Barbara, Santa Barbara, CA, USA

© Springer International Publishing Switzerland 2017

L. Tilley, A.A. Schrenk (eds.), *New Developments in the Bioarchaeology of Care*, Bioarchaeology and Social Theory, DOI 10.1007/978-3-319-39901-0_9

abrasion of the bone in consistent, small drill holes; and (4) linear cutting, or the removal of bone in a sawing motion. Technique preference varies by era, regions, and even community. Trepanation is most commonly described as a medical response to cranial trauma, as cranial fractures associated with surgical apertures provide a bioarchaeologically observable motive for surgery. Some trepanations are thought to be in response to infections, neurological disorders like epilepsy, and post-traumatic seizures, although these tend to be less visible in the skeletal record (Verano, 2003; Kurin, 2013; Burneo, 2003; Clower & Finger, 2001). Other authors have considered religio-magical roles of trepanation, such as for the acquisition of amulets (Erdal & Erdal, 2011).

By explicitly defining trepanation as a form of care, its analysis using the bioarchaeology of care interpretive framework (Tilley, Chap. 2 this volume) nuances our understanding of how and why these techniques developed. It also allows us to illuminate the physical effects of trepanation on individuals, the impacts on the community that supports them, and the prehistoric logic of healing. Furthermore, by using trepanation as direct evidence of care for trauma, we can test this framework's suitability for theorizing care for traumatic injuries by considering the possibility of care and accommodation for non-life-threatening injuries in the past.

Case Study: The Chanka of Andahuaylas Peru

The first skeletal evidence of trepanation in the Andes appears around 400 BC (Verano, 2003). In other areas, such as the Andahuaylas region of south-central Peru – the focus of this study – the first known trepanation appears relatively late, during the Late Intermediate Period [LIP], dating to AD 1000–1400 (Fig. 9.1). The LIP was a period of social balkanization and the highest levels of conflict in the prehistoric Andes. This instability is thought to be a consequence of the concurrent collapses of the Wari and Tiwanaku empires circa AD 1000, compounded by an intensifying drought (Arkush & Tung, 2013; Bauer, Kellett, & Silva, 2010). One of the most infamous societies to emerge during this era was the Chanka, a formidable and bellicose polity which was ultimately vanquished by the emergent Inca Empire (Bauer et al., 2010). Like other contemporaneous groups, the Chanka organized themselves into *ayllus*, which are ranked, nested social units founded on real and/or imagined kinship, whose members trace descent from a common ancestor and maintain communal landholdings (Isbell, 1997). Recent archaeological evidence has presented a view of the Chanka as a group of highly decentralized communities with little evident social hierarchy, who would have been unable to pose a legitimate threat to the expansion of the Inca state (Bauer & Kellett, 2010; Kellett, 2010).

Sometime around AD 1000–1050, villages nested on the valley floors of Andahuaylas were abandoned, as people abruptly moved to high altitude, ridge-top settlements. Occupying such mountainous terrain offers natural defenses in terms of steep slopes, barriers, increased visual range, and the creation of buffer zones.

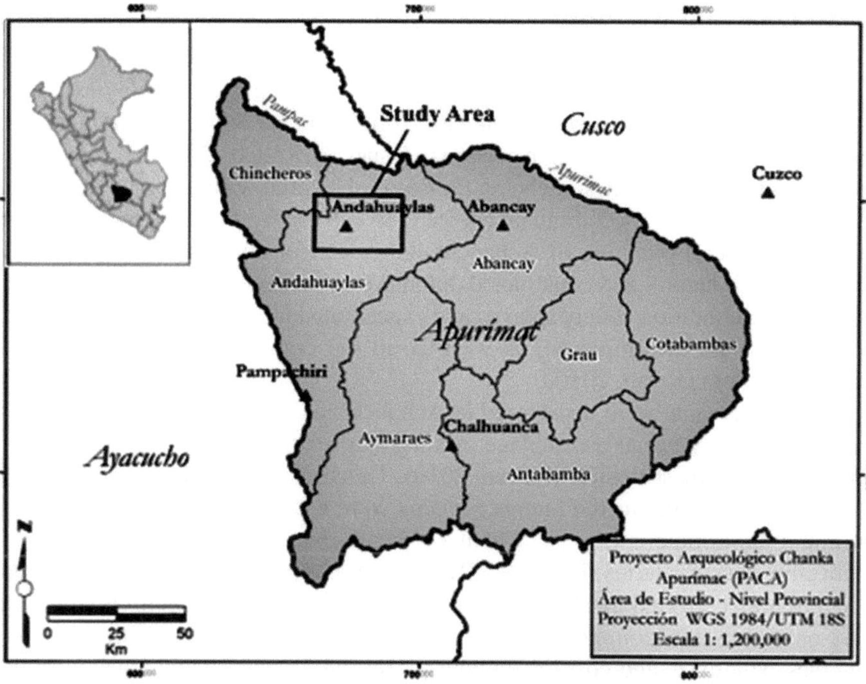

Fig. 9.1 Map of the Andahuaylas region in south-central Peru. The study area includes the site of Achanchi, where the primary skeletal remains discussed in this chapter were excavated

However, in such settlements, the agglutinated living spaces, distance from vital resources, and requisite changes in subsistence practices provide indirect evidence that warfare significantly affected and constrained life for the Chanka. This is confirmed by the bioarchaeological data, which demonstrate significant increases in cranial trauma and stress indicators, as well as the advent of trepanation (Kurin, 2016a; Kellett, Jolly, Kurin, & Monteagudo, 2015).

The bioarchaeological data from the Chanka provide a case study with which to explore the relationship of warfare, in-group identity, and care. Skeletal data from the region indicate that violence was not experienced equally. Certain social groups, whose identity was marked by artificial cranial modification, were overwhelmingly targeted for violence (Kurin, 2014). The data clearly show that social identity was a decisive factor in violence and victimization, but may have also structured life in other ways. One such domain likely included access to therapeutic intervention and care following accidental or intentional traumatic injury. Evidence of care in the form of cranial surgery could have had significant implications for how social identities and group affiliations (i.e., "auspicious survivors," "the disabled," and "wounded warriors") were renegotiated, as well as illuminating the social effects of endemic warfare.

Materials and Methods

Located at approximately 4000 m above sea level, the archaeological site of Achanchi is the largest known Chanka hill-fort, with over 300 small circular houses on densely occupied habitation terraces (Bauer & Kellett, 2010). Achanchi was permanently occupied, despite being far from substantial water sources and agricultural fields, indicating a communal choice to live in a safer, but less productive, area. The architectural planning of Achanchi shows a clear concern with defensibility, utilizing both natural and constructed defensive measures (Kellett, 2010). Such difficult living conditions likely spurred and exacerbated health concerns by increasing the burdens on the impaired, as well as on the communities who might have supported them (Kurin, 2016b).

Human remains were discovered at Achanchi in 2006, in a highly commingled and fragmentary burial assemblage eroding out of the hillside and located in the midst of domestic structures (Kellett, 2010). This burial assemblage is unique in the Andahuaylas region, as the human remains were excavated from an unmarked pit within a domestic context. The Chanka typically buried their dead in *machays*, or collective cave ossuaries (Kurin, 2012). Another common burial context is in *chullpas*, or above ground mortuary monuments. In Andahuaylas, *chullpas* were small and only able to accommodate two or three adult burials in the form of mummy bundles. Their size and position on windy, arid saddles suggest that they were used for the desiccation of human remains (Kurin, 2012). Machays and highly visible chullpas were important ritual spaces, but were also used to mark territory and delimit the boundaries of social groups (Kurin, 2012; Mantha, 2009). Therefore, the lack of evident superstructure marking the Achanchi burial is unusual.

While the Achanchi individuals may not have been afforded the "proper" Chanka burial, the patterns of commingling and fragmentation, as well as types of grave goods in the assemblage, are consistent with other burial contexts in Andahuaylas (Kellett et al., 2015). At Achanchi, two complete individuals were found at the bottom of the pit, with a collection of highly commingled remains above them. The inclusion of grave goods suggests that this is not a context marked strictly by violation of the human remains (i.e., a mass grave) (Duncan, 2005). The differences between pit and cave burials remain unclear, although the uniqueness of this burial assemblage may be, in part, due to the general lack of settlement excavations in this region. With future research we may be able to better infer the social identities of those interred in the Achanchi burial pit.

Analysis of the highly commingled skeletal assemblage in the Achanchi pit yielded a minimum number of individuals [MNI] of 39. When possible, age and sex were determined using established standards for osteological analysis (Buikstra & Ubelaker, 1994). Efforts were made to distinguish antemortem, perimortem, and postmortem trauma (Lovell, 1997), and pathological lesions were recorded according to the established standards (Buikstra & Ubelaker, 1994). Of note, one of the two complete skeletons recovered, termed ACH 3, demonstrates multiple trepanations. When positioned within the overall community health profile and archaeological data, the case of ACH 3 can be used to reconstruct the experience of physical impairment and its impact on life for the injured Chanka living at Achanchi.

Results

Osteobiographic Profile

ACH 3 is a remarkable find, as it represents the only complete and articulated skeleton with trepanation excavated in Andahuaylas. Therefore, this individual's osteobiography provides significant insights into the embodied experience of trepanation. The body of ACH 3 was originally deposited on sterile soil, as these remains were excavated from the bottom of the burial assemblage. This position in the pit is typical of apical ancestor inhumations observed elsewhere (Kurin, 2012). ACH 3 was placed in a flexed position, with the knees tucked inside the thoracic cavity, a placement that strongly implies postmortem curation and evisceration of the thoracic viscera. The only grave good directly associated with the skeleton was a worked human rib pendant, with a hole drilled for suspension. Isotopic research suggests that such rib pendants represent trophies, as they were taken from nonlocal individuals (Kurin, 2016a).

ACH 3's skeleton was complete but extensively fragmented by root damage. Morphological characteristics of the pelvis indicate that ACH 3 was male (Buikstra & Ubelaker, 1994). His third molars had erupted, and the ischial tuberosity and iliac crest epiphyses were in the process of fusing, suggesting that he was between 18 and 22 years old at the time of his death (Buikstra & Ubelaker, 1994). The cranium was reconstructed to the extent possible and shows clear signs of artificial modification. During infancy, when the cranial bones were unfused and malleable, ACH 3's head was tightly bound to mark in-group identity (Torres-Rouff, 2002), a conspicuous form of group affiliation that likely increased his risk for targeted violence. ACH 3's skeleton evinces several cranial and postcranial fractures, signs of impaired mobility, and multiple trepanations, although, remarkably, all of these wounds bear evidence of long-term healing. Without a single differential diagnosis to unify the symptoms of his exhibited pathologies, it is necessary to explore the impact of each before reconstructing the full-body experience of impairment and need for care.

Cranial Trauma

ACH 3 has a total of four healing cranial wounds. First, the frontal bone bears a healed scraped trepanation above the supraorbital ridge that is fairly small, measuring 11 mm wide by 13 mm tall (medio-lateral by supero-inferior) (Fig. 9.2). A radiating fracture line with some healing extends posteriorly from the superior margin of the trepanation. This extant fracture line strongly suggests that the surgery was a response to blunt force trauma, even though the impact site was obliterated by the trepanation.

The second head wound is on the left parietal. The impact pattern of a star-headed mace – defined by two connected impact sites of the same size – is visible, and is associated with a scraped trepanation (Fig. 9.3). Star-headed stone maces are common weapons in the Andes, used in close-contact assaults (Arkush & Tung, 2013).

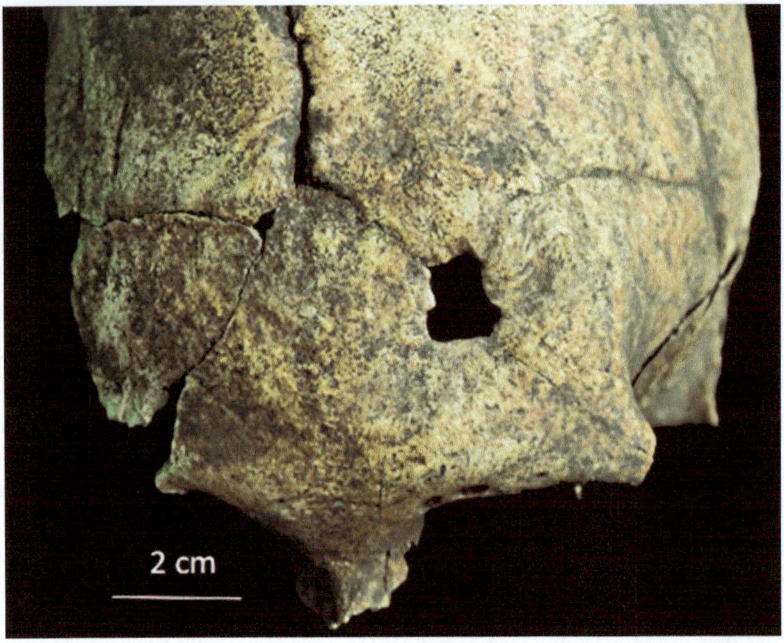

Fig. 9.2 Healed trepanation with a radiating fracture above left orbit (ACH 3)

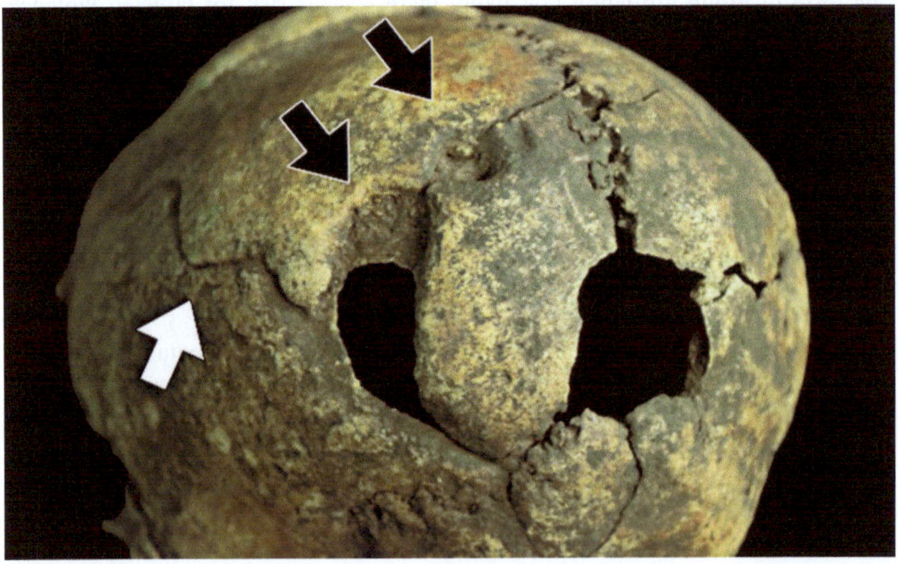

Fig. 9.3 Impact sites of star-headed mace (*black arrows*) with healing radiating fractures (*white arrow*) on the left parietal. Healed trepanation superposes the inferior impact site (ACH 3)

This wound is superposed with a scraped trepanation, larger than the first at 28 mm wide by 48 mm tall, with a healing radiating fracture extending anteriorly, terminating in the fracture line from the frontal bone wound. Another healing fracture line from this mace wound extends through the sagittal suture.

The third wound is a blunt force injury to the zygomatic process of the right temporal bone. This wound shows long-term healing, although there is malunion of the two sides of the process. Finally, the fourth wound is a blunt force injury to the right parietal bone and a third scraped trepanation, comparably sized to that on the frontal. This injury shows a lesser degree of healing than the others.

The extent of the radiating fracture lines associated with two of these wounds suggests that these were high velocity weapons blows and, furthermore, indicates a violent etiology. Additionally, due to the differential degrees of healing on these cranial wounds, ACH 3 qualifies as an injury recidivist, or a victim of consecutive violent attacks. Based on their associations with blunt force trauma, ACH 3's trepanations were surgical responses to what was perceived by the Chanka as life-threatening injuries received in violent contexts.

Temporary and longer term side effects from high velocity cranial wounds could have had wide-ranging consequences for ACH 3's ability to undertake activities, potentially affecting all facets of daily life. The combined onslaught of blunt force trauma and trepanation likely compounded the side effects ACH 3 experienced. The clinical impacts of serious or concurrent cranial wounds and the risks of neurosurgery are difficult to predict even now, so it is impossible to reconstruct precisely the extent to which ACH 3 was affected. Nevertheless, research has consistently shown that head trauma has significant physiological effects, as symptoms can last from days, to months, to even years. Side effects include headaches, dizziness, concussions, amnesia, unusual behavior, seizures, nerve damage, loss of motor skills, and failing mental functions (Karrar, Mansour, & Bhansali, 2011). Concussions, while not identifiable bioarchaeologically, occur relatively frequently with cranial trauma and may take the form of headaches, dizziness, malaise, cognitive problems, and depression. The symptoms of post-concussive syndrome can last for days up to several years. Frequent head trauma is also associated with chronic traumatic encephalopathy, a condition commonly associated with modern-day athletes, in which an individual faces progressive deterioration in cognitive functions that can result in cognitive dysfunction, dementia, and Parkinson's disease (McKee et al., 2009). Although ACH 3 was young, and thus more likely to recover faster than an older adult, receiving multiple head wounds likely slowed his recovery times and posed significantly higher risks of more serious side effects.

Postcranial Trauma

In addition to clearly life-threatening cranial wounds ACH 3 displays multiple postcranial pathologies and injuries, although none of these would be classified as potentially fatal. Postcranial pathologies are briefly described below.

ACH 3 evinces mild osteoarthritis on the left superior articular facets of his fifth and sixth cervical vertebrae. This could have resulted in pain or neck stiffness, or it could have restricted movement of the neck. This osteoarthritis may relate to his cranial injuries, as 10 % of modern severe head injuries have an associated spine injury, most commonly on the cervical vertebrae (Karrar et al., 2011).

ACH 3 also exhibits bilateral osteochondritis dissecans [OCD] on the glenoid fossae of his scapulae. OCD is a fracture of the joint surface, particularly affecting active adolescents, most commonly males. OCD is most commonly caused by repetitive microtrauma involving shearing and compressive forces on a joint surface, leading to the loss of the blood supply to part of the bone which then chips off and moves into the joint (Hixon & Gibbs, 2000 *ibid.*). Unilateral OCD is uncommon in modern populations and so this bilateral occurrence is exceptionally rare, especially considering that the glenoid fossa is an infrequent location of the pathology. It may suggest that ACH 3 had repetitive trauma to both his shoulders, was subject to genetic predisposition, or had ischemia (restricted blood supply), all of which have been suggested as possible causes of the condition. OCD causes mild persistent or intermittent pain related to activity, stiffness, catching sensations as the bone chip locks into the joint, restricted movement, and joint weakness, all of which worsen with weight-bearing. These fractures typically resolve themselves after 10–18 months without significant intervention beyond resting, stretching, range-of-motion exercises, and immobilization (Hixon & Gibbs, 2000).

In the last year or so of ACH 3's life it is likely that he would have experienced some difficulty with the use of both of his arms, most likely mild soreness or pain that would have worsened with activity. Regardless of the ongoing degree of pain, it is likely that OCD fractures would have made daily tasks (i.e., canal cleaning, wall building, sowing and harvesting, and stone slinging) more challenging or bothersome. Additionally, he has pitting behind the sternal end of his right clavicle, further attesting to a stressed shoulder joint. In sum, these stress markers on the shoulder girdle support a characterization that ACH 3 was actively engaged in strenuous activities, so it is likely that he was still working in community labor projects following initial injuries.

ACH 3 has a well-healed fracture on the posterior aspect of his left 12th rib, just past the rib angle. Single rib fractures have been found to occasionally result in so much pain that an individual cannot work; minimally it lowers the afflicted individual's quality of life until it heals (Kara, Dikmen, Erdal, Simsir, & Kara, 2003). Fractures to the floating ribs are especially damaging, as they are not connected to cartilage and can more easily damage the liver, spleen, kidneys, and diaphragm (Brickley, 2006). ACH 3's injury is healed, so if any internal organs were damaged, they healed enough to allow him to survive, albeit with consequences that remain unobservable. Nevertheless, ACH 3 would have faced weeks of persistent pain and discomfort.

ACH 3 displays periostitis on the distal shafts of the right radius and ulna. While periostitis is the mildest nonspecific bone infection (Larsen, 1997), it may be suggestive of a chronic wrist problem, or possibly a very well healed fracture with minimal bone distortion. ACH 3's left tibia also evinces periostitis, suggestive of a

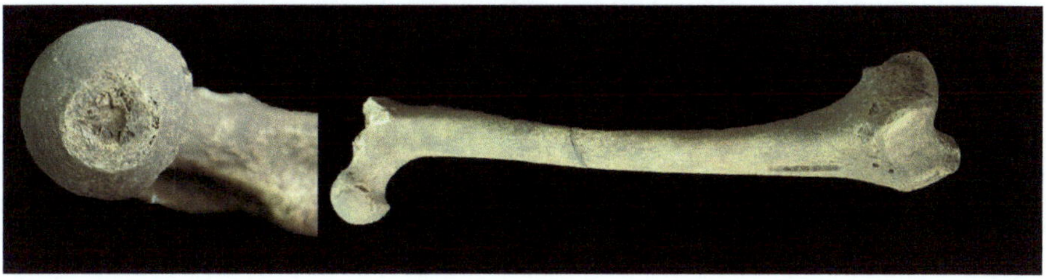

Fig. 9.4 Left femoral head evincing a fibrotic response of the ligamentum teres (*on left*) and significant torsion of the distal shaft (*on right*) (ACH 3)

bothersome limb. However, he has bilateral tibial musculoskeletal stress markers on the attachment site of the Sartorius muscle. This muscle is involved in flexing and laterally rotating the hip joint and flexing the knee, suggesting that this muscle was used extensively enough to develop enthesophytes on both sides.

ACH 3's left femoral head displays a traumatic injury, with a flattened ring around the fovea capitis and torsion of the distal shaft (Fig. 9.4). This is characteristic of an excessive fibrotic response of the *ligamentum teres*. This pathology tends to have an accidental etiology, caused by a tear of the ligament through overextension or flexion of the joint and compounded by excessive post-traumatic scar tissue (arthrofibrosis). Minimally, ACH 3 would have walked with a limp. Leg injuries of this sort would have been a particular challenge at the mountainous site of Achanchi.

Despite his numerous ailments and injuries, there is no clear cause of death apparent in the remains of ACH 3. In addition to the evidence for pathology discussed above a piece of the posterior cranium is missing, although this most likely relates to postmortem damage and taphonomic fragmentation. ACH 3's skeleton also bears a series of perimortem cutmarks on several bones. These are present on the lateral distal shafts of both femora, possibly cutting the popliteus or gastrocnemius muscles, and on the lateral side of the left fibula under the proximal epiphysis. The cutmarks most likely relate to postmortem processing of the body for mummification, allowing the knees to be inserted into the thoracic cavity. There are also extensive cutmarks on the shafts of both ulnae and radii; these are shallower and more numerous than those on the lower limb, and the "chattermark" appearance is most consistent with observed cases of defleshing. While motivations remain unclear, this activity also most likely relates to postmortem processing of the body.

Overall, ACH 3's paleopathological analysis presents the image of an athletic youth, who was targeted for violence that left him with permanent bodily damage and, plausibly, mental damage as well. With wounds from violent events, and a worked human rib around his neck, he certainly fits the ethno-historically documented image of the ferocious Chanka warrior. Even if this combatant status was temporary, injury recidivism from weapons-based trauma suggests that he engaged in multiple violent encounters, either as the raider of an enemy site, the defender of Achanchi, or as a noncombatant victim – the latter especially likely after his initial injuries.

ACH 3 faced several life-threatening cranial wounds that the Chanka identified as injuries meriting surgical treatment and acute care. His physical conditions likely left him with a degree of impairment that placed him within a complex sociomedical system of longer term care for the duration of his short lifespan. Furthermore, we can hypothesize that such a system of care in the Achanchi community extended to postcranial as well as cranial injuries.

Discussion

The overall sample of skeletal remains from Andahuaylas establishes the regional patterns of health, trauma, and trepanation that assist in our understanding of ACH 3's survival by informing on the demographic and status variables affecting ACH 3's risk of exposure to violence and access to care. Additionally, such data enable a reconstruction of the Chanka logic of healing, through comparing the unique perspective gained from one complete set of individual remains to the trepanation data gathered from the disarticulated skulls more commonly found in Andahuaylas mortuary contexts.

A Regional View of Trepanation Practices

Besides ACH 3, 32 other trepanned crania from the Andahuaylas region have been analyzed, and these provide a baseline of data for comparison with ACH 3's surgeries. Local patterns must be identified, as considerable regional variation has been documented in Andean trepanation practices in terms of technique, time of adoption, and success rates with various techniques (Toyne, 2015; see Nystrom, 2007; Andrushko & Verano, 2008; Kurin, 2013). Each of ACH 3's trepanations was performed with a scraping technique. Scraped trepanations are the most common technique in Andahuaylas, although all four methods have been documented on crania. Scraped trepanations have been noted on 27 in Andahuaylas individuals and, remarkably, have 100 % survival rates, appearing to be much more successful than other methods (Kurin, 2013). Scraping maintains lower and slower forces penetrating the bone, allowing for greater precision and reducing the risk of hitting underlying tissues. Therefore, technique was important in structuring patient outcomes. ACH 3 received only scraped trepanations, so multiple wounds did not always necessitate riskier, more experimental techniques. The consistent use of scraped trepanation on this individual may represent an attempt to minimize risk in the face of compounding side effects.

Regional patterns of trepanation can also identify the social factors that mediated access to care. While subadults in Andahuaylas demonstrate both antemortem and perimortem cranial trauma, no subadult crania from the region evidence trepanations, suggesting that this form of care was restricted to adults (Kurin, 2012).

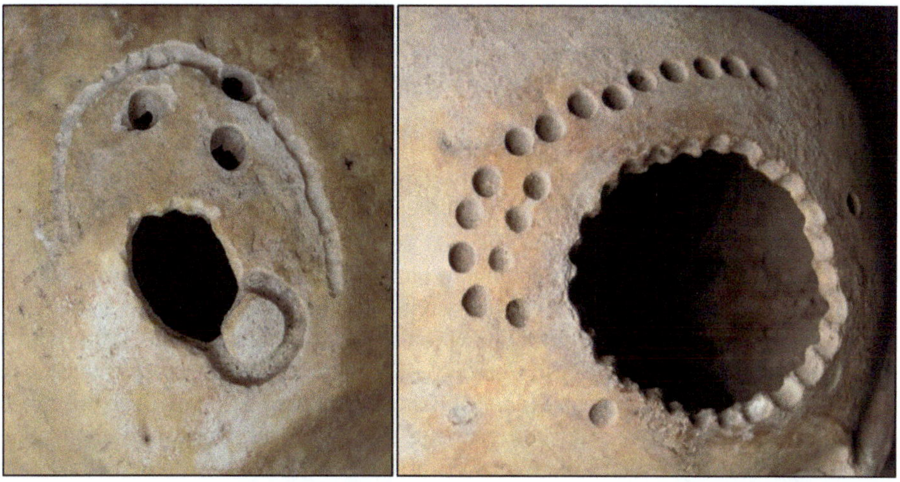

Fig. 9.5 Experimental trepanations: *left*, postmortem drill holes using various techniques; *right*, postmortem bore holes increasing in depth posteriorly

Furthermore, while Chanka males and females experienced trauma at similar rates, they did not have the same access to care, as 79 % (25/33) of trepanned individuals were males. This care differential may correspond to male combatant status, as receiving injuries as an altruistic warrior may have justified reciprocal support from his community. However, males tend to receive trepanations more commonly than females throughout the Andes (Andrushko & Verano, 2008), so access to trepanation may correspond to another aspect of male status more universal throughout time and place.

Crania from Andahuaylas indicate that medical practitioners were experimenting on deceased individuals to improve their knowledge of cranial anatomy and to advance their technical skills (Kurin, 2012; Kurin, 2013). Two crania display a series of postmortem drill holes, one systematically increasing in depth in order to test the thickness of the parietal bone and the other experimenting with drill bits and techniques (Fig. 9.5). Another cranium shows linear cutting on the endocranial surface. This interest in refining treatment procedures suggests that the Chanka were invested in the survival of their community members. Furthermore, experimental trepanations help to explain why Chanka medical practitioners so rapidly achieved such success with scraping, as well as suggesting that they recognized the need to focus on treatment efficacy in response to high levels of conflict.

A general awareness of anatomy in Chanka communities may also have developed from their experience with camelid husbandry and butchery (Kellett, 2010). The Chanka made *charki* (jerky) by naturally "mummifying" llama meat using a combination of salt and cold temperatures. Similarly, Chanka mummification of deceased humans involved the severing of leg muscles in order to insert the legs into the thoracic cavity and a process for drying out the remaining soft tissue. The Chanka may have gained some anatomical familiarity through these experiences, even though none of these techniques match the surgical precision apparent in trepanation. As in the trepanations on ACH 3's cranium, most trepanations from Andahuaylas occur on parts of the cranium without musculature, suggesting that Chanka medical practitioners were selective about the kinds and locations of wounds on which they chose to operate.

In-group identity became increasingly important to the Chanka, as illustrated by the increasing ubiquity of cranial modification in Andahuaylas (Kurin, 2012). Individuals with modified crania, like ACH 3, had significantly higher cranial trauma rates than their unmodified counterparts (Kurin, 2012). Eighty-two per cent (27/33) of trepanned individuals exhibit cranial modification (Kurin, 2012). Because targeted violence and collective victimization reaffirms in-group identity, this would have created solidarity within the perceived group and have structured access to community-based care systems. Increasing medical awareness may have prompted increased availability of advanced treatment, albeit only for select individuals with certain types of injuries. While Chanka warrior status may have reflected a more temporary status than an "elite" class, the community members they served might have been more willing to provide them with care.

Coping with Trauma and Trepanation

Cranial trauma can have significant physical, emotional, and economic effects on an individual, their family, and their community. In contexts with high rates of violence, such as in LIP Andahuaylas, the effects of cranial trauma should be considered in terms of how these affected both the individual and the wider community. Forty-one percent (9/22) of adult individuals over the age of 15 at Achanchi bear evidence of cranial trauma. Despite the small sample size, this rate is consistent with overall frequencies in Andahuaylas, as 57 %, (138/243) of LIP crania from other excavated Andahuaylas sites have at least one traumatic cranial wound. Of the nine adults from Achanchi, there are a total of 18 wounds, 10 of which are antemortem and eight of which are perimortem. Antemortem trauma affected 23 % of the Achanchi burial population ($n = 5$), including ACH 3. From the broader Andahuaylas context, 35 % (85/243) of individuals experienced sublethal wounds (Kurin, 2012). Even though ACH 3's cranial injuries are severe, such wounds were relatively common both at the Achanchi site and in the region, suggesting that the functional impacts of these wounds placed strain on the community over time.

Even in modern populations, head trauma takes a high emotional, psychosocial, and economic toll and results in comparatively long hospital stays, as even mild head wounds and fractures require a full 24 h of monitoring (Sainsbury & Sibert, 1984). In modern clinical settings, patients presenting with moderate head injuries and traumatic brain injury require an average of nine days in the intensive care unit (ranging between 2 and 36 days) for a total average hospitalization of 16 days (ranging between 4 and 58 days) (Vitaz, Jenks, Raque, & Shields, 2003). Ultimately, 5–10 % of individuals with head injuries require discharge to a long-term care facility (Karrar et al., 2011).

While modern contexts of head injury may be very different to those in the past, cranial injuries, regardless of their historical context, can have significant impacts on motor, sensory, and reflex abilities resulting from neurological defects following trauma. Complications are frequent with severe brain injuries, and long-term care usually requires rehabilitation by physical, occupational, vocational, speech, and recreational therapies. The outcome of head trauma depends on the initial level of injury, but even "mild" head injuries can greatly decrease life expectancy and can increase the likelihood of developing depression following head trauma (Karrar et al., 2011).

In communities like Achanchi, cranial trauma would have become increasingly familiar as conflict during the LIP persisted. Ancillary effects, such as change in life expectancy and mental health disorders, would have had long-lasting impacts on social organization and social relations arising from the short- and long-term outcomes of trauma on community members and pressures to care for increasing numbers of patients..

Traumatic Brain Injury

Another common complication of cranial trauma is traumatic brain injury [TBI], which has become a major research interest of modern medicine. TBI is defined as an injury to the head from blunt force trauma, the mildest symptoms of which result in one or more of the following: a period of confusion, disorientation, or impaired consciousness; any dysfunction of the memory around the time of injury; loss of consciousness lasting less than 30 min; and/or the onset of observed signs or symptoms of neurological or neurophysiological dysfunction (Corrigan, Selassie, & Orman, 2010). Side effects range from mild concussion, headache, and dizziness to moderate, severe, or potentially fatal consequences. "Mild" TBI does not describe an inconsequential injury, but merely indicates that the effects of the injury are temporary and/or of a lesser grade of severity than "severe" TBI. While TBI affects soft tissue unavailable in the archaeological record, Corrigan et al. (2010) define skull fractures as a form of (minimally) mild TBI, thereby enabling bioarchaeologists to include common TBI complications when considering the possible health effects of skeletally visible cranial fractures.

Seventy-five percent of modern TBI cases are diagnosed as mild, and these can have a substantial impact on an individual's physical, emotional, and economic capacities, and lessen their quality of life. Ten to twenty percent of patients with mild TBI continue to experience psychosocial problems such as depression and mood disorders, which contribute to extended recovery periods and poor outcomes after injury (Valente & Fisher, 2011). We cannot rule out the possibility that factors associated with poor recovery from TBI may have contributed to ACH 3's early death, or at least reduced his quality of life.

The failure to provide appropriate treatment for TBI can result in amnesia, confusion, or loss of consciousness, and even in permanent damage to the brain. Fifteen percent of people with mild TBI have symptoms that last a year or more. Twenty percent of people with mild TBI suffer depression or mood disorders, including anger, poor concentration, physical violence, and sexually offensive behavior, as decreased inhibitions, anxiety disorders, and depression are commonly seen for at least a year following trauma (Valente & Fisher, 2011). Cognitive difficulties, associated with learning, memory, information processing, communication, and reasoning, are also commonly affected.

Even when treatment is given, one study found that among patients in the United States diagnosed with TBI and discharged from the hospital, 43 % develop long-term disabilities related to TBI, with disability defined broadly as the individual being unable to perform, or having difficulty in performing, daily life activities; unable to achieve personal goals; or having poor cognitive and mental health scores based on standard measures. Furthermore, 40 % of males diagnosed with TBI were assessed as having a long-term disability after 1 year (Corrigan et al., 2010). Given the clinical research, ACH 3 (and many of the other injured Chanka) probably faced some degree of long-term impairment from TBI.

TBI, when combined with other factors like family history of violence and substance abuse, may predispose patients to violence (Linton, 2015; Fazel, Lichtenstein, Grann, & Långström, 2011). In a study of Swedish patients diagnosed with TBI, Fazel et al. (2011) found that 9 % committed a violent crime after their diagnosis, a significantly higher rate than found in the general population, although the causal relationship between TBI and violence has not been conclusively shown. Additionally, patients with TBI acquired from violent physical assault often demonstrate antisocial behavior and poorer community integration than survivors with TBI from unintentional causes (Kim, Colantonio, Dawson, & Bayley, 2013). TBI resulting from violence may therefore have consequences that affect a community long past the initial injury.

The increasing frequencies of cranial trauma amongst the Chanka would inevitably lead to a correspondingly increased awareness of the individual physical and psychological symptoms and side effects of this injury. The complications of TBI may have also influenced general community operation in important ways – for example, helping to perpetuate violent interpersonal behaviors and values; it is possible that the Chanka viewed wounds acquired through violence as a "badge of honor." It is unknown whether and how trepanation affected Chanka experience of TBI, as modern medicine still struggles to identify the exact neurological mechanism behind this pathology.

Treatment Procedures

Regardless of whether trepanation was performed in response to cranial trauma, most head injuries would have required some sort of nursing care, over time, to assist recovery. Short- and long-term physical and mental effects of cranial trauma, occurring as these did within a general environment of sustained conflict, likely resulted in dynamic and possibly challenging relationships between the afflicted individuals, their caregivers, and the broader community. Therefore, this may have had a significant impact on general community mental health at Achanchi.

While trepanation may have offered health benefits to patients with TBI, it also posed dangers. Injuries to the underlying dura or venous sinuses would have been catastrophic, as would have been hitting major blood vessels. Both during and after surgery the patient could easily have gone into shock, or faced further edema (swelling) of the brain. Reducing the risk of these consequences would have been especially critical to the success of trepanation in the past, and would have required anatomical knowledge. Bioarchaeologists cannot reconstruct the timing of performance of trepanation after injury, but early response would support better patient outcomes.

The pain of cutting through the scalp and periosteum would have been intense (Weber & Czarnetzki, 2001), and it has been suggested that alcohol, narcotics, or even coca would have been used to alleviate this (Liu & Apuzzo, 2003). In some instances the patient might lose consciousness during surgery in response to pain, or be unconscious at the beginning of the procedure due to their initial injury. Maintaining a stable surface for operating would be necessary to reduce the risk of error, and it is likely that the medical practitioner would need assistance in keeping an unanesthetized patient motionless. Ready availability of such assistance would also have been required in case an unconscious patient regained consciousness during surgery (Liu & Apuzzo, 2003). This need for helpers may have provided an opportunity for training new practitioners.

It is likely that stone tools were used to trepan in Andahuaylas (Kurin, 2012). Studies have found that freshly knapped flint is a sterile surgical instrument (Löwen, 1997 in Weber & Wahl, 2006). Modern neurosurgical practices typically involve clipping the scalp back and cauterizing major blood vessels to avoid excessive bleeding, especially when cutting through the scalp and periosteum (Weber & Wahl, 2006). Fast operating times are important in modern neurosurgical practice in order to limit blood loss and minimize pain. Smaller trepanations might have been a prehistoric solution to these problems (Weber & Wahl, 2006). Two of ACH 3's trepanations were small, supporting this hypothesis. The small scraped trepanations may also be dictated by wound size, as larger trepanations might have unnecessarily introduced risk. The trepanation associated with the star-shaped mace injury was much larger, possibly in response to its multiple impact sites and more devastating impact. The two better-healed trepanations (Fig. 9.3) could conceivably have been done contemporaneously, as they are both on the left side of the skull and were probably accessible to the practitioner at the same time, but such a conclusion awaits future paleohistological and radiographic analysis.

Even if no underlying tissues were affected, postsurgical infection in trepanation patients would have been a particular risk. Previous research has found possible evidence of the use of poultices on a mummified trepanned individual to reduce the risk of postoperative infection (Kurin, 2013). Poultice use and bandaging would also prevent the wounds from being left open to contaminants. Even without direct evidence on skeletonized remains, it is likely that poultices were used, suggesting close monitoring for signs of infection. Assuming that practitioners performed trepanations with such frequency as to hone their craft, it seems likely that communities would have postoperative systems in place to assist those in recovery as standard practice. Even in the face of resource constraints, trepanned individuals would likely have been allowed extensive convalescence periods to recover, as too much physical activity too soon after surgery can increase the risk of damage to the brain, nullifying any beneficial effects of trepanation.

Ultimately, any bioarchaeological approach can only approximate the physical impacts of trauma and trepanation, and cannot determine the emotional and mental fallout of these events. Modern doctors view emotional support for TBI patients as integral to their recovery as temporary or chronic depression, ranging from mild to severe, is common after head trauma; informal support by caregivers is recommended, unless the patient exhibits signs of severe clinical mental disorders (Karrar et al., 2011). During recovery this can place additional strain on caregivers who are faced with attempting to respond to, or manage, a patient's emotional response to debilitating head trauma. Such may have been the case in the ancient past as well.

Caregiver Experience

It is likely that the stresses of surgery and postoperative recovery processes were not only felt by the care-recipients but by the practitioners and caregivers as well. Despite the difficulty of identifying caregivers archaeologically, here we identify possibly stressors acting on these care providers in order to model a holistic experience of care and caregiving at Achanchi.

Ethnographic research from Andean Colombia depicts caregiving in this region as a form of unpaid, domestic labor, usually assigned on a gender basis. Women are typically assigned duties of caregiving for elderly parents, disabled adults, or the chronically ill, and these duties may generate stress, anxiety, and depression (Friedemann-Sánchez, 2012). While the gender of the trepanation specialist cannot be determined, the burden of more general caregiving may have fallen on the women at Achanchi. The responsibilities of patient care in clinical settings have been associated with raised levels of stress, burnout, and interpersonal problems. In modern practice, surgeons are known to experience increased risks of hypertension and cardiovascular disease (Klimo & Couldwell, 2008; Klimo et al., 2013). Prehistoric trepanation practitioners may not have had the workload of modern neurosurgeons, but an intensely felt pressure to realize successful surgery may have placed substantial stress on practitioners, leading to other health consequences and significantly affecting their quality of life.

Although caregiving at Achanchi may not have been as intertwined with economic pressures and employment stressors as in modern ethnographically studied populations, the increased need for caregiving for impaired individuals (reflecting changes in social, economic, and political contexts) may have added to carers' stress. Mental health disorders following cranial trauma, the normal stresses of caregiving, the anxiety induced by endemic warfare, and the basic needs of labor-intensive subsistence, could together have exacerbated a climate of diminished community mental health – called *manchayrisqa* in Quechua – at Achanchi and at other Chanka sites.

Theorizing Trauma and Care

While the Chanka seem to have had a long-term perspective on cranial wound care, we cannot be sure that less-than-life-threatening injuries were so intensively supported; however, accommodation is not always mediated by threat to life. For a thorough discussion of what constitutes care versus accommodation, refer to Tilley (Chap. 2). The choices of settlement type and location that the Chanka made suggest that they selected for defense, not convenience of lifestyle and access to resources. Considering that at least 20 % of Achanchi residents had a debilitating leg pathology or fracture, they may have negotiated a flexible strategy of labor dependent on degree of short-term impairment. Alternately, impaired individuals may have struggled up and down the mountain for daily labor tasks, walking 2–4 km one-way to agricultural fields or water sources. The prevalence of injury and disease would have compounded the problems of accommodating the requirements of quotidian activities, both for the afflicted individuals and for the broader community.

Reducing and splinting fractures may be a fairly commonsense medical practice, but trepanation goes far beyond this. Extrapolating from Chanka skills in trepanation suggests the Chanka were likely capable of developing complex care practices for other traumatic injuries. However, one radius recovered from the Achanchi site displays a healed fracture with significant malunion and deformation of the bone, suggesting that it was not properly treated. Because fractures that could have been splinted were so rarely documented in this assemblage, it is difficult to determine whether the poor treatment associated with this radius fracture was common amongst postcranial injuries. Ultimately, there are too few healed postcranial fractures noted in this highly commingled and fragmentary collection to identify other patterns of trauma care at Achanchi.

Trepanation, and the long-term survival of physically impaired persons, shows an investment in care amongst the Chanka. These data speak to the value of an individual's life, even that of the impaired, regardless of resource constraints or fear of attack. It is unknown exactly how the care afforded to trepanned individuals extended to other types of disease or injury, or whether "war wounds" had a different status, in terms of being a medical crisis requiring response, to that of symptoms of nonviolence-related disease. For example, those Chanka individuals with afflicted legs may very well have been left to struggle with daily tasks, as it is difficult to be certain what care they received. However, the practice of cranial surgery and the provision of the necessary recovery and convalescence periods for head trauma do suggest a social organization designed to respond to the need for intensive care.

Theorizing care for traumatic injuries in the bioarchaeological record requires different considerations than those required in theorizing past care either in response to infectious and/or systemic diseases or for chronic conditions. Trauma has an observable mechanism of injury, whose etiology is usually subject to less speculation and stigma. Many traumatic injuries are nonfatal, and have positive prognoses if allowed the proper time and support. Therefore some forms of traumatic wounds likely resulted in different social experiences to those elicited by nontraumatic diseases, especially where these latter had life-long consequences.

Because ACH 3 evinces multiple afflictions, there is no single, unifying differential diagnosis. Therefore, the problems of approximating functional constraints are increased. Although we can identify a range of possible, and even probable, complications associated with cranial injury there is no direct evidence of these in his remains. Furthermore, it is difficult to sequence ACH 3's injuries, so we cannot tell when each occurred and what their implications were for care and recovery. Some of ACH 3's postcranial pathologies may have been sequelae of cranial injuries. For example, it is possible that the vertebral arthritis was associated with his cranial trauma, although we cannot determine whether ACH 3 experienced symptoms of this arthritis and, if so, how he or his community responded to any limitations associated with it. Ultimately, details of the type and the extent of accommodation provided to ACH 3 in response to impairments from his cranial and/or postcranial pathologies may be unknowable.

Conclusions

This in-depth exploration of how trauma and trepanation affected an individual and his community elucidates aspects of changing social organization and identity in a period of high rates of interpersonal violence. Despite any short- or long-term side effects, ACH 3's life remained valuable to his community and merited repeated interventions. Patients who are bedridden following trepanation would be entirely dependent on caregivers for the initial weeks to months following surgery, and would be unable to contribute to the ongoing needs of the community. ACH 3's carers were willing to support him through more than one surgery, as well as possibly other episodes of care. Ultimately, he, like other trepanation patients, was buried with non-trepanned individuals, suggesting that his surgeries did not affect his burial treatment or ancestor status.

While ACH 3's group identity may have predisposed him to an increased risk for violence, group solidarity also structured his access to care. However, the relationship between the afflicted individual and his caregivers would have been dynamic, imbued with all the subtleties of human interaction. An interest in survival does not necessarily equate to a high quality of life. Over time Achanchi residents were becoming increasingly familiar with the side effects of cranial trauma and trepanation. Just as increasing cranial trauma rates catalyzed improvements to trepanation procedures, they could also have led to the development of techniques of care that are less archaeologically visible. Not all those recovering from injury would have been able to contribute equally – or "pull their weight" – in terms of resource acquisition and physical labor obligations within their society, but they may still have been able to participate in other forms of community activity.

Reconstructing this logic of healing is important to the consideration of how interpersonal violence affected community organization and of the ways communities responded to this violence. The dataset discussed in this chapter reveals the sophisticated, community-based, sociomedical structures that were developed in order to manage the consequences of the violence commonly faced in Late intermediate Period Peruvian highlands, and it speaks to the degree of complex social organization present in a time long thought to lack any meaningful social hierarchy. The focus on healthcare and impairment at Achanchi illuminates the ramifications of warfare and conflict for community decision-making.

The changes in post-traumatic injury brain function that are beginning to be noted in modern populations may have had significant and long-lasting effects on afflicted individuals, caregivers, and community members at Achanchi. As bioarchaeologists, we need to go beyond defining recovery from cranial fracture in terms of skeletal healing from proximate injury, expanding our analysis to include the recovery of the brain itself – a concept which has physical, emotional, and social implications. For example, TBI is now recognized as being associated with poor social integration and violent behavior in recovering individuals, and this may have contributed to intra-societal discord amongst the Chanka. Furthermore, continuing complications faced by survivors of cranial trauma may have played a role in reaffirming the societal fragmentation and persistent conflict that defined the LIP.

While bioarchaeological studies of warfare have contributed many insights to our understanding of the effects of conflict in the past, a care-based perspective illuminates details of the physical effects of interpersonal violence *and* the social organization required to manage these. A focus on Chanka care elucidates aspects of a community that was both accustomed to violence and, at the same time, constantly adjusting to it, experimenting with new solutions to manage the pervasive consequences of conflict. Ultimately, just as in the present, social identity had very real effects both in structuring violence and in structuring access to care, shaping the health outcomes of group members.

Acknowledgements We gratefully acknowledge the support of the Curtiss T. & Mary G. Brennan Foundation Grant, the National Science Foundation, Fulbright-Hays Fellowship, the University of Pittsburgh, Vanderbilt University, and the University of California, Santa Barbara. We thank Lorna Tilley and Alecia A. Schrenk for organizing this inventive and thought-provoking session and volume (as well as providing tremendously insightful feedback throughout this process), as well as Margaret Judd, Elizabeth Arkush, and two anonymous reviewers for their helpful comments on this chapter. Further thanks are given to Emanuel Gomez Choque, Soccoro Ouispe, and members of the Andahuaylas Bioarchaeology Project. All errors are our own.

References

Andrushko, V. A., & Verano, J. W. (2008). Prehistoric trepanation in the Cuzco region of Peru: A view into an ancient Andean practice. *American Journal of Physical Anthropology, 137*(1), 4–13.

Arkush, E. N., & Tung, T. A. (2013). Patterns of war in the Andes from the archaic to the late horizon: Insights from settlement patterns and cranial trauma. *Journal of Archaeological Research, 21*(4), 307–369.

Bauer, B. S., & Kellett, L. C. (2010). Cultural transformations of the Chanka homeland (Andahuaylas, Peru) during the late inter- mediate period (ad 1000–1400). *Latin American Antiquity, 21*, 87–111.

Bauer, B. S., Kellett, L. C., & Silva, M. A. (2010). *The Chanka: Archaeological research in Andahuaylas (Apurimac), Peru*. Los Angeles: UCLA Cotsen Institute of Archaeology.
Brickley, M. (2006). Rib fractures in the archaeological record: A useful source of sociocultural information? *International Journal of Osteoarchaeology, 16*(1), 61–75.
Buikstra, J. E. & Ubelaker, D. H. (Eds). (1994). *Standards for data collection from human skeletal remains. Proceedings of a Seminar at the Field Museum of Natural History*. Fayetteville: Arkansas Archaeological Survey. Research Series, No. 44.
Burneo, J. G. (2003). Sonko-Nanay and epilepsy among the Incas. *Epilepsy & Behavior, 4*(2), 181–184.
Clower, W. T., & Finger, S. (2001). Discovering trepanation: The contribution of Paul Broca. *Neurosurgery, 49*(6), 1417–1426.
Corrigan, J. D., Selassie, A. W., & Orman, J. A. L. (2010). The epidemiology of traumatic brain injury. *The Journal of Head Trauma Rehabilitation, 25*(2), 72–80.
Duncan, W. N. (2005). Understanding veneration and violation in the archaeological record. In *Interacting with the dead: Perspectives on mortuary archaeology for the new millennium* (pp. 207–227).
Erdal, Y. S., & Erdal, Ö. D. (2011). A review of trepanations in Anatolia with new cases. *International Journal of Osteoarchaeology, 21*(5), 505–534.
Fazel, S., Lichtenstein, P., Grann, M., & Långström, M. (2011). Risk of violent crime in individuals with epilepsy and traumatic brain injury: A 35-year Swedish population study. *PLoS Medicine, 8*(12), e1001150.
Friedemann-Sánchez, G. (2012). Caregiving patterns in rural Andean Colombia. *Feminist Economics, 18*(3), 55–80.
Hixon, A. L., & Gibbs, L. M. (2000). Osteochondritis dissecans: A diagnosis not to miss. *American Family Physician, 61*(1), 151–156.
Isbell, W. H. (1997). *Mummies and mortuary monuments: A postprocessual prehistory of central Andean social organization*. Austin: University of Texas Press.
Kara, M., Dikmen, E., Erdal, H. H., Simsir, I., & Kara, S. A. (2003). Disclosure of unnoticed rib fractures with the use of ultrasonography in minor blunt chest trauma. *European Journal of Cardio-Thoracic Surgery, 24*(4), 608–613.
Karrar, E. E., Mansour, N., & Bhansali, A. (2011). Cranial and spinal trauma: Current concepts. *Disease-a-Month, 57*(10), 543–557.
Kellett, L. C. (2010). *Chanka settlement ecology: Hilltop sites, land use, and warfare in late Prehispanic Andahuaylas, Peru*. University of New Mexico. Unpublished Ph.D. dissertation.
Kellett, L. C., Jolly, S. A., Kurin, D. S., & Monteagudo, G. (2015). *Life at Achanchi: A high altitude Chanka burial site from the Andahuaylas Region of Southern Peru*. Poster presented at the 80th Annual Meeting of the Society for American Archaeology, San Francisco, CA.
Kim, H., Colantonio, A., Dawson, D. R., & Bayley, M. T. (2013). Community integration outcomes after traumatic brain injury due to physical assault. *Canadian Journal of Occupational Therapy, 80*(1), 49–58.
Klimo, P., Jr., & Couldwell, W. T. (2008). Stress and burnout: Insidious influences. *AANS Neurosurgeon in Action, 17*(1), 17–18.
Klimo, P., DeCuypere, M., Ragel, B. T., McCartney, S., Couldwell, W. T., & Boop, F. A. (2013). Career satisfaction and burnout among US neurosurgeons: A feasibility and pilot study. *World Neurosurgery, 80*(5), e59–e68.
Kurin, D. S. (2012). *The Bioarchaeology of Collapse: Ethnogenesis and Ethnocide in Post- imperial Andahuaylas, Peru (AD 900–1200)*. Vanderbilty University. Unpublished Ph.D. dissertation.
Kurin, D. S. (2013). Trepanation in south-central Peru during the early Late Intermediate period (ca. AD 1000–1250). *American Journal of Physical Anthropology, 152*(4), 484–494.
Kurin, D. S. (2014). Conflict and ethnic identity among the post-collapse Chanka of Andahuaylas, Peru (ca. AD 1000–1400). In D. L. Martin & C. Anderson (Eds.), *Forensic and bioarchaeological approaches to interpreting violence* (pp. 151–173). New York: Cambridge University Press.
Kurin, D. S. (2016a). *The bioarchaeology of societal collapse and reorganization in ancient Peru*. New York: Springer.

Kurin, D. S. (2016b). Trauma, nutrition, and malnutrition in the Andean highlands during Peru's dark age (1000–1250 C.E.). In A. M. VanDewarker & G. D. Wilson (Eds.), *The archaeology of food and warfare: Food insecurity in prehistory* (pp. 229–257). New York: Springer.

Larsen, C. S. (1997). *Bioarchaeology: Interpreting behavior from the human skeleton* (Vol. 70). Cambridge: Cambridge University Press.

Linton, K. F. (2015). Interpersonal violence and traumatic brain injuries among Native Americans and women. *Brain Injury, 29*(5), 639–643.

Liu, C. Y., & Apuzzo, M. L. (2003). The genesis of neurosurgery and the evolution of the neurosurgical operative environment: Part I—Prehistory to 2003. *Neurosurgery, 52*(1), 3–19.

Lovell, N. C. (1997). Trauma analysis in paleopathology. *Yearbook of Physical Anthropology, 40*, 139–170.

Löwen, H. (1997). Ein neurochirurgischer Eingriff an einem Schädel aus dem Grossteingrab Warburg IV, Kreis Höxter. Archäologische Beitraöge zur Geschichte Westfa- lens; 73–76.

Mantha, A. (2009). Territoriality, social boundaries and ancestor veneration in the central Andes of Peru. *Journal of Anthropological Archaeology, 28*(2), 158–176.

McKee, A. C., Cantu, R. C., Nowinski, C. J., Hedley-Whyte, E. T., Gavett, B. E., Budson, A. E., et al. (2009). Chronic traumatic encephalopathy in athletes: Progressive tauopathy following repetitive head injury. *Journal of Neuropathology and Experimental Neurology, 68*(7), 709–718.

Nystrom, K. C. (2007). Trepanation in the Chachapoya region of northern Perú. *International Journal of Osteoarchaeology, 17*(1), 39–51.

Sainsbury, C. P., & Sibert, J. R. (1984). How long do we need to observe head injuries in hospital? *Archives of Disease in Childhood, 59*(9), 856–859.

Torres-Rouff, C. (2002). Cranial vault modification and ethnicity in Middle Horizon San Pedro de Atacama, Chile1. *Current Anthropology, 43*(1), 163–171.

Toyne, J. M. (2015). Tibial surgery in ancient Peru. *International Journal of Paleopathology, 8*, 29–35.

Valente, S. M., & Fisher, D. (2011). Traumatic brain injury. *The Journal for Nurse Practitioners, 7*(10), 863–870.

Verano, J. W. (2003). Trepanation in prehistoric South America: Geographic and tem- poral trends over 2000 years. In R. Arnott, S. Finger, & C. U. M. Smith (Eds.), *Trepanation: History, discovery theory* (pp. 223–236). Lisse: Swets and Zietlinger.

Vitaz, T. W., Jenks, J., Raque, G. H., & Shields, C. B. (2003). Outcome following moderate traumatic brain injury. *Surgical Neurology, 60*, 285–291.

Weber, J., & Czarnetzki, A. (2001). Trepanations from the early medieval period of southwestern Germany—Indications, complications and outcome. *Zentralblatt für Neurochirurgie, 62*(1), 10–14.

Weber, J., & Wahl, J. (2006). Neurosurgical aspects of trepanations from Neolithic times. *International Journal of Osteoarchaeology, 16*(6), 536–545.

Part II
New Directions for Bioarchaeology of Care Research

Chapter 10
Mummy Studies and the Soft Tissue Evidence of Care

Kenneth Nystrom and Dario Piombino-Mascali

Introduction

In a series of articles, Lorna Tilley and colleagues (Tilley, 2015; Tilley & Cameron, 2014; Tilley & Oxenham, 2011) introduced an analytical framework through which researchers can attempt to estimate the level of care or accommodation an individual may have required based on the presence of paleopathological evidence. Tilley and Oxenham (2011, p. 36) discuss two broad circumstances in which skeletal and/or mummified remains could provide evidence of care: (1) long-term survival with disability "rendering functional independence impossible" and (2) healed/healing trauma or illness that would have necessitated intervention or care to ensure recovery and survival. These reflect relatively serious and potentially disabling diseases that manifest in the skeleton and thus would presumably provide the clearest opportunity to observe care in the bioarchaeological record. As the diagnosis of pathological conditions based on skeletal material is hampered by bone's limited ability to respond to pathogens, the analysis of mummified soft tissue, as well as other sources of data commonly associated with mummified remains, such as coprolites and intestinal contents, has the potential to provide valuable insight into this aspect of human behavior.

K. Nystrom, Ph.D. (✉)
Department of Anthropology, State University of New York at New Paltz,
New Paltz, NY, USA
e-mail: nystromk@newpaltz.edu

D. Piombino-Mascali, Ph.D.
Department of Cultural Heritage and Sicilian Identity, Sicilian Region, Palermo, Italy

© Springer International Publishing Switzerland 2017

L. Tilley, A.A. Schrenk (eds.), *New Developments in the Bioarchaeology of Care*, Bioarchaeology and Social Theory, DOI 10.1007/978-3-319-39901-0_10

The goal of this chapter, therefore, is to consider how the field of mummy studies may contribute to this effort. The following discussion will focus on three areas where mummy researchers have most explicitly considered some aspects of intervention and care: surgical intervention, therapeutic tattooing, and the use of medicinal plants. To date, while there is a disciplinary focus on the reconstruction of health, differential diagnosis, and epidemiology, the field has not truly engaged with the human and societal response to disease. The hope is that through synthesis and critical evaluation further research will be stimulated in this area, as these behaviors may "reflect some of the most fundamental aspects of a culture" (Tilley & Oxenham, 2011, p. 35) and thus can provide a more holistic perspective on health and disease in the past.

Surgical Intervention

The most common forms of ante- or perimortem surgical procedures that leave traces on the bone include trepanation (e.g., Jolly and Kurin, Chap. 9 this volume; O'Donnabháin, 2003; Toyne, 2015) and amputation (e.g., Dupras et al., 2010; Owsley, 1995; Verano, Anderson, & Franco, 2000). Both have long been recognized as forms of surgical intervention and treatment in traumatic and life-threatening situations (see Clower & Finger, 2001 and Kirkup, 2007 for discussions of the history of these procedures).

There are some examples of this type of skeletal evidence in mummified remains where the authors have suggested that the procedure was conducted as a form of treatment. In their examination of the mummified remains of a young adult male from the Rimac Valley of coastal Peru, Zimmerman et al. (1981, p. 499) observed several partially healed cranial fractures and a trepanation that "may have been done in an effort to relieve the effects of a new fracture…" Further, the researchers recovered a small twig within the cranium that possibly belonged to a genus of plants that has antibacterial properties; the authors suggest that "the twig might be interpreted as a post-trephination medicinal agent, perhaps used as a dressing during life…" (Zimmerman et al., 1981, p. 499). In their discussion of evidence for the intra-vital amputation of the big toe of a 21st/22nd Dynasty Egyptian mummy, Nerlich and colleagues (2000) suggest that the motivation for the procedure may have ischemic gangrene.

The latter study is particularly pertinent for our discussion because of the amount of information available regarding Egyptian medical practices, the extent and sophistication of which is well established based on the Medical Papyri (Aboelsoud, 2010; Campbell, 2008; David, 2008). Despite this level of documentary evidence, in addition to the number of publications that discuss the existence of various surgical practices (e.g., Barr, 2014; Ascaso, Lizana, & Cristóbal, 2009; see Blomstedt, 2013, 2014a, 2014b for counterargument), the investigation of human remains "have provided scant evidence regarding medical practices and treatment" (David, 2008, p. 181). Indeed, Rowling (1989) states that out of the 30,000 Egyptian mummies that have been reported in the literature there is not a single example of antemortem surgery.

Therapeutic Tattooing

Skin is composed of two primary layers: the dermis, which consists principally of collagen, and the epidermis, which is composed of epithelial cells. The latter will usually decompose rapidly, though it is occasionally observed in mummified remains (e.g., Cersoy, Richardin, Walter, & Brunelle, 2012; Chang et al., 2006). The high collagen content of the dermis, however, makes it much more resistant to decay. In some instances preservation of the skin has allowed researchers to identify the presence of tattoos (see Deter-Wolf, Robitaille, Krutak, & Galliot, 2016 for a list of sites where tattoos have been reported). The discussion of tattoos has been structured by the interpretation of function, with a division established between communicative/symbolic and therapeutic tattoos. Function is inferred based on the design elements of the tattoo and its visibility. Communicative or symbolic tattoos are representational or abstract in form, depicting animals or geometric shapes, and are located such that they would have been visible during life. Tattoos that are not representational, often consisting of simpler dots and/or dashes located in areas of the body that would not be visible are, almost by default, considered to be therapeutic in nature. This functional interpretative framework was established very early on in the literature and continues to structure current research and interpretation.

In his publication on the Pazyryk mummies from Siberia, Rudenko (1970) differentiates between the elaborate animal tattooing on the arms and legs of the Pazyryk individual from barrow two and the two rows of "disks" that run parallel to the vertebral column (Fig. 10.1). Rudenko concludes, citing ethnographic data and personal observation, that the latter "were probably put there with a therapeutic aim" (Rudenko, 1970, p. 112).

Very early in the research on Ötzi the Tyrolean Iceman (Fig. 10.2), the presence of tattoos was linked to a noncommunicative, therapeutic function.

> *In the Val Senales mummy, the pigmented marks are located in regions of the body that would normally have been covered (back, knee, ankle). This would exclude a 'communicative' function for these tattoos...In our case, the pigmented marks on the skin are geometric, without curved segments, are simple, and contain neither anthropomorphic nor zoomorphic motifs. This allows us to rule out an ornamental function for the tattoos found on the Val Senales mummy* (Capasso, 1993, pp. 179–180).

Dorfer and colleagues (1999, p. 1023) conclude that Ötzi's tattoos "do not seem to have decorative importance because they have a simple linear geometric shape and are located on the less visible parts of the body." These functional assumptions have structured nearly all of the subsequent work on Ötzi's tattoos, as well as influencing this type of investigation in other mummies as well.

Capasso (1993, p. 181) also concluded that there was a "generalized correspondence between the locations of the tattoos and joints" and that Ötzi's tattoos were applied for therapeutic reasons. Over twenty years later, Kean and Kean (2014) identify what they consider to be a narrowing of the discs between L4/L5 and L5/S1, with L5 assuming a transitional position. Based on this, Kean and Kean (2014, p. 13) conclude that "[t]he right and left lower lumbar tattoos correspond to sites of lower lumbar mechanical back pain possibly related to the disc narrowing at L4/5 and L5/S1, and local nerve root irritation …."

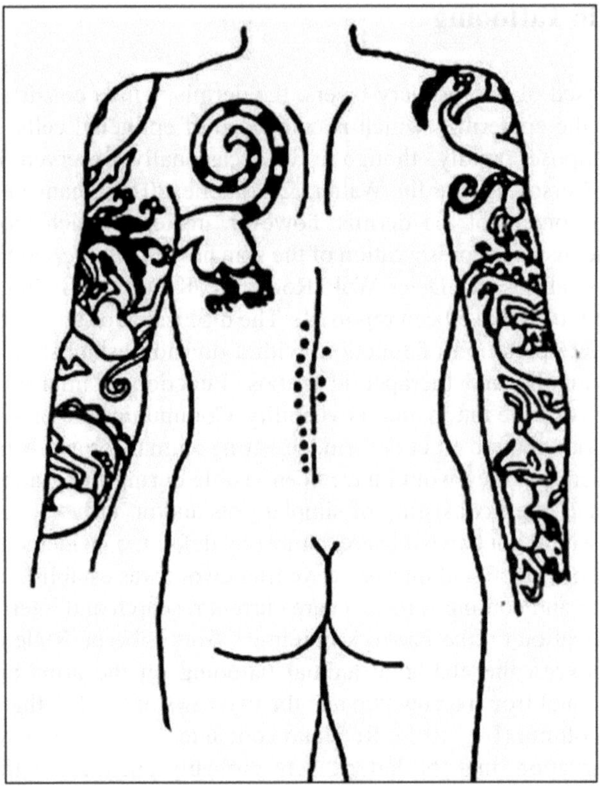

Fig. 10.1 Posterior view of the tattoos observed on the Pazyryk male mummy from barrow 2 (Adapted from Argent, 2013)

Even in instances in which tattoos are not located near joints, or where there is no evidence of osteoarthritic development, a therapeutic function is still offered. For instance, Dorfer et al. (1999) suggest several of the tattoos on Ötzi's right and left legs are associated with known acupuncture points for the gallbladder, spleen, or liver that are used by modern practitioners to treat abdominal disorders. Referring to these same tattoos, Kean and Kean (2014, p. 13) suggest that these may "correspond to possible sites of sciatic nerve referred pain." Samadelli, Melis, Miccoli, Vigl, and Zink (2015) recently identified new tattoos on Ötzi's chest, and suggest that these may be related to chest pain due to gallstones, atherosclerosis, and whipworm infection. There are also parts of Ötzi's body where researchers have observed musculoskeletal damage related to injury or osteoarthritic development, but where there are no tattoos; these include the cervical and lumbar vertebra, right sacroiliac joint and pubic symphysis, right hip, fractured ribs, and left little toe (Murphy et al., 2003). Kean and Kean (2014) suggest that these locations may not have resulted in significant pain or may have been asymptomatic.

In their description of a Chiribaya mummy, Pabst and colleagues (2010, p. 3257) differentiate between two different types of tattoos: ornamental tattoos that "[represent] birds, apes, reptiles, and symbols" and a series of overlapping circles on the

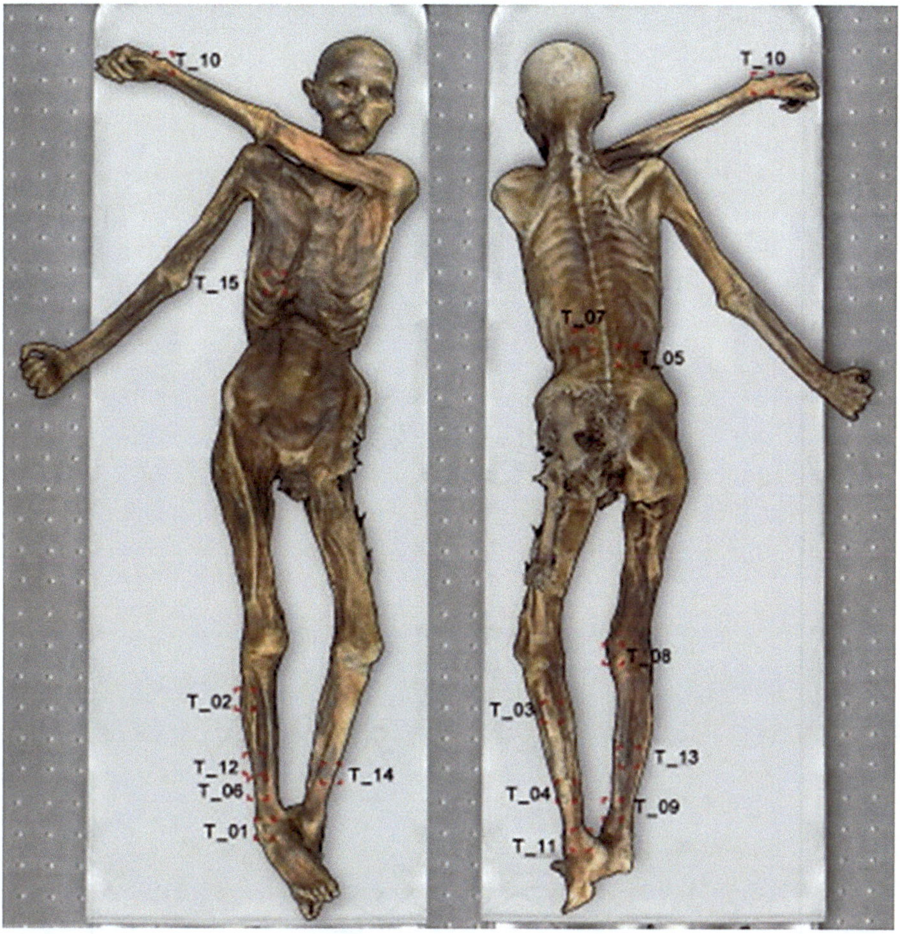

Fig. 10.2 The location of the tattoos on Ötzi. Reproduced from Samadelli et al. Complete mapping of the tattoos of the 5300-year-old Tyrolean Iceman. Journal of Cultural Heritage 2015; 16(5): 753–758. Copyright ©2015. Elsevier Masson SAS. All rights reserved

neck that are potentially therapeutic in function (Fig. 10.3). The latter are located on the posterior of the neck and thus "would have been hidden by the neck hairs and the clothing during the lifetime of the bearer" (Pabst et al., 2010, p. 3257).

Pabst and colleagues (2010, p. 3262) note that the location of the tattoos on the neck corresponds to meridians identified in Chinese acupuncture, and conclude that in relation to "the possible medical intention lying behind the circle tattoos, we assume local problems of the upper spine or headaches as possible reasons for treatment by the tattooing." The connection to Chinese acupuncture reflects previous statements that have been advanced to explain the location of the tattoos observed on Ötzi, as well (Dorfer et al., 1999). However, there is no CT or X-ray data presented by Pabst and colleagues which would indicate the presence of any pathological or degenerative process in the neck region that may have necessitated the application of a therapeutic tattoo.

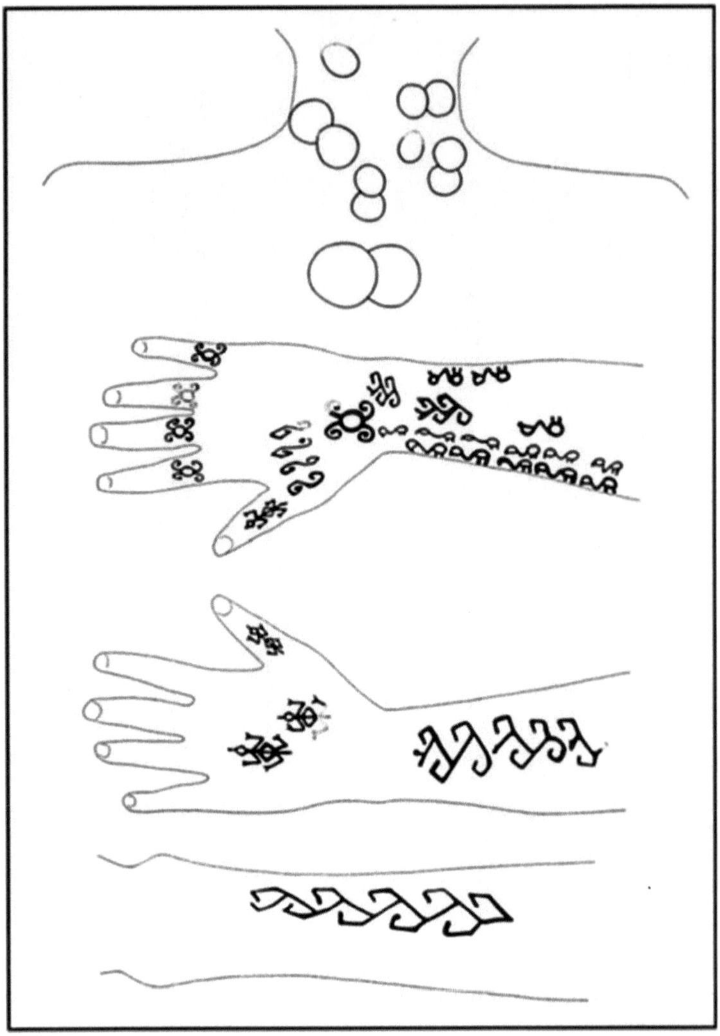

Fig. 10.3 Representation of the tattoos examined by Pabst et al. (2010). Reprinted from Journal of Archaeological Science, 37, Pabst et al., Different staining substances were used in decorative and therapeutic tattoos in a 1000-year-old Peruvian mummy, 3256–3262, Copyright (2010), with permission from Elsevier

Medicinal Plants

In the mummy studies literature, the use of plants with medicinal properties has been linked to pain management, the treatment of parasitic infection, and possibly to combat cancer. The following examples come from a range of time periods and cultural contexts, and the data are derived from both microscopic and biochemical assays of coprolites, intestinal contents, hair, and/or soft tissue. In all instances, the authors articulate the presence of plant material or its metabolites as "medicine" or "therapy," and are therefore, at least implicitly, discussing evidence of care.

Beginning in the early 1990s, several researchers started testing hair samples from South American mummies for the presence of cocaine or its metabolite benzoylecgonine (BZE). Cartmell and colleagues (1991) analyzed the hair of 163 individuals from a number of different cultural phases in northern Chile spanning some 4500 years' worth of time, and found that 76 (46.6 %) tested positive for the presence of BZE. A decade later, Cartmell and colleagues (2001) reported the results of testing soft tissue samples from some of the same mummies.

The analysis of hair provides a longer term record of coca-use, while the higher turnover rate of most soft tissues means that presence of BZE indicates ingestion occurred closer to the time of death, reflecting what Cartmell and colleagues (2001, p. 80) consider "acute exposure."

The researchers conclude that the detection of high levels of cocaine in soft tissue samples taken from infants is the result of acute exposure and reflects the use of a coca-leaf tea as a form of "therapeutic treatment" (Cartmell, Aufderheide, Lorentz, Wittmers, & Weems, 2001, p. 80). Among adult females high levels of cocaine in soft tissue samples, in combination with low levels of cocaine in hair, are also interpreted as evidence of drinking coca-leaf tea for medicinal purposes. Similarly, Rivera and colleagues (2005, p. 458) suggest that the detection of cocaine metabolites in the hair of a 3- to 4-year-old child from the site of Pisagua-7 (3000–1450 BP) in northern Chile is most likely due to "coca leaf tea administered as a therapeutic agent to combat what proved to be her terminal illness."

Hair from mummies has also been used to consider the medicinal use of ayahuasca. As commonly known, ayahuasca is a hallucinogenic drink derived from a mixture of the plants *Banisteriopsis caapi* and *Psychotria viridis* (Luna, 2011). When ingested independently, the hallucinogenic alkaloids (*N*, *N*-dimethyltryptamine or DMT) in *Psychotria* are normally inactivated by enzymes in the stomach. The ingestion of *Banisteriopsis*, which contains harmine, inhibits this enzymatic activity and thus facilitates the metabolism of DMT. Ogalde, Arriaza, and Soto (2009) analyzed hair samples from 32 mummies from the Azapa Valley of Chile dating to the middle Tiwanaku period, testing for evidence of *Banisteriopsis caapi* consumption. The authors detected the presence of harmine, but not DMT, leading them to conclude that "the consumption of *Banisteriopsis* was part of a medicinal practice, perhaps as Ayahuasca infusion" (Ogalde et al., 2009, p. 471).[1]

[1] While ayahuasca is a term that is commonly applied to both the hallucinogenic drink and the *Banisteriopsis* plant from which it is partially derived, the term is perhaps best reserved just for the drink. Luna (2011) refers to the plant and the preparation made solely from it as *caapi* (Luna, 2011). Based on this nomenclature, the detection of harmine by Ogalde and colleagues (2009) in mummified remains, coupled with the absence of DMT, would point to the drinking of *caapi* rather than the hallucinogenic drink ayahuasca.

The Egyptian Medical Papyri provide information on pharmacology and herbal medicine, and while several authors (Aboelsoud, 2010; Campbell, 2008; Counsell, 2008) discuss evidence for drug use in Egypt, there is very little evidence from human remains that directly speaks to the therapeutic use of these substances. In 1995, Nerlich and colleagues (1995) report histochemical findings from a 21st Dynasty Egyptian mummy that indicate extensive depositions of hemosiderin within collapsed, but otherwise normal, lung tissue. While the authors run through a differential diagnosis that includes chronic pulmonary hypertension, pulmonary parasitosis, pulmonary arteriosclerosis, trauma, mycobacterial infection, and vasculitis, ultimately they could only conclude the "patient suffered from possibly recurrent pulmonary bleeding during life" (Nerlich, Wiest, Löhrs, Parsche, & Schramel, 1995:427). The authors tested several tissue samples from the skin, bone, tendon, liver, lung, stomach, and intestines for the presence of nicotine, cocaine, and delta-9-tetrahydrocannabinol (THC) and/or its metabolites. Based on the differential concentration levels in these sample tissues, the authors suggest that the nicotine and cocaine were ingested, while the THC was inhaled, and conclude that the presence of these drugs "provides evidence that multidrug therapy was given to relieve his pain" (Nerlich et al., 1995, p. 428).

Paleoparasitological research on mummies has clearly and convincingly demonstrated that we have had a long history with a variety of ecto- and endoparasites (Lee, Shin, & Seo, 2011; Reinhard & Buikstra, 2003; Searcey et al., 2013). Some researchers have also discussed evidence that may indicate attempts to treat parasitic infection. Aspöck and colleagues (1996) identified *Trichuris trichiura* (whipworm) eggs in samples taken from Ötzi's colon. Among Ötzi's possessions were the fruit of the bracket fungus *Piptoporus betulinus*, which Capasso (1998, p. 1864) describes as containing "toxic resins and an active compound, agaric acid, which are powerful purgatives and result in strong though short-lived bouts of diarrhea. *Piptoporus betulinus* also contains oils that are toxic to metazoans and have antibiotic properties, acting against mycobacteria." This leads Capasso to conclude that Ötzi was carrying the fungus to combat the *Trichuris* infection. Several authors were quick to point out that Capasso was incorrect in his description of *P. betulinus*' medicinal properties (Peintner, Pöder, & Pümpel, 1998; Pöder & Peintner, 1999; Tunón & Svanberg, 1999), with Pöder (2005, p. 358) ultimately concluding that researchers "have to admit that we simply do not know the Ice Man's intentions concerning these mushrooms."

Additionally, results of microbotanical analyses of gut samples taken from Ötzi have been interpreted as indicating the intentional consumption of the bracken *Pteridium aquilinum* (Oeggl, Kofler, & Schmid, 2005). Oeggl and colleagues (2005) conclude that the bracken was most likely used as an anthelmintic, in light of the results reported above on the presence of human whipworm eggs in Ötzi's colon.

There is a large body of literature on the paleopathological analysis of historic Italian mummies (e.g., Fornaciari, 1999; Piombino-Mascali et al., 2015), in several of which it may be possible to infer or observe evidence of care. In their investigation of the mummified remains of Mary of Aragon (1503–1568) Gino Fornaciari and colleagues (1989) noted the presence of a small ulcerous lesion wrapped by a

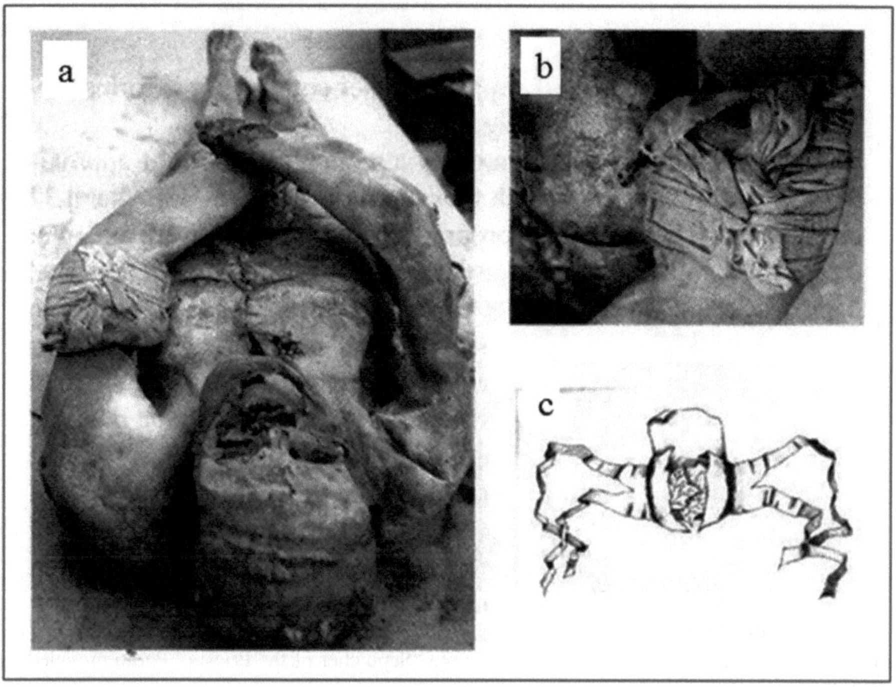

Fig. 10.4 The mummified remains of Mary of Aragon with (**a**) a bandage on her proximal left arm, (**b**) close-up of the bandage, and (**c**) graphic depiction of the bandage with ivy leaves contained within small internal pocket. Figure modified from Giuffra et al. (2008, p. 171)

bandage on her proximal left arm (Fig. 10.4). Contained within a small pocket on the underside of the bandage were ivy leaves, while inside the lesion itself was a small round mass that, when analyzed, was found to consist of sulfur. Historical sources indicate ivy could be used to purify, desiccate, and stimulate the regeneration of flesh, while sulfur has "the virtue of healing moderately; it conglutinates and consolidates the ulcers and sores, and it rapidly and marvelously recreates the flesh" (Giuffra, Marinozzi, Vultaggio, & Fornaciari, 2008, p. 178).

Expanded Case Study: Piraino 1

The following case study is presented in slightly greater detail than preceding examples in an effort to demonstrate how the confluence of multiple data sources can be considered within the context of care. As part of the Sicily Mummy Project, Kumm, Reinhard, Piombino-Mascali, and Araújo (2010) and Piombino-Mascali et al. (2013) examined the mummified remains of 26 individuals dating to approximately the late eighteenth to mid-nineteenth century AD from the Piraino Mother Church

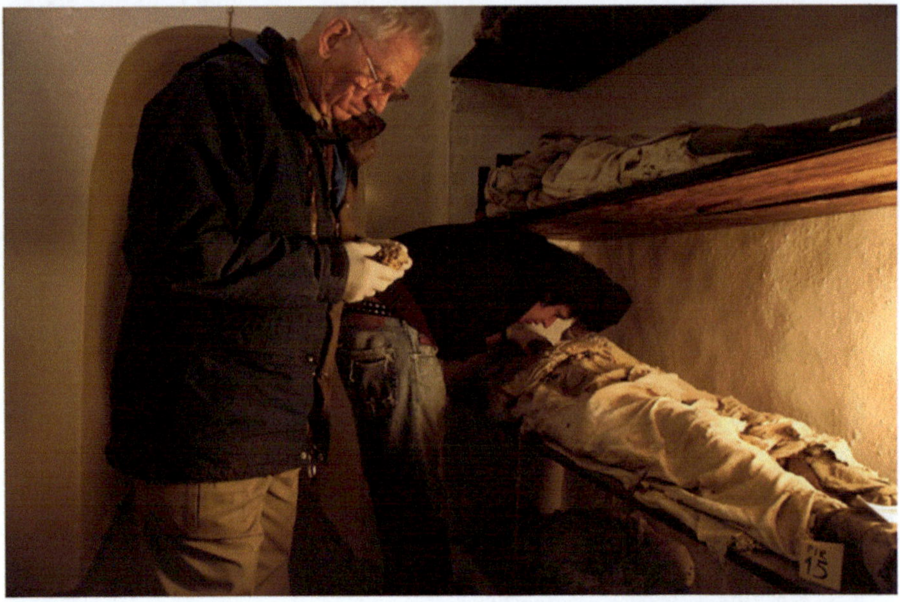

Fig. 10.5 Arthur Aufderheide (*left*) and Dario Piombino-Mascali (*right*) examining one of the mummies from the Piraino Mother Church in the "Sepulcher of the Priests." Photo provided by second author

in the province of Messina, Sicily (Fig. 10.5). In particular, multiple lines of evidence observed in the individual identified as Piraino 1, an adult male, point to several different pathological conditions that would likely have necessitated some degree of care in order to ensure survival and continued functioning.

Multiple small osteolytic changes were noted on the skull, the right distal humerus, the left proximal humerus, the right pubic bone, and possibly on the distal part of the right scapula of Piraino 1. Chest radiographs revealed distinct osteolytic lesions, with fracture of the second and fifth rib, an expansive osteolytic lesion of the eighth rib, and small osteolytic lesions of the ninth and tenth rib in the left hemithorax. Possible osteolytic changes were observed in the fifth and sixth rib of the right hemithorax, while the fourth and seventh rib exhibited fractures without the presence of osteolytic changes. Both proximal femora exhibited a distinct nonhomogeneous bone structure with possible small osteolytic changes. There was no evidence of any osteoblastic activity.

The described osteolytic changes are compatible with the diagnosis of multiple myeloma or skeletal metastases. Multiple myeloma, also called plasma cell myeloma, is a malignant neoplastic proliferation of the plasma cells in the bone marrow and is the most common primary malignant bone tumor. Skeletal metastases are the most common secondary bone tumor. They can be classified as purely osteolytic, purely osteosclerotic, and mixed osteolytic-osteosclerotic (Ortner, 2003). A differential diagnosis between multiple myeloma and the lytic form of metastatic carcinoma is difficult. Both processes affect the same age group (older age group, particularly after the age of 50 years) and involve essentially the same areas of the skeleton, which are the vertebral column, the ribs, the pelvis, the skull, and the proximal femur and humerus (Chhem & Brothwell, 2008; Resnick, 2002; Steinbock, 1976). In Piraino 1, osteolytic changes in the skull, the ribs, the humeri, and the pelvis were clearly seen. The second and fifth ribs on the left side exhibit antemortem fractures. An adequate evaluation of the spine, which might have enabled possible discrimination between multiple myeloma and skeletal metastases, was not possible. Based particularly on the involvement of the skull, the lack of new bone formation, and the punched-out character of the lesions, the authors favored the diagnosis of multiple myeloma.

Symptoms associated with multiple myeloma include constipation, nausea, bone pain particularly centered in the chest and back, loss of appetite, and increased susceptibility to infection. Renal failure and pathological fractures are also commonly associated with the disease. Prognosis is grim as the disease is progressive and ultimately incurable, and before the introduction of alkylating agents and chemotherapy median survival was less than 1 year (Kumar et al., 2008).

In addition to this, paleoparasitological analysis of coprolites recovered from Piraino 1's viscera recorded a very high concentration of *Trichuris trichiura* eggs (Kumm et al., 2010). Further, investigation of the body revealed evidence of several disease processes, including degenerative joint disease in the spine and pleural adhesions possibly resulting from pneumonia.

Evidence that Piraino 1 was receiving some form of health care is based on palynological and macrobotanical analyses. Palynological analysis of the coprolites indicated the presence of several plant residues, which Piombino-Mascali and colleagues (2013) suggest may have had medicinal functions. The pollen spectrum was dominated by Polygalaceae, the Milkwort Family. Based on comparison to published keys, it was determined that the pollen came from a species of *Polygala.* The absence of plant parts attributable to the *Polygala* species indicates that the pollen was not eaten with food, but was most likely imbibed as an infusion derived from foliage or flowers (Chaves & Reinhard, 2006; Reinhard, Hamilton, & Hevly, 1991). Of the species in the *P. vulgaris* type, *P. vulgaris* itself was used as a medicinal tea in Turkey for several purposes, including as an expectorant and as treatment for lung problems (Johnson, 1999), and it also contains antitumor cytotoxic compounds (Dall'Acqua et al., 2002).

The macrobotanical remains from a succulent fruit with a yellowish pulp and peel of a Rosaceae were found, most likely belonging to the *Prunus* sp., which includes peaches, plums, cherries, and apricots. Members of this genus are an effective laxative and stomachic, while the bark can be used as a febrifuge. They also contain amygdalin and prunasin, which break down in water to form hydrocyanic acid (cyanide or prussic acid) and in small amounts can stimulate respiration, improve digestion, and promote a sense of well-being (Bown, 1995; Chiej, 1984; Grieve, 1971). Their antioxidant and anticancer properties have recently been described (Jabeen & Aslam, 2011).

The grape residues of seeds, fruit skin, and pedicles are more difficult to interpret. It appears that these were crushed, and may therefore be by-products of juice production. The general antioxidant properties of skin and seeds have been well defined (Vitseva, Varghese, Chakrabarti, Folts, & Freedman, 2005), while flavonoids found in fruit skin and seeds are useful in treating some cancers and cardiovascular disease (Yilmaz & Toledo, 2004).

In sum, the example of Piraino 1 provides an excellent example of how the analysis of mummified soft and hard tissue, as well as data sources often encountered with mummy remains (e.g., gut contents), can be mobilized to discuss evidence of care. By considering the known prognosis and symptoms associated with multiple myeloma, as well as modern research on the medical properties of various plants, researchers have the potential to examine the cultural context of living with, and treating, a terminal illness.

Discussion

Efforts to reconstruct evidence of care, accommodation, disability, and social stigma associated with disease have so far been exclusively based on the analysis of skeletal material (e.g., Knüsel, 1999; Marsteller, Torres-Rouff, & Knudson, 2011; Roberts, 1999, 2011; Tilley, 2015; Tilley & Oxenham, 2011); indeed, this chapter is the only contribution to the current volume that considers soft tissue. As the diagnosis of pathological conditions based on skeletal material is hampered by bone's limited ability to respond to pathogens, the analysis of mummified soft tissue has great potential to contribute to the discussion of care and provisioning in the past.

This potential, of course, has to be tempered by the fact that soft tissue is much more susceptible to postmortem taphonomic changes than osseous tissue. As the rate of decomposition is influenced by the metabolic activity of the tissue, tissues such as epithelial, heart muscle, and cells that have secretory/absorption functions, decay more quickly than connective tissues such as collagen and cartilage. Organs such as the liver and kidneys decay rapidly, while such seemingly delicate structures as the lungs are commonly well preserved (Aufderheide 2003). Therefore, while the preservation of soft tissue offers the promise of identifying a wider range of pathological conditions, and by extension more opportunities to infer the presence of care or accommodation, caution must be exercised.

Up to this time, research in soft tissue paleopathology has been more focused on detection and diagnoses, and while advances in biomedical imaging and molecular analyses have facilitated the diagnosis of a wider range of pathological conditions, the discussion of what level of care or provisioning an individual may have required in order to live with a particular condition has been limited. It is interesting that, despite the fact that mummies have been characterized as "deceased patients" (Dageförde, Vennemann, & Rühli, 2014, p. 214), the antemortem care that the individual may have received has not been addressed; the analytic focus is on the disease process itself and not on the individual, culturally contingent disease/health experience.

The most explicit engagement with evidence that could be considered associated with health care has been in the discussion of surgical intervention, therapeutic tattooing, and the use of medicinal plants. In truth, evidence in the first category is limited to surgical procedures that affect bone, such as trepanation and amputation, and is well documented in both skeletonized and mummified remains. These procedures reflect relatively extreme, life-or-death circumstances, while other less acute forms of surgical intervention such as cataract surgery, circumcision, blood-letting, and suturing have not been documented in mummy research. It is difficult to imagine circumstances, even given the number of examples in the literature where soft tissue preservation is exceptional, where it might be possible to observe such evidence. In light of the structural changes in the epidermis and dermis associated with decomposition, evidence for healing of an antemortem surgical incision would likely be quite ephemeral and difficult to identify.

Discussion of the potential therapeutic function of tattoos has been structured by two factors: the perceived complexity of the tattoos, and their location. Ethnographic descriptions of the therapeutic benefits of tattoos have been documented among modern groups, with Krutak (2013) providing examples from a number of different regions including the St. Lawrence Island Yupiget, native Greenlanders, the Ainu, Aleuts/Unangan in Alaska, and the Chippewa of the Great Lakes area in North America. Krutak notes similarities in location (often at major joints) and form (small series of dots, incised lines) between these ethnographic examples and the tattoos that have been observed on the Pazyryk burials, Ötzi, and others. It is certainly possible that some tattoos observed on mummified remains were therapeutic in nature. What is of concern, however, is that the categorization of tattoos as either decorative or therapeutic has been fairly simplistic, based on culturally laden concepts of what constitutes decorative and communicative versus non-decorative. Therefore it is argued that a more holistic approach to tattoos would consider what the function of the tattoos is likely to have been in their particular context.

As an example, and specifically referencing the Chiribaya mummy examined by Pabst and colleagues (2010), it is worthwhile engaging more deeply with the significance of the tattoos by contextualizing them in relation to what is known about the body, its metaphorical linkages with the physical landscape, and cosmology in Andean groups. Akin to the reconstruction of sickness ideology (Marsteller et al., 2011), it is possible to describe a general "body ideology" in Andean prehistory. Among the Kallawayan healers of Bolivia, Bastien (1978) describes how the components of the body are mapped onto geography; the head is the mountain peak, while the trunk and legs are the central and lower slopes of the mountain. The villages that comprise the communities and the human body are linked by water and blood flow. Considering the potential time depth of the body-mountain metaphor (Bastien, 1978), it may be possible to provide a more holistic discussion of the location and possible function of the tattoos based upon archaeological and bioarchaeological knowledge of the Chiribaya and the metaphorical connections between the geographical and cosmological landscape and the body.

Further, the notion that sickness results from some internal physiological disruption is grounded in the Western conception of health. Among the Kaata, Bastien (1978, p. 129) reports that sickness was considered to be a "malfunctioning of the social and ecological order." As the mountain and the body are intimately linked, sickness in one reflects sickness in the other. In the case of the Kaata, sickness was often linked to land disputes, and healers therefore sought to redress the underlying conflict to effect a cure. While this is necessarily a bit speculative, the point remains that we cannot limit ourselves to simplistic divisions between what is decorative and what is therapeutic, nor approach sickness from the Western tradition as something exclusively internally generated.

The preservation of stomach and gut contents in mummified remains offers unique opportunities to investigate a wide range of research questions, including dietary reconstruction (Reinhard, LeRoy-Toren, & Arriaza, 2011), parasitic infection (Seo, Araujo, Reinhard, Chai, & Shin, 2014), and even daily mobility (Oeggl et al., 2007). The isolation and identification of macro- and microbotanicals from gut contents has led a number of researchers to suggest that certain plants were ingested as a form of medical treatment. These interpretations are based on known medicinal properties and/or the fact that the plant in question is not a standard food item. For instance, based on the quantity of bracken (*Pteridium aquilinum*) spores detected in samples taken from Ötzi's gut Oeggl and colleagues (2005) suggest it is likely he ingested the fronds, which the authors propose may have been used to treat indigestion. Similarly, palynological analysis of a coprolite from Piraino 1 revealed the presence of several plants with documented medicinal properties (Piombino-Mascali et al., 2013). It is crucial in such instances to demonstrate that the plant matter has been intentionally introduced as some form of medicine or treatment. For example, in their discussion Piombino-Mascali and colleagues go to great pains to demonstrate that the pollen that they suggest indicates medicinal use of certain plants could not have been part of the pollen rain which is naturally present in the environment.

While the chemical analysis of hair facilitates the reconstruction of diet (Turner et al., 2013), mobility (Knudson, Pestle, Torres-Rouff, & Pimentel, 2012), exposure to environmental toxins (Byrne et al., 2010, and short-term systemic physiological stress (Webb et al., 2010), it can also register the ingestion, inhalation, or imbibing of nonfood items. In the South American Andes, researchers have identified evidence that indicates the use of coca-leaves and ayahuasca, and in some instances have suggested that their administration was therapeutic in nature. In the cases discussed above, it is important to note that the authors do not report any evidence of pathology that may have required or necessitated the administration of medicine.

Both coca-leaves and ayahuasca are known to have medicinal or therapeutic properties. Coca-leaves (*Erythroxylum* sp.) have been used to treat dysentery, indigestion, cramps, diarrhea, toothaches, and rheumatism (Martin, 1970; Plowman, 1986). While ayahuasca is used by Amazonian groups to diagnose illness and to combat the agents responsible for sending the sickness (Luna, 2011; Schultes & Hofmann, 1980), researchers are exploring its efficacy in treating depression (de Lima et al., 2011; Palhano-Fontes et al., 2014; Santos, Landeira-Fernandez, Strassman, Motta, & Cruz, 2007). Ethnohistoric and ethnographic literature provides considerable insight into the role that coca-leaves and ayahuasca play in society (e.g., Allen, 2002; Schultes, 1982). Coupled with the reconstruction of Andean sickness ideology, "the shared system of ideas and beliefs associated with disease and illness" (Marsteller et al., 2011, p. 26), there is fertile ground for discussing prehistoric evidence of care – even in the absence of gross pathology.

Conclusion

To date, engagement with evidence of health care in mummy studies has been limited. The goal of this chapter, therefore, has been to synthesize and critically evaluate how researchers in mummy studies have engaged with this aspect of paleopathology, in the hope that it will stimulate further research in this area. It is our opinion that the reconstruction of health care represents a significant and worthwhile avenue of investigation, one that will complement current foci in the field while fostering a more holistic approach to the investigation of prehistoric disease.

This also speaks to a broader issue that may be facing mummy studies. Arthur Aufderheide (2013, p. 134) once cautioned that the continued vitality of the field necessitated finding a disciplinary home:

> *[i]t is possible but unlikely that the field of mummy studies will ever be large enough to be an independent scientific discipline. Thus, to survive and flourish, the field will need to join a related discipline* (Aufderheide, 2013, p. 134).

Mummy studies have always been deeply connected with the biomedical and natural sciences, and based on current publication trends there is evidence to suggest that this connection is becoming stronger. Alternatively, research that explicitly engages with archaeological data or social theory is less frequent. The investigation of care and accommodation is a prime example where the synergy between the disciplines can be accentuated. As advances in medical imaging and molecular analyses improve our ability to identify, diagnose, and discuss the evolution and impact of disease in the past, the reconstruction of health care can contribute significantly to our understanding of the human and cultural response to disease.

Acknowledgements The authors thank Alecia A. Schrenk and Lorna Tilley for organizing the 2015 Society for American Archaeology session where this material was originally presented. We also thank Stephanie Panzer and Karl Reinhard for all their work on the remains from the Piraino Mother Church. Lastly, the comments and suggestions of two external reviewers were very much appreciated and helped improve the focus of the chapter.

References

Aboelsoud, N. (2010). Herbal medicine in ancient Egypt. *Journal of Medicinal Plants Research, 4*, 82–86.
Allen, C. J. (2002). *The hold life has: Coca and cultural identity in an Andean community*. Washington: Smithsonian Institution.
Argent, G. (2013). Inked: Human-horse apprenticeship, tattoos, and time in the Pazyryk world. *Society and Animals, 21*(2), 178–193.
Ascaso, F. J., Lizana, J., & Cristóbal, J. A. (2009). Cataract surgery in ancient Egypt. *Journal of Cataract & Refractive Surgery, 35*(3), 607–608.
Aspöck, H., Auer, H., & Picher, O. (1996). Trichuris trichiura Eggs in the Neolithic Glacier Mummy from the Alps. *Parasitology Today, 12*(7), 255–256.
Aufderheide, A. C. (2003). *The scientific study of mummies*. Cambridge: Cambridge University Press.
Barr, J. (2014). Vascular medicine and surgery in ancient Egypt. *Journal of Vascular Surgery, 60*(1), 260–263.
Bastien, J. W. (1978). *Mountain of the Condor: Metaphor and ritual in an Andean Ayllu*. Illinois: Prospect Heights.
Blomstedt, P. (2013). Dental surgery in ancient Egypt. *Journal of the History of Dentistry, 61*(3), 129–142.
Blomstedt, P. (2014a). Orthopedic surgery in ancient Egypt. *Acta Orthopaedica, 85*(6), 670–676.
Blomstedt, P. (2014b). Cataract surgery in ancient Egypt. *Journal of Cataract & Refractive Surgery, 40*(3), 485–489.
Bown, D. (1995). *Encyclopaedia of herbs and their uses*. London: Dorling Kindersley.
Byrne, S., Amarasiriwardena, D., Bandak, B., Bartkus, L., Kane, J., Jones, J., et al. (2010). Were Chinchorros exposed to arsenic? Arsenic determination in Chinchorro mummies' hair by laser ablation inductively coupled plasma-mass spectrometry (LA-ICP-MS). *Microchemical Journal, 94*(1), 28–35.
Campbell, J. M. (2008). Pharmacy in ancient Egypt. In A. R. David (Ed.), *Egyptian mummies and modern science* (pp. 216–233). Cambridge: Cambridge University Press.
Capasso, L. (1993). A preliminary report on the tattoos of the Val Senales mummy (Tyrol, Neolithic). *Journal of Paleopathology, 5*, 173–182.
Capasso, L. (1998). 5300 years ago, the Ice Man used natural laxatives and antibiotics. *The Lancet, 352*(9143), 1864.
Cartmell L, Aufderheide AC, Lorentz, E., Wittmers, J., & Weems C. (2001). The predictive value of cocaine hair/visceral tissue ratios in Andean mummies—A pilot study. *Proceedings of the Fourth World Congress on Mummy Studies* (pp. 79–81). Nuuk, Greenland.
Cartmell, L. W., Aufderheide, A. C., & Weems, C. (1991). Cocaine metabolites in pre-Columbian mummy hair. *Journal of the Oklahoma State Medical Association, 84*, 11–12.
Cersoy, S., Richardin, P., Walter, P., & Brunelle, A. (2012). Cluster TOF-SIMS imaging of human skin remains: Analysis of a South-Andean mummy sample. *Journal of Mass Spectrometry, 47*, 338–346.
Chang, B. S., Uhm, C. S., Park, C. H., Kim, H. K., Lee, G. Y., Cho, H. H., et al. (2006). Preserved skin structure of a recently found fifteenth-century mummy in Daejeon, Korea. *Journal of Anatomy, 209*, 671–680.
Chaves, S., & Reinhard, K. J. (2006). Critical analysis of coprolite evidence of medicinal plant use, Piauí, Brazil. *Palaeogeography Palaeoclimatology Palaeoecology, 237*(1), 110–118.
Chhem, R. K., & Brothwell, D. R. (2008). *Paleoradiology: Imaging mummies and fossils*. Berlin: Springer.
Chiej, R. (1984). *Encyclopaedia of medicinal plants*. Edinburgh: MacDonald.
Clower, W. T., & Finger, S. (2001). Discovering trepanation: The contribution of Paul Broca. *Neurosurgery, 49*(6), 1417–1426.

Counsell, D. J. (2008). Intoxicants in ancient Egypt? opium, nymphaea, coca and tobacco. In A. R. David (Ed.), *Egytpian mummies and modern science* (pp. 195–215). Cambridge: Cambridge University Press.

Dageförde, K. L., Vennemann, M., & Rühli, F. J. (2014). Evidence based palaeopathology: Meta-analysis of Pubmed®-listed scientific studies on pre-Columbian, South American mummies. *HOMO Journal of Comparative Human Biology, 65*(3), 214–231.

Dall'Acqua, S., Innocenti, G., Viola, G., Piovan, A., Caniato, R., & Cappelletti, E. M. (2002). Cytotoxic compounds from Polygala vulgaris. *Chemical & Pharmaceutical Bulletin, 50*, 1499–1501.

David, A. R. (2008). The ancient Egyptian medical system. In A. R. David (Ed.), *Egyptian mummies and modern science* (pp. 181–194). Cambridge: Cambridge University Press.

de Lima, O. F., de Macedo, L. R. H., de Sousa, J. P. M., Pinto, J. P., Quevedo, J., de Souza Crippa, J. A., et al. (2011). The therapeutic potential of harmine and ayahuasca in depression: Evidence from exploratory animal and human studies. In R. G. dos Santos (Ed.), *The ethnopharmacology of ayahuasca* (pp. 75–85). Transworld Research Network: Trivandrum, India.

Deter-Wolf, A., Robitaille, B., Krutak, L., & Galliot, S. (2016). The world's oldest tattoos. *Journal of Archaeological Science: Reports, 5*, 19–24.

Dorfer, L., Moser, M., Bahr, F., Spindler, K., Egarter-Vigl, E., Guillén, S., et al. (1999). A medical report from the stone age? *The Lancet, 354*(9183), 1023–1025.

Dupras, T. L., Williams, L. J., De Meyer, M., Peeters, C., Depraetere, D., Vanthuyne, B., et al. (2010). Evidence of amputation as medical treatment in ancient Egypt. *International Journal of Osteoarchaeology, 20*(4), 405–423.

Fornaciari, G. (1999). Renaissance mummies in Italy. *Medicina nei Secoli, 11*, 85–105.

Fornaciari, G., Castagna, M., Tognetti, A., Tornaboni, D., & Bruno, J. (1989). Syphilis in a renaissance Italian mummy. *The Lancet, 8663*, 614.

Giuffra, V., Marinozzi, S., Vultaggio, C., & Fornaciari, G. (2008). A medical bandage in an Italian renaissance mummy (Naples, XVI century). *Medicina nei Secoli, 20*, 169–181.

Grieve, M. (1971). *A modern herbal: The medicinal, culinary, cosmetic and economic properties, cultivation and folk-lore of herbs, grasses, fungi, shrubs & trees with their modern scientific uses*. New York: Dover Publications.

Jabeen, Q., & Aslam, N. (2011). The pharmacological activities of prunes: The dried plums. *Journal of Medicinal Plant Research: Planta Medica, 5*(9), 1508–1511.

Johnson, T. (1999). *CRC ethnobotany desk reference*. Boca Raton: CRC Press.

Kean, W. F., & Kean, M. (2014). The mechanical back pain and leg neurosensory pain of the Similaun Iceman: Relationship to 'Medicinal' tattoos. *Yearbook of Mummy Studies, 2*, 7–14.

Kirkup, J. R. (2007). *A history of limb amputation*. London: Springer.

Knudson, K. J., Pestle, W. J., Torres-Rouff, C., & Pimentel, G. (2012). Assessing the life history of an Andean traveler through biogeochemistry: Stable and radiogenic isotope analyses of archaeological human remains from Northern Chile. *International Journal of Osteoarchaeology, 22*(4), 435–451.

Knüsel, C. (1999). Orthopaedic disability: Some hard evidence. *Archaeological Review from Cambridge, 15*(1), 31–53.

Krutak L. (2013). The power to cure: A brief history of therapeutic tattooing. In P. Della Casa & C. Witt (Eds.), *Tattoos and body modification in antiquity proceedings of the Sessions at the EAA annual meetings: Zurich studies in archaeology* (pp 27–34).

Kumar, S. K., Rajkumar, S. V., Dispenzieri, A., Lacy, M. Q., Hayman, S. R., Buadi, F. K., et al. (2008). Improved survival in multiple myeloma and the impact of novel therapies. *Blood, 111*(5), 2516–2520.

Kumm, K., Reinhard, K. J., Piombino-Mascali, D., & Araújo, A. (2010). Archaeoparasitological investigation of a mummy from Sicily (18th-19th century AD). *Anthropologie, 48*, 177–184.

Lee, H.-J., Shin, D.-H., & Seo, M. (2011). Discovery of Taeniid Eggs from a 17th Century Tomb in Korea. *Korean Journal of Parasitology, 49*(3), 327–329.

Luna, L. E. (2011). Indigenous and mestizo use of ayahuasca: An overview. In R. G. dos Santos (Ed.), *The ethnopharmacology of ayahuasca* (pp. 1–21). Trivandrum, India: Transworld Research Network.

Marsteller, S. J., Torres-Rouff, C., & Knudson, K. J. (2011). Pre-Columbian Andean Sickness Ideology and the social experience leishmaniasis: A contextualized analysis of bioarchaeological and paleopathological data from San Pedro de Atacama, Chile. *International Journal of Paleopathology, 1*, 24–34.

Martin, R. T. (1970). The role of coca in the history, religion, and medicine of South American Indians. *Economic Botany, 24*(4), 422–438.

Murphy, W. A., Jr., Dz, N., Gostner, P., Knapp, R., Recheis, W., & Seidler, H. (2003). The iceman: Discovery and imaging. *Radiology, 226*(3), 614–629.

Nerlich, A. G., Wiest, I., Löhrs, U., Parsche, F., & Schramel, P. (1995). Extensive pulmonary haemorrhage in an Egyptian mummy. *Virchows Archiv, 427*(4), 423–429.

Nerlich, A. G., Zink, A., Szeimies, U., & Hagedorn, H. G. (2000). Ancient Egyptian prosthesis of the big toe. *The Lancet, 356*(9248), 2176–2179.

O'Donnabháin, B. (2003). Trepanations and pseudotrepanations: Evidence of cranial surgery from prehistoric and early historic Ireland. In R. Arnott, S. Finger, & C. U. M. Smith (Eds.), *Trepanation: History, discovery, theory* (pp. 79–94). Lisse: Swets & Zietlinger.

Oeggl, K., Kofler, W., Schmidl, A., Dickson, J. H., Egarter-Vigl, E., & Gaber, O. (2007). The reconstruction of the last itinerary of 'Ötzi', the Neolithic Iceman, by pollen analysis from sequentially sampled gut extracts. *Quaternary Science Reviews, 26*, 853–861.

Oeggl, K., Kofler, W., & Schmidl, A. (2005). New aspects to the diet of the Neolithic Tyrolean iceman 'Ötzi'. *Journal of Biological Research, 80*, 344–347.

Ogalde, J. P., Arriaza, B. T., & Soto, E. C. (2009). Identification of psychoactive alkaloids in ancient Andean human hair by gas chromatography/mass spectrometry. *Journal of Archaeological Science, 36*(2), 467–472.

Ortner, D. J. (2003). *Identification of pathological conditions in human skeletal remains* (2nd ed.). San Diego: Academic.

Owsley, D. W. (1995). Contributions of bioarchaeological research to knowledge of nineteenth-century surgery. In S. R. Saunders & A. Herring (Eds.), *Grave reflections: Portraying the past through cemetery studies* (pp. 120–151). Toronto: Canadian Scholars' Press Inc.

Pabst, M. A., Letofsky-Papst, I., Moser, M., Spindler, K., Bock, E., Wilhelm, P., et al. (2010). Different staining substances were used in decorative and therapeutic tattoos in a 1000-year-old Peruvian mummy. *Journal of Archaeological Science, 37*(12), 3256–3262.

Palhano-Fontes, F., Alchieri, J. C., Oliveira, J. P. M., Soares, B. L., Hallak, J. E., Galvao-Coelho, N., et al. (2014). *The therapeutic potentials of ayahuasca in the treatment of depression* (pp. 23–39). The Therapeutic Use of Ayahuasca: Springer.

Peintner, U., Pöder, R., & Pümpel, T. (1998). The iceman's fungi. *Mycological Research, 102*(10), 1153–1162.

Piombino-Mascali, D., Jankauskas, R., Zink, A. R., Todesco, M. S., Aufderheide, A. C., & Panzer, S. (2015). Paleoradiology of the Savoca mummies, Sicily, Italy (18th-19th centuries AD). *The Anatomical Record, 298*, 988–1000.

Piombino-Mascali, D., Zink, A. R., Reinhard, K. J., Lein, M., Panzer, S., Aufderheide, A. C., et al. (2013). Dietary analysis of Piraino 1, Sicily, Italy: The role of archaeopalynology in forensic science. *Journal of Archaeological Science, 40*, 1935–1945.

Plowman, T. (1986). Coca chewing and the botanical origins of coca (Erythroxylum spp.) in South America. *Coca and cocaine: Effects on people and policy in Latin America* (pp. 5–34).

Pöder, R. (2005). The ice man's fungi: Facts and mysteries. *International Journal of Medicinal Mushrooms, 7*(3), 357–359.

Pöder, R., & Peintner, U. (1999). Laxatives and the ice man. *The Lancet, 353*(9156), 926.

Reinhard, K. J., & Buikstra, J. (2003). Louse infestation of the Chiribaya culture, Southern Peru: Variation in prevalence by age and sex. *Memórias do Instituto Oswaldo Cruz, 98*, 173–179.

Reinhard, K. J., Hamilton, D. L., & Hevly, R. H. (1991). Use of pollen concentration in paleopharmacology: Coprolite evidence of medicinal plants. *Journal of Ethnobiology, 11*, 117–134.
Reinhard, K. J., LeRoy-Toren, S., & Arriaza, B. T. (2011). Where have all the plant foods gone? The search for refined dietary reconstruction from Chinchorro mummies. *Yearbook of Mummy Studies, 1*, 139–151.
Resnick, D. (2002). *Diagnosis of bone and joint disorders* (4th ed.). Philadelphia: W.B. Saunders Company.
Rivera, M. A., Aufderheide, A. C., Cartmell, L. W., Torres, C. M., & Langsjoen, O. (2005). Antiquity of coca-leaf chewing in the south central Andes: A 3,000 year archaeological record of coca-leaf chewing from northern Chile. *Journal of Psychoactive Drugs, 37*(4), 455–458.
Roberts, C. A. (1999). Disability in the skeletal record: Assumptions, problems and some examples. *Archaeological Review from Cambridge, 15*(2), 79–97.
Roberts, C. A. (2011). The bioarchaeology of leprosy and tuberculosis: A comparative study of perceptions, stigma, diagnosis, and treatment. In S. C. Argarwal & B. A. Glencross (Eds.), *Social bioarchaeology* (pp. 252–281). West Sussex: Wiley-Blackwell.
Rowling, J. T. (1989). The rise and decline of surgery in dynastic Egypt. *Antiquity, 63*(239), 312–319.
Rudenko, S. I. (1970). *Frozen tombs of Siberia: The Pazyryk burials of iron age horsemen*. Tr. M. W. Thompson. Berkeley and Los Angeles: University of California Press.
Samadelli, M., Melis, M., Miccoli, M., Vigl, E. E., & Zink, A. R. (2015). Complete mapping of the tattoos of the 5300-year-old Tyrolean Iceman. *Journal of Cultural Heritage, 16*(5), 753–758.
Santos, R., Landeira-Fernandez, J., Strassman, R., Motta, V., & Cruz, A. (2007). Effects of ayahuasca on psychometric measures of anxiety, panic-like and hopelessness in Santo Daime members. *Journal of Ethnopharmacology, 112*(3), 507–513.
Schultes, R. E., & Hofmann, A. (1980). *The botany and chemistry of hallucinogens*. Springfield, IL: Charles C. Thomas.
Schultes, R. E. (1982). The beta-carboline hallucinogens of South America. *Journal of Psychoactive Drugs, 14*(3), 205–220.
Searcey, N., Reinhard, K. J., Egarter-Vigl, E., Maixner, F., Piombino-Mascali, D., Zink, A. R., et al. (2013). Parasitism of the Zweeloo Woman: Dicrocoeliasis evidenced in a Roman period bog mummy. *International Journal of Paleopathology, 3*, 224–228.
Seo, M., Araujo, A., Reinhard, K., Chai, J. Y., & Shin, D. H. (2014). Paleoparasitological studies on mummies of the Joseon Dynasty, Korea. *Korean Journal of Parasitology, 52*, 235–242.
Steinbock, R. T. (1976). *Paleopathological diagnosis and interpretation: Bone disease in ancient human populations*. Springfield: Charles C. Thomas.
Tilley, L. (2015). Accommodating difference in the prehistoric past: Revisiting the case of Romito 2 from a bioarchaeology of care perspective. *International Journal of Paleopathology, 8*, 64–74.
Tilley, L., & Cameron, T. (2014). Introducing the index of care: A web-based application supporting archaeological research into health-related care. *International Journal of Paleopathology, 6*, 5–9.
Tilley, L., & Oxenham, M. F. (2011). Survival against the odds: Modeling the social implications of care provision to seriously disabled individuals. *International Journal of Paleopathology, 1*, 35–42.
Toyne, J. M. (2015). Tibial surgery in ancient Peru. *International Journal of Paleopathology, 8*, 29–35.
Tunón, H., & Svanberg, I. (1999). Laxatives and the ice man. *The Lancet, 353*(9156), 925–926.
Turner, B. L., Klaus, H. D., Livengood, S. V., Brown, L. E., Saldaña, F., & Wester, C. (2013). The variable roads to sacrifice: Isotopic investigations of human remains from Chotuna-Huaca de los Sacrificios, Lambayeque, Peru. *American Journal of Physical Anthropology, 151*(1), 22–37.
Verano, J. W., Anderson, L. S., & Franco, R. (2000). Foot amputation by the Moche of ancient Peru: Osteological evidence and archaeological context. *International Journal of Osteoarchaeology, 10*(3), 177–188.
Vitseva, O., Varghese, S., Chakrabarti, S., Folts, J. D., & Freedman, J. E. (2005). Grape seed and skin extracts inhibit platelet function and release of reactive oxygen intermediates. *Journal of Cardiovascular Pharmacology, 46*, 445–451.

Webb, E., Thomson, S., Nelson, A., White, C. D., Koren, G., Rieder, M., et al. (2010). Assessing individual systemic stress through cortisol analysis of archaeological hair. *Journal of Archaeological Science, 37*, 807–812.

Yilmaz, Y., & Toledo, R. (2004). Health aspects of functional grapeseed constituents. *Trends in Food Science and Technology, 15*, 422–433.

Zimmerman, M. R., Trinkaus, E., LeMay, M., Aufderheide, A. C., Reyman, T. A., Marrocco, G. R., et al. (1981). Trauma and trephination in a Peruvian mummy. *American Journal of Physical Anthropology, 55*, 497–501.

Chapter 11
Towards a Bioarchaeology of Care of Children

Marc Oxenham and Anna Willis

Introduction

One of the key case studies used in the development, both theoretical and practical, of the bioarchaeology of care model (see Tilley & Oxenham, 2011) was the adult Man Bac Burial 9 (MB9), who as it turns out was severely physically (at least) incapacitated from childhood (Oxenham et al., 2009). In many ways the current staged approach to exploring the issue of care in the past (see Chap. 2, this volume and references therein) can assess any individual from any time period and/or cultural background regardless of their final age-at-death. Indeed, the care model should, at face value, be able to be trained on children, adults and the very old to great effect. In the case of MB9 care commenced while he was a young child, although an exact age of onset of his condition cannot be determined with any specificity, and continued throughout childhood, into his teens and onto his mid to late twenties – at which time he died.

The chief aim of this chapter is not so much to develop a complete, robust, theoretical and operational approach to the bioarchaeology of care of children, as we do not think this is necessary (see below), but rather to raise a series of questions regarding the study of children in potential care contexts in the past and to provide a case study that explores some of the implications of looking at children in contexts of potential care. This case study focuses on the children that lived, potentially received health care, and died at Man Bac some 4000 years ago in northern Vietnam.

M. Oxenham, Ph.D. (✉) • A. Willis, Ph.D.
School of Archaeology and Anthropology, Australian National University, Canberra, ACT, Australia
e-mail: marc.oxenham@anu.edu.au

© Springer International Publishing Switzerland 2017

L. Tilley, A.A. Schrenk (eds.), *New Developments in the Bioarchaeology of Care*, Bioarchaeology and Social Theory, DOI 10.1007/978-3-319-39901-0_11

Health Care and Parental Nurturing Care

In considering a bioarchaeology of care for children it is worth examining Tilley's (2015, pp. 99–100) distinction between a bioarchaeology of care model and parental (maternal for the most part) nurture, while appreciating that her views are developed within the context of explanatory models for the potential biological basis (evolutionary) of care behaviours:

> *Under normal circumstances the state of pregnancy and period of infant dependency are not pathological. Some of the skillsets used in health-related care giving undeniably overlap with some of those employed in assisting healthy women around pregnancy and in raising dependent infants ... Nevertheless, caring for an individual with a specific, continuing disability entails qualitatively different sets of actions and motivations...This does not deny that some pregnant women, some mothers and probably many infants may be candidates for healthcare at various times. However, to explain health-related care provision as an extension of infant nurturing is to ignore the quite different, and perhaps more complex, cognitive demands involved in caring for an individual suffering from the impacts of disease.*

While we are not entirely sure we would agree that parental care during the period of infant dependency is necessarily less cognitively demanding, it is the case, albeit highly contingent, that infant care will follow a predictive pattern, unlike the situation with health care where the care needed and the requirements and status of the care receiver will often vary in an unpredictable manner. Further, for the most part parental nurturing will be associated with an expectation of positive outcomes during the infant dependency period. Such may not necessarily be the case with health-related care, and may consequently add to the stress, and ultimately the health, of the caregiver(s).

It could be argued that parental nurturing, and even pregnancy itself, can and does have negative health implications. There is a large literature on the health costs of pregnancy (e.g. see Lukacs, 2008; Lukacs & Largaespada, 2006), and it has also been suggested that fluctuations in rates of oral health over the past 6000 years in Southeast Asia are directly related to fluctuating fertility rates (see Willis & Oxenham, 2013 for instance). Dependency ratios, of the very old and very young relative to the working age cohort in a community, have been used by bioarchaeologists for years as a quick, if blunt, measure of potential levels of social stress in an ancient community (e.g. Oxenham et al., 2008). Somewhat paradoxically, communities witnessing elevated levels of fertility are recognised as such by way of relatively high infant mortality, a factor that will artificially increase perceived dependency rates. Notwithstanding, elevated rates of newborns, even if their lives are somewhat short, will add to community stress and impact on community health outcomes. The host of potential infant diseases will obviously also have a negative social impact on the affected infant(s), immediate parental nurturer(s), associated family and the community at large, particularly if epidemic in proportion. However, does this necessitate a child-specific model of health care, or is the current bioarchaeology of care model sufficient?

In answering that question a recent comment by Matsumoto and colleagues (2015, p. 2), in the context of a study of non-human primates, is relevant: 'Research on maternal care of disabled infants is useful for developing our understanding of maternal investment and behavioural flexibility in a context in which the amount, type, and duration of care do not fit the usual patterns associated with infant development'. Without recourse to such an approach we are left in the indefensible position of interpreting an infant's inability to perform the basic tasks of daily living (see discussion of the bioarchaeology of care Stage 2, Chap. 2 this volume) as clinical and functional impacts of disability, with equally bizarre flow on effects into Stages 3 and 4 of the care model. Tilley (2015, p. 164) clearly, and explicitly, recognises this problem: '[t]he natural dependency of infants and young children will make it difficult to distinguish, empirically and conceptually, between 'normal' altricial care and '*ab*normal' health-related care'.

Defining Our Children

How we define children has relevance, particularly in the context of non-pathologically oriented normal parental nurturing as opposed to health-related care. Clearly children can be defined biologically, if not chronologically, with recourse to their skeletal and dental state of maturation. Defining children socially or culturally is as fraught as any other age class: when are the elderly 'elderly', for instance (Cave & Oxenham, 2014; Ross & Oxenham, 2016)? This question is particularly problematic in the context of health-related caregiving: would it ever be possible to disentangle health-related care and maternal care and nurturing in the case of babies? We would suggest not, although we know the maternal bond and care-nurturing imperative can be tested, as examples of infanticide would seem to suggest (see a discussion of infanticide, in the context of Man Bac, in Oxenham et al., 2008). Further, where the remains of severely physically disabled infants are retrieved archaeologically, and regardless of mortuary treatment, it would be difficult to determine if the premature death was natural or deliberately engineered (particularly with regard to infant neglect, although overt infanticide 'almost always occurs at birth or very shortly thereafter' [Scrimshaw, 1984, p. 449] and may therefore be possible to identify), let alone if some form of health-related care was provided.

Is some level of independence of mobility a useful defining category of childhood for health-related care purposes? A child's ability to crawl and place objects in its mouth is certainly a time for increased risk of misadventure and contact with pathogenic organisms, and such behaviours associated with this developmental stage have been linked to at least one dental pathology, localised primary canine hypoplasia (McDonnell & Oxenham, 2014). At a minimum, attendant child carers would need to be more vigilant, and at a maximum would need to provide immediate post trauma or other forms of care associated with coughs, colds, fevers, diarrhoea and so forth. But again, such forms of care, although clearly health related, are presumably universal and part of the everyday child raising energy and time budget.

While enormously variable cross-culturally, and presumably also through time, the period of increasing independence in physical and cognitive abilities is perhaps when we may have the greatest success in distinguishing between an extension of normal parental nurturing and health-related care. When it comes to older children, the question may become more about the bioarchaeology of care of adults than of children, although this is complicated by wide variations in the biological and/or chronological age at which children transition into adulthood; for instance, Crawford (1991) notes that 10 year-olds were legally adult in seventh century Anglo-Saxon England. This still leaves us with the question of how to define 'children' in the context of the bioarchaeology of care. Such a definition will be highly contingent on a range of factors, including temporal period, sociocultural complexity, demography and so on, and is therefore sample or site specific, although our discussion has suggested some general guidelines.

It is perhaps time to look at a specific case study in order to explore some of the issues dealt with so far. The study sample is, as previously mentioned, the ancient community in which MB9 was born, raised and intensively cared for over much of his childhood and early adulthood. In the context of identifying children at Man Bac, and because this is essentially an exploratory exercise (we are not testing any particular hypothesis), we have chosen to focus on all subadults 8 years old or younger in order to capture a range of more altricial to more precocial (older) individuals, although we will broaden this definition if and where appropriate. The archaeology of the site, including aspects of its demographic composition, local environment, subsistence economy and its basic human health background, has been dealt with extensively elsewhere (e.g. see contributions in Oxenham, Matsumura, & Nguyen, 2011). Moreover, aspects of the bioarchaeology of childhood and the children of Man Bac have also been reported on (e.g. Oxenham et al., 2008). Notwithstanding, a summary is given here.

Man Bac: A Biosocial Background

Man Bac represents a community that flourished during the emergence and development of farming in the context of regionally massive and profound population mobility. The site itself, located in the karstic landscape of Ninh Binh province, on the southern edge of the Red River Delta, is in a climatically subtropical zone, albeit in one of the most species diverse regions of Southeast Asia. The subsistence of the inhabitants was focused on a combination of rice farming (Willis & Oxenham, 2013) and possibly domestic pig husbandry, and associated with hunting and gathering a wide range of terrestrial and aquatic animals and also, presumably, plant resources. Indeed, it is arguable that the vast majority, if not all, Southeast Asian Neolithic communities included equally significant farming and hunter-gathering components in their subsistence strategies and diets (see Oxenham & Buckley, 2016). Man Bac is aligned with a broadly defined early Neolithic culture operating in northern Vietnam between c. 4000–3500 BP named the Phung Nguyen culture or period. The Phung Nguyen itself had extensive trading networks, which included southern China. Socially, there appears to be a somewhat egalitarian political structure, while status seems to be more of an acquired commodity than an inherited one. Indeed, there is some evidence to suggest increasing age attracted greater levels of social status or recognition. Aspects of what we know of health and disease at Man Bac are detailed below.

Man Bac: The Bioarchaeology of Care Model

Stage 1 of the Bioarchaeology of Care Model

Health

In outlining the clinical and functional impacts of disease and/or disability at Man Bac we proceed from a population rather than individual perspective, and as such we will not explore specific cases of potential childhood disability. The following summary is based on Oxenham and Domett's (2011) account unless otherwise stated. In terms of oral health, 3.7 % of all deciduous dentition (27.8 % of subadult individuals) had carious lesions. While linear enamel hypoplasia (LEH) was not observed in deciduous teeth, 64.9 % of adult anterior teeth (canines and incisors) displayed at least one instance of LEH, with relatively higher frequencies of LEH seen in young males and females compared to older males and females. The ubiquity of LEH and the higher percentage in younger adults suggests many children suffered physiological insult severe enough to cause LEH, and that the causes of LEH may have placed individuals at a higher risk of death in early adulthood.

Children did suffer from localised primary canine hypoplasia (LPCH), and McDonell and Oxenham (2014) found that 41.7 % of children with deciduous canines (or 20.9 % of all deciduous canines) exhibited this defect. These authors go on to suggest that LPCH has a complex multifactorial aetiology, but that 'the reasonably high prevalence of this condition at Man Bac suggests depressed maternal and neonatal health' (McDonnell & Oxenham, 2014, p. 531).

The frequency of cribra orbitalia, a condition believed to develop in childhood and differentially remodel in adulthood, affected 73.1 % of all adults, although the majority of cases displayed remodelled lesions (Oxenham & Domett, 2011). Of the children themselves, 90.6 % showed evidence for cribra orbitalia, with 75 % of these cases having an active form of the lesion. By any comparison, the entire community was suffering from the effects of at least one, although more likely multiple, physiological stressors.

Data not previously published on childhood health at Man Bac indicate that of those subadults aged from perinate through to 12 years with preserved cranial and/or postcranial remains 9/36 (25 %) suffered from long bone periostitis, 4/31 (12.9 %) from cranial periostitis, 3/31 (6.5 %) from cranial lytic lesions and 2/31 from premature cranial synostosis. Collectively, 12/29 (41.4 %) suffered from cranial and/or postcranial periostitis, while 15/29 (51.7 %) displayed cranial and/or long bone lytic or periosteal lesions (a figure which excludes the two individuals with premature

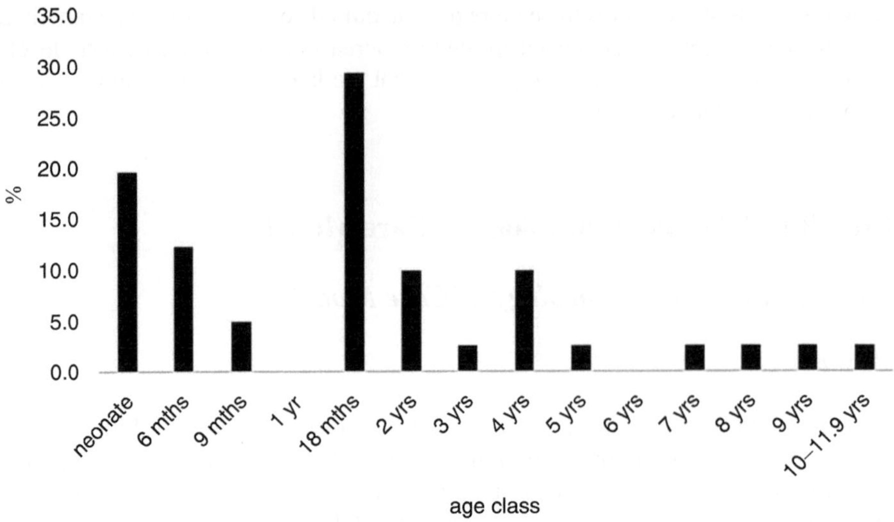

Fig. 11.1 Man Bac subadult mortality profile, $n=41$ (adapted from Domett & Oxenham, 2011)

suture closure). With one exception, all instances of these pathologies occurred in children aged 8 years old or less, suggesting an extraordinarily elevated rate of serious morbidity in the Man Bac subadult sample.

Demography

A range of demographic descriptors for Man Bac indicates very high levels of fertility (JA ratio 0.25; D20+/D5+ ratio 0.737; MCM 0.097) (Domett & Oxenham, 2011), which essentially equates with very elevated levels of subadult mortality. Indeed, some 52 % of the entire sample is aged 14 years or less. Further, the subadult mortality distribution is somewhat unusual (see Fig. 11.1) in that three mortality peaks can be observed: the first is the expected high perinate mortality rate, a second occurs between 1 and 2 years with a peak at 1.5 years, while the third peak occurs at 4 years of age.

Burial Treatment

While all individuals in the Man Bac cemetery show evidence of deliberate burial and orientation in a preferred direction (east–west for the most part), children were treated differently to adults in as much as the inclusion of non-perishable grave goods varied by age (with all adults receiving grave goods). As Fig. 11.2 demonstrates, perinates had a 50:50 chance of receiving grave furnishings, rising to 71.4 % of all 6–9 month-olds receiving grave goods, 83.5 % of 3–5 year-olds and 100 % of all individuals aged 7 years and older.

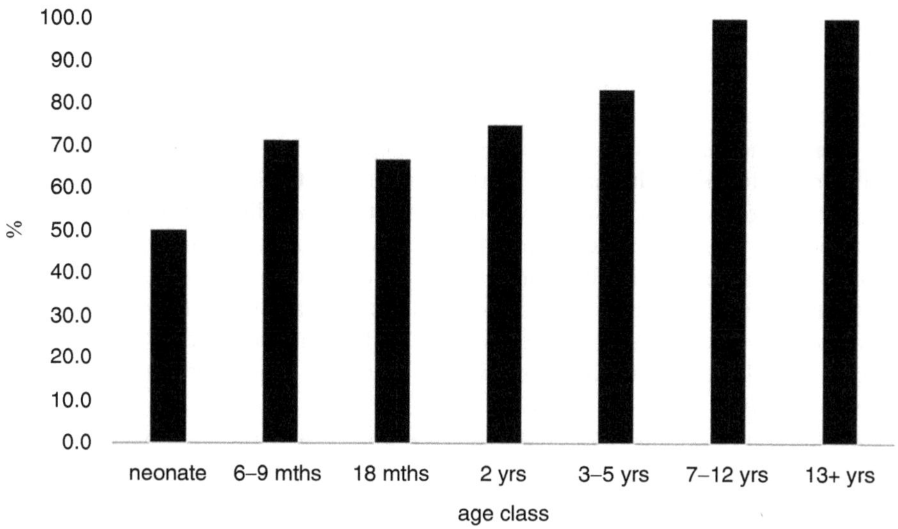

Fig. 11.2 Man Bac: Proportion of each age class with grave goods ($n=60$)

The type of grave good also appears to have varied by age class. While bivalve shells occur at virtually any age, these shells occur among 40 % of perinates and 18–24 year-olds, compared to 20–25 % of most other age classes, except for the 25+ year group where only 4.5 % of these adults had bivalves. Tools do not appear as grave goods in burials of individuals aged younger than 3 years, but occur in 20–25 % of all burials in the age classes between 4 and 24 years (interestingly, only 9.1 % of burials in the 25+ year age class contained tools). The inclusion of nephrite beads also varies by age class, with such beads first occurring at 18–24 months (25 %), peaking at 3–5 years (60 %), and not occurring again in any graves until 18–24 years (20 %) and 25+ years (31.8 %).

Looking at the distribution of grave goods in the context of the mortality profile of Man Bac several observations can be made: (a) high perinate mortality is associated with lower mortuary investment; (b) the 18 month-old mortality peak is associated with the earliest age at which nephrite beads are used as grave goods and (c) the smaller mortality peak at 4 years is associated with the introduction of tools as graves goods.

Stage 2 of the Bioarchaeology of Care Model

Looking at health care from a population level, and in the context of children, means that only generalisations regarding potential clinical and functional impacts of the described status of childhood health and disease is possible. The high levels of childhood physiological disruption identified in adult skeletons (e.g. cribra orbitalia and LEH), along with the very high frequencies of active cribra orbitalia in children's remains and the elevated frequency of localised primary canine hypoplasia, suggest poor childhood health in general. The poor level of oral health in addition to the high frequency of cranial and postcranial periosteal lesions, as well as several instances of lytic cranial lesions, all point to extremely depressed levels of childhood health at Man Bac.

One of the main issues in dealing with non-specific disease signatures (LEH, cribra orbitalia, periostitis and so forth) is our inability to identify which, of an enormous range of pathogens, were responsible for the morbidity and mortality we see in ancient Southeast Asian children. Here we review a range of conditions and their causes that more than likely contributed to, if not accounted for, the poor health outcomes seen at Man Bac. The following is based on recent work by Willis (2015) and the literature is focused on current or modern day conditions, although it is highly probable the same conditions were as prevalent, if not more so, in the past as they are today.

Respiratory tract infections, diarrhoeal disease and malaria are the leading causes of childhood mortality in tropical countries today (Lozano et al., 2012; Webb, 1991). Although the effects of these do not tend to leave skeletal signatures, they have the potential to contribute to increased childhood, and later adult, frailty and susceptibility. Pneumonia can be caused by a number of bacteria, viruses and fungi. *Streptococcus pneumoniae* and *Haemophilus influenza* are common causes of bacterial pneumonia in children in Vietnam, particularly in those less than 2 years old (Anh et al., 2009), with symptoms including coughs, breathing difficulties and sometimes fever. Diarrhoea is a common symptom of a range of bacterial, viral and parasitic infections. Bacterial *Campylobacter, Shigella, Enterohaemorrhagic Escherichia coli* and *Salmonella* are common food-borne pathogens found in children in Vietnam, particularly in those less than 1 year of age (Isenbarger et al., 2001; Thompson et al., 2015), and symptoms can include diarrhoea, fever and vomiting. Rotavirus and norovirus are also commonly found in modern Vietnamese children (Thompson et al., 2015), and symptoms include vomiting and diarrhoea, often associated with fever and abdominal pain.

In Vietnam, parasitic zoonotic infections from food-borne pathogens include trematodes (liver flukes) such as *Opisthorchis viverrine* and *Clonorchis sinensis* (Nguyen et al., 2003). The trematodes reside in the bile ducts, and symptoms of mild infections include general feelings of illness sometimes associated with abdominal pain. Chronic infections can result in inflammation of the infected organs, fibrosis of tissues and cholangiocarcinoma (the latter a form of bile duct cancer). Eating raw fish, a major source of parasitic infection, is common in Vietnam, although predominantly an adult male activity in present times (Nguyen, 2004). While the effects of trematodes likely have a smaller impact on children, cross-contamination during shared meals or the consumption of associated sauces or garnishes mean that individuals who do not themselves eat raw fish are also commonly infected (Phan, Ersbøll, Do, & Dalsgaard, 2010).

Intestinal parasitic infections from soil-transmitted helminths such as hookworm *(Necator americanus* and *Ancylostoma duodenale)*, whipworm *(Trichuris trichiura)* and roundworm *(Ascaris lumbricoides)* are common in Vietnam (Needham et al., 1998; van der Hoek et al., 2003; Verle et al., 2003). Infections from these parasites cause diarrhoea, loss of appetite, reduced absorption of micronutrients, abdominal pain and fatigue. Hookworms can cause chronic blood loss within the intestine that can result in anaemia, while roundworm may compete for vitamin A within its host. Vietnamese adults generally have a higher prevalence of helminths than infants (Trang, Mølbak, Cam, & Dalsgaard, 2007; Verle et al., 2003). Roundworm is the most common helminth affecting children under 5 years of age (Trang et al., 2007; Verle et al., 2003), although one study found a very high frequency of whipworm and roundworm in children by 5 years of age (Needham et al., 1998), while hookworm was present in lower rates in young children but at increasing levels with increasing age (Needham et al., 1998; Verle et al., 2003).

Malaria is a particularly important disease in terms of both child and adult health, and potentially played a major role in the depressed levels of childhood health in Vietnam. Malaria is a parasitic infection caused by the protozoan *Plasmodium* spp. transmitted by female *Anopheles* mosquitos. *P. falciparum* and *P. vivax* are the most common species of *Plasmodium* in Southeast Asia and Vietnam (Erhart et al., 2005; Thang et al., 2008). Symptoms of malaria include headache, fever and vomiting. Males appear to suffer more during blood stage malaria due to hormonal influences (Bernin & Lotter, 2014; Cernetich et al., 2006), whereas females appear to have some level of immunity to malaria (Klein, Easterbrook, Lalime, & Klein, 2008); however, this is compromised during pregnancy (Reubin, 1992; Vlassoff & Bonilla, 1994). Pregnant women who contract malaria are more predisposed to anaemia and hypoglycaemia, and are more likely to suffer miscarriage, stillbirth, premature delivery, infants of low birth weight and maternal death (Chongsuphajaisiddhi, 1991).

Anaemia, common in contemporary Vietnam, can be caused by deficiencies in iron folate and vitamin A or B_{12}, while other causes include chronic inflammation, parasitic infections (including malaria and also genetic conditions that protect against malarial infection) or inherited conditions. The symptoms include fatigue, weakness and general cognitive impairments. Traditionally, the Vietnamese diet is low in bioavailable iron and high in absorption inhibitors, significantly increasing the prevalence of iron deficiency (Nguyen et al., 2006). The Vietnamese environment has a high presence of parasitic intestinal pathogens that may increase anaemia risk. Anaemia is highest in women and children, particularly in pregnant women and children <2 years of age (Nguyen et al., 2006). A study of school children in Vietnam suggested that anaemia was high, although not necessarily associated with iron deficiency, suggesting that other proximate causes, particularly coinfection with intestinal parasites, were contributing to anaemia (Le, Brouwer, Verhoef, Nguyen, & Kok, 2007) and perhaps competing for essential vitamins. The youngest group of children at 5 years had the highest prevalence of anaemia, and boys had a higher prevalence of anaemia, and lower haemoglobin concentrations, than girls (Le et al., 2007).

The last two sections have outlined (a) the extremely high frequency of both non-specific skeletal and dental lesions among the children of Man Bac, (b) associated high fertility rates and elevated child mortality, (c) a range of plausible diseases, all affecting modern Vietnamese and other Southeast Asian communities today, potentially responsible for the elevated rates of childhood morbidity and mortality and (d) a series of symptoms ranging from debilitating to severe that individuals suffering from these conditions would likely have suffered. All of these factors in combination strongly suggest (e) a clear case for health-related care, in many instances extended care, for the children of Man Bac.

Stage 3 of the Bioarchaeology of Care Model

The previous section indicates that poor childhood health, if not maternal health, would seem to be the expectation of Man Bac parents and carers from the outset. When dealing with non-specific signatures of poor and chronic ill health it is necessarily difficult to infer specific sets of care models. It is fair to say that a majority of Man Bac children would have required an elevated level of care and nurturing beyond that normally provided to non-ill children of an equivalent age cohort in this community. For particularly young children, perinates through to 1 year-olds, extra care would likely have not been noticeably elevated over and above the level of care and nurturing any healthy infant would receive as a matter of course, given the 24/7 attention healthy infants normally receive. There may have even been an expectation of a poor outcome in the case of poor perinate health, which may be reflected in the reduced mortuary investment in such children (such a fatalistic approach is discussed below with reference to an African ethnographic case study). For less altricial children care requirements would have been differentially elevated over and above normal care and nurturing requirements, and presumably the more precocial the child the greater, or more obvious, the extra care investment required. The sheer level of poor subadult health in this community, much of this potentially being associated with fevers, diarrhoea, dehydration, lethargy, listlessness and varying degrees of pain, may have necessitated a community-level response to care requirements (the idea of a community level involvement in care is discussed in the second part of the Stage 4 bioarchaeology of care analysis below).

It is also worth noting the potentially synergistic effects between normal parental care and nurturing behaviours and negative health outcomes and/or negative intervention outcomes. For instance, weaning and the introduction of solids may have been a factor that catalysed or facilitated certain childhood illnesses at Man Bac, as well as exacerbated a child's physiological responses to the pathogens responsible for a given illness. In a similar vein, particular cultural behaviours, for instance food taboos that were either gender or age based, may have facilitated or exacerbated a range of childhood illnesses. Oxenham (2001, p. 377) notes:

> *Food taboos, prohibitions and avoidances are common in many societies, present and past ... [and] ... many of these food prohibitions can occur even in the face of a great variety and abundance of food-stuffs. Furthermore, pregnant and postpartum mothers are commonly the target of these food taboos and avoidances.*

In terms of weaning, or the process of the reduction in breastfeeding in combination with the introduction of solid foods (which can take place over a shorter or longer period of time), the Man Bac peak in childhood mortality at or around 18 months (with a range of between 1 and 2 years of age) is intriguing. If weaning, or some other unknown cultural behaviour, is in part responsible for this peak in child mortality, it suggests that a major change in the care relationship between parent and child may have triggered the need for an increase in *health* care-related activities. Instead of a reduction in the intensity and necessity of normal parental care and nurturing the opposite occurs, which may also have had negative health consequences for the primary carer. An examination of Gray's (1996) ethnography of weaning practices among the nomadic Turkana pastoralists of Kenya may have some relevance here.

Gray (1996) noted the very early introduction of non-breast milk foods, a practice beginning around the middle of the first post-partum month that saw different foods introduced as the infant developed, and a relatively abrupt cessation of breastfeeding, often around 18 months old, was traumatic both for the mother and the infant. Gray (1996, p. 455) also noted that '[d]uring their first 15–18 months, Turkana children are in almost constant physical contact with their mothers…', but that this behaviour changes markedly at around 18 months, often in association with a new pregnancy. The reasons for cessation of breastfeeding aside, Gray (1996, p. 457) suggests that the decision to introduce non-breast milk foods so early and in a continuous and staged manner is a trade-off between the energetic benefits of food supplements and the lower risks of disease associated with exclusive breastfeeding. Meehan and Roulette (2013) have forwarded a similar argument in explaining early supplementation of breast milk by the Aka, central African foragers. Moreover, Gray (1996, p. 458) notes, in the context of an adaptive scenario, that:

> *Mothers apparently believe that they can do little about infant exposure to illness and disease, but they might nevertheless have some effect on infant susceptibility or recovery by ensuring positive energy balance in young children for as long as possible.*

However, Gray (1996, p. 459) suggests that ecological uncertainties this community has to deal with on a day-by-day basis ensures a variability in maternal responses to weaning and that, '[u]ltimately, high fertility is the best strategy where survival cannot be assured'.

Clearly, we cannot know what maternal strategies were invoked 4000 years ago in northern Vietnam. Notwithstanding, both Man Bac and these Turkana pastoralists experienced ecologically volatile environments, high disease loads, elevated levels of infant morbidity and mortality, and perhaps similar ages of weaning. Minimally, the Turkana experience provides one possible scenario for approaching an understanding of infant health and the potential consequences of decisions relating to weaning at Man Bac.

Before moving onto the Stage 4 discussion of the bioarchaeology of care it is worth noting, in the context of the discussion of weaning, that the first appearance of nephrite beads with children's burials occurs during the peak period of infant mortality and, presumably, a peak period of morbidity as well, if we assume an absence of specific skeletal signatures for most childhood illnesses at Man Bac. Minimally, the death of a child at this stage of their development would have been particularly psychologically traumatic for parents or carers, a feeling expressed in the mortuary treatment the child received. However, can we take another step and infer that this was a particularly important biosocially constructed stage in an infant's life cycle? A life stage that may have been recognised in terms of cognitive and physical development, risk of death and, perhaps, culturally prescribed behaviours such as a (terminal?) stage in the weaning process?

We have seen in this discussion that the age, or developmental stage, of a child will potentially inform the nature and level of health-related care within the context of the type, severity and duration of a child's illness. We have also explored the possibility that carers made decisions about their children, sick or otherwise, in terms of a form of cost-benefit analysis, with a potentially complex interplay between the needs of the child and the requirements of the mother and the community at large. This, of course, does not trivialise the enormous emotional, psychological and even physical investment carers had in their charges, but rather reifies these motivations into operationally viable (if not adaptive) behaviours. The next stage of this discussion is clearly to explore the issue of agency.

Stage 4 of the Bioarchaeology of Care Model

Tilley (2015, p. 177) notes that '[t]he central premise of Stage 4 analysis is that the behaviours making up the giving and receiving of health-related care express the agency of all concerned, and that this agency has the potential to illuminate aspects of group and individual identity'. Clearly the aims and motivations of health-related care in the context of children will be inextricably intertwined with the underlying (whether biologically and/or culturally based) aims and motivations of normal parental care and nurturing. Moreover, the question of agency, or choice if you like, in the context of the health-related care of a perinate or even 18 month old is perhaps moot from the perspective of both carer and care-receiver. The same argument can be plausibly applied to a child of any age, although agency may play a more substantive role in the dialogue between carer and care-receiver the older the child is.

Indeed, agency can be explored in the context of older children at Man Bac in as much as there is ample evidence for children engaging in important social and economic roles from a very early age (see discussion of this regarding Man Bac children in Oxenham, 2012; Oxenham et al., 2008). Moreover, the introduction of tools within mortuary contexts at around 4 years of age and the presence of a mortality peak at this age is intriguing. Increasing social and economic responsibilities at this age, in concert with increased levels of mobility and potentially reduced supervision due to normal nurturing care being diverted to younger (ill?) children, may be relevant here, albeit in the sense of negative agency outcomes. Notwithstanding, the issue of agency was specifically explored, to some extent, with the case of MB9 (Tilley & Oxenham, 2011), although the issue of MB9's agency during the early (childhood) stage of his condition was not explicitly addressed in this paper.

From a community level perspective (see discussion of this below), particularly in the context of children's health-related care, agency will be a difficult issue to address. However, it can, and has been, explored in the context of the mortuary treatment of children at Man Bac. In work based on approximately half of the current Man Bac assemblage, Oxenham et al. (2008, p. 204) concluded that:

> *In what is otherwise a relatively egalitarian community, deferential mortuary behaviour may be indicative of choice in individual mortuary treatment open to parents and/or carers of deceased children. As long as certain conventions were maintained, relatives of dead children may have had considerable flexibility in what was interred, if anything at all, with their young.*

Looking at a much enlarged sample, we see no need to change our opinion. If agency, if only in terms of choices in how to grieve, is difficult to explore in the context of a bioarchaeology of children's health-related care, and aims and motivations are likely universal to some degree, can a population approach to children's health and care provide any surprises? We would suggest it can, and that Man Bac is important in showing what must have been a community-wide response to the care and support of, and subsequent grieving for, severely ill children, even if in each circumstance this response was only enacted by a small number of caregivers. At a minimum, this community was psychologically equipped to deal with and respond to extremely high levels of childhood morbidity. Rather than respond negatively to poor childhood health outcomes, which the sheer number of subadult deaths attest to, they treated their dead children with respect and imbued them with individual identities, some based on gender and others on age cohort. In this sense, they provided even the youngest children with their own agency, even if one that the children themselves were unable to exercise directly.

We have referred to the idea of 'community level' responses in both the Stage 3 and 4 components of the bioarchaeology of care model. Here we explore this idea in a little more detail. Clearly this is a speculative exercise, but it may provide another avenue through which we can approach an understanding of a bioarchaeology of care for children in ancient Man Bac. We have discussed agency in terms of the immediate carers and the cared-for children within a framework of individual and/or family responses to both the living sick child and the dead child. However, we now wish to explore what community level care might have been like, if indeed such a thing existed some four millennia ago in Vietnam.

The implicit assumption for health-related care of children in this chapter has been that parents or family members performed the required care. It is not a stretch to assume that older children, siblings and other genetically or affinally related children, were also involved to a greater or lesser extent in the care of sick children. In this context it is important to remember, as stressed by Meehan and Roulette (2013, p. 113), that '...cross-culturally, humans cooperatively rear children ... and non-maternal caregivers are active feeders of infants and young children'. Clearly, alloparenting in all its forms (sibling, aunt, father, grandmother and non-genetically related family and community members) has the capacity to affect infant health both positively and negatively, but can also impact on the degree of agency of the parental carers themselves. Alloparenting aside, an intriguing question is: were other community members specifically involved in the care of sick children at Man Bac? A way in which non-family members may have been involved with the care of ill children is in the context of individuals tasked with specific forms of medical care and/or assistance in the care of mothers and infants. Midwifery is perhaps one avenue through which such non-family-related care could have occurred. Writing on the case of Lucretia, a late nineteenth century African-American midwife, Wilkie (2003, pp. 140–141) notes:

> *As a midwife, she was able to support herself transmitting the knowledge of her first and truest profession, motherhood ... Lucretia would have been teaching pregnant women how to care for themselves during pregnancy, what to expect during the ordeal of childbirth, and, afterward, how to care for their newborns. After experiencing 11 pregnancies ... and enduring the deaths of six of her children ... Lucretia was also especially able to respond empathetically to women who experienced the loss of pregnancies or babies.*

Knowledge gained through experience, as well as through some form of training from older women in the community, would have provided our hypothetical midwives in ancient Man Bac with both practical skills and a sense of empathy for those they cared for. Marland (1993, p. 1) notes '…it is generally recognised that the midwife has been with us since biblical times, and that midwifery is the oldest female occupation and without doubt one of the most important', although we would suggest a much longer pedigree than biblical times. While the chief role of midwives, cross-culturally, has been to attend to pregnant women and assist in births, their role in eighteenth century Italy, for instance, also included consultations regarding 'irregular menstrual cycles, breastfeeding, sterility, rape or venereal disease' (Filippini, 1993, p. 155).

Assuming midwifery in some form was a part of the social fabric of Neolithic communities in Vietnam, would their skills or knowledge have extended further than pregnancies and deliveries? Knowledge of women and 'women's maladies' in general would have made midwives an important resource in a community like Man Bac. They may have had knowledge of a range of remedies (*materia medica*), therapies and interventions to treat both general and specific medical problems. There is a long history for the effective use of various plant, animal and mineral remedies as contraceptives, abortifacients and emmenagogues (Riddle, 1992), while the use of herbal remedies in general dates back to at least 1100 BCE in East Asia (Leung, 2006). Little is known of potential drug therapies in Neolithic Vietnam, although the use of betel nut has been suggested as a therapy for the pain associated with rampant childhood caries at Man Bac (Oxenham et al., 2008). Notwithstanding the cross-cultural diversity in approaches to pregnancy and childbirth (see contributions in Davis-Floyd & Sargent, 1997), we suggest it is not such a stretch in credulity to believe that women filled the role of midwives at Man Bac some 4000 years ago. Moreover, the incredibly high rates of subadult morbidity and mortality would have ensured such specialists, if indeed they existed, were kept very busy and were well respected in this community (a question many may wish to ask of other prehistoric communities).

Conclusions

At the outset we stated that we wished to explore the idea of a bioarchaeology of care of children, and not necessarily attempt to develop a child-specific version of this approach. We delved into a number of issues, including the difficulty in distinguishing between normal parental nurturing and health-related care in the case of infants, and the fact that parental nurturing, and even pregnancy itself, can negatively impact on the health of mother and child. We also stressed that the way in which we define the subject of interest (i.e. the children) will mould the sorts of questions we can ask, the nature of the evidence we can access, and the inferences we may be able to make about health-related care of children in the past. Much of the substance of our discussion, however, was in the context of an extended case study focussing on the children of Man Bac, for the most part perinates through to 8 year-olds, representing the extremities of the more altricial to more precocial spectrum.

This case study effectively employed the stages outlined by Tilley as a framework in which to investigate health-related care of children in the past. The way in which Stage 2 of the bioarchaeology of care model is approached is clearly crucial in a model that was originally, and explicitly, designed to deal with adults. The younger the child the more difficult it will be to tease out specific health-related care from normal parental nurturing care. This will also be the case with the identification of serious physical disability in infants. Notwithstanding, the Man Bac example has demonstrated that inferences regarding health-related care can be made (at both Stages 3 and 4 of the model) even with respect to perinates and infants, where the rates of subadult morbidity and mortality are so high that one can only conclude a serious impact on the community and, potentially, a community-level response.

The Man Bac example has also demonstrated the importance of interpreting potential responses to subadult health and disease in the context of mortuary behaviour. We must be alert to any demographic signals in our cemetery samples that correlate with changes in the way in which children were treated in death. Clearly, while correlation does not equate with causation, it does provide a starting point for investigating behaviours that may have been influenced by the rate and nature of subadult illness and death in the past. Similarly, we also need to be aware of the potential for synergistic interactions between subadult morbidity and mortality and 'normal' parental nurturing care: timing of the introduction of non-breast milk foods and weaning behaviours are a case in point. It is not necessarily the case that all facets of parental nurturing care will necessarily be in the immediate interests of the child in question, with adults having their own agency in terms of the decisions they make as carers (e.g. redirecting resources to a new pregnancy as a way to offset increased chances of existing infant mortality). The care of sick children will clearly add to the psychological and physical burden on a carer already potentially stretched with the demands of normal nurturing care. It would be unrealistic to suppose that carers in such circumstances are not constantly making decisions regarding the distribution of finite resources and the probabilities of return for expenditure, even in the face of an overwhelming emotional investment in their charges.

The bioarchaeology of care model can be very effectively trained on children of all ages. However, children are quite clearly not adults, and the sorts of inferences we can make about them in the context of each stage of the care model will be heavily dependent on their age, their particular illness or disability, and the community and environment in which they existed.

References

Anh, D. D., Kilgore, P. E., Slack, M. P. E., Nyambat, B., Tho, L. H., Yoshida, L. M., et al. (2009). Surveillance of pneumococcal-associated disease among hospitalized children in Khanh Hoa province, Vietnam. *Clinical Infectious Diseases, 48*(2), S57–S64.

Bernin, H., & Lotter, H. (2014). Sex bias in the outcome of human tropical infectious diseases: Influence of steroid hormones. *Journal of Infectious Diseases, 209*(suppl 3), S107–S113.

Cave, C., & Oxenham, M. F. (2014). Identification of the archaeological 'invisible elderly': An approach illustrated with an Anglo-Saxon example. *International Journal of Osteoarchaeology, 26*, 163–175.

Cernetich, A., Garver, L. S., Jedlicka, A. E., Klein, P. W., Kumar, N., Scott, A. L., et al. (2006). Involvement of gonadal steroids and gamma interferon in sex differences in response to blood-stage malaria infection. *Infection and Immunity, 74*(6), 3190–3203.

Chongsuphajaisiddhi, T. (1991). Malaria. In P. Stanfield, M. Brueton, M. Chan, M. Parkin, & T. Waterston (Eds.), *Diseases of children in the subtropics and tropics* (pp. 657–674). Kent: E. Arnold.

Crawford, S. (1991). When do Anglo-Saxon children count? *Journal of Theoretical Archaeology, 2*, 17–24.

Davis-Floyd, R. E., & Sargent, C. F. (1997). *Childbirth and authoritative knowledge: Cross-cultural perspectives*. Berkeley: University of California Press.

Domett, K. M., & Oxenham, M. F. (2011). The demographic profile of the Man Bac cemetery sample. In M. Oxenham, H. Matsumura, & N. K. Dung (Eds.), *Man Bac: The excavation of a Neolithic site in Northern Vietnam. The biology* (Vol. 33, pp. 9–20). Canberra: ANU Epress.

Erhart, A., Thang, N. D., Van Ky, P., Tinh, T. T., Van Overmeir, C., Speybroeck, N., et al. (2005). Epidemiology of forest malaria in central Vietnam: A large scale cross-sectional survey. *Malaria Journal, 4*(1), 58.

Filippini, N. M. (1993). The Church, the State and childbirth: The midwife in Italy during the eighteenth century. In H. Marland (Ed.), *The art of Midwifery: Early modern midwives in Europe* (pp. 152–175). London: Routledge.

Gray, S. J. (1996). Ecology of weaning among nomadic Turkana pastoralists of Kenya: Maternal thinking, maternal behavior, and human adaptive strategies. *Human Biology, 68*(3), 437–465.

Isenbarger, D. W., Hien, B. T., Ha, H. T., Ha, T. T., Bodhidatta, L., Pang, L. W., et al. (2001). Prospective study of the incidence of diarrhoea and prevalence of bacterial pathogens in a cohort of Vietnamese children along the Red river. *Epidemiology and Infection, 127*(02), 229–236.

Klein, P. W., Easterbrook, J. D., Lalime, E. N., & Klein, S. L. (2008). Estrogen and progesterone affect responses to malaria infection in female C57BL/6 mice. *Gender Medicine, 5*(4), 423–433.

Le, H. T., Brouwer, I. D., Verhoef, H., Nguyen, K. C., & Kok, F. J. (2007). Anemia and intestinal parasite infection in school children in rural Vietnam. *Asia Pacific Journal of Clinical Nutrition, 16*(4), 716–723.

Leung, A. Y. (2006). Traditional toxicity documentation of Chinese Materia Medica: An overview. *Toxicologic Pathology, 34*, 319–326.

Lozano, R., Naghavi, M., Foreman, K., Lim, S., Shibuya, K., Aboyans, V., et al. (2012). Global and regional mortality from 235 causes of death for 20 age groups in 1990 and 2010: A systematic analysis for the Global Burden of Disease Study 2010. *The Lancet, 380*(9859), 2095–2128.

Lukacs, J. R. (2008). Fertility and agriculture accentuate sex differences in dental caries rates. *Current Anthropology, 49*(5), 901–914.

Lukacs, J. R., & Largaespada, L. L. (2006). Explaining sex differences in dental caries prevalence: Saliva, hormones, and 'life-history' etiologies. *American Journal of Human Biology, 18*(4), 540–555.

Marland, H. (1993). Introduction. In H. Marland (Ed.), *The art of Midwifery: Early modern midwives in Europe* (pp. 1–8). London: Routledge.

Matsumoto, T., Itoh, N., Inoue, S., & Nakamura, M. (2015). An observation of a severely disabled infant chimpanzee in the wild and her interactions with her mother. *Primates, 57*(1), 3–7.

McDonnell, A., & Oxenham, M. F. (2014). Localised primary canine hypoplasia: Implications for maternal and infant health at Man Bac, Vietnam, 3500-4000 years BP. *International Journal of Osteoarchaeology, 22*, 235–244.

Meehan, C. L., & Roulette, J. W. (2013). Early supplementary feeding among central African foragers and farmers: A biocultural approach. *Social Science and Medicine, 96*, 112–120.

Needham, C., Thi Kim, H., Viet Hoa, N., Dinh Cong, L., Michael, E., Drake, L., et al. (1998). Epidemiology of soil-transmitted nematode infections in Ha Nam Province, Vietnam. *Tropical Medicine & International Health, 3*(11), 904–912.

Nguyen, V. D. (2004). Fish-borne trematodes in Vietnam. *Southeast Asian Journal of Tropical Medicine and Public Health, 35*, 299–301.

Nguyen, V. D., Murrell, K. D., Le, D. C., Phung, D. C., Le, V. C., Nguyen, D. T., et al. (2003). The food-borne trematode zoonoses of Vietnam. *The Southeast Asian Journal of Tropical Medicine and Public Health, 34*(Suppl 1), 12–34.

Nguyen, P. H., Nguyen, K. C., Le Mai, B., Nguyen, T. V., Ha, K. H., Bern, C., et al. (2006). Risk factors for anemia in Vietnam. *The Southeast Asian Journal of Tropical Medicine and Public Health, 37*(6), 1213–1223.

Oxenham, M. F. (2001). *Health and behaviour during the Mid-Holocene and Metal period of Northern Vietnam*. Ph.D. Thesis, Northern Territory University.

Oxenham, M. F. (2012). Kids through adult eyes: The bioarchaeology of children. *The SAA Archaeological Record, 12*(2), 35–37.

Oxenham, M. F., & Buckley, H. R. (2016). Meta-themes in the bioarchaeology of the Asia pacific region. In M. F. Oxenham & H. Buckley (Eds.), *The routledge handbook of bioarchaeology in Southeast Asia and the Pacific* (pp. 655–662). London: Routledge.

Oxenham, M. F., & Domett, K. (2011). Palaeohealth at Man Bac. In M. Oxenham, H. Matsumura, & N. K. Dung (Eds.), *Man Bac: The excavation of a Neolithic site in Northern Vietnam. The biology* (Vol. 33, pp. 77–93). Canberra: ANU Epress.

Oxenham, M. F., Matsumura, H., Domett, K., Nguyen, K. T., Nguyen, K. D., Nguyen, L. C., et al. (2008). Health and the experience of childhood in late Neolithic Vietnam. *Asian Perspectives, 47*(2), 190–209.

Oxenham, M. F., Matsumura, H., & Nguyen, K. D. (2011). *Man Bac: The excavation of a Neolithic site in Northern Vietnam. The biology*. Canberra: ANU Press.

Oxenham, M. F., Tilley, L., Matsumura, H., Nguyen, L. C., Nguyen, K. T., Nguyen, K. D., et al. (2009). Paralysis and severe disability requiring intensive care in Neolithic Asia. *Anthropological Science, 117*(2), 107–112.

Phan, V. T., Ersbøll, A. K., Do, D. T., & Dalsgaard, A. (2010). Raw-fish-eating behavior and fish-borne zoonotic trematode infection in people of Northern Vietnam. *Foodborne Pathogens and Disease, 8*(2), 255–260.

Reubin, R. (1992). Women and malaria. In P. Wijeyaratne, E. M. Rathgeber, & E. St-Onge (Eds.), *Women and tropical diseases* (pp. 41–53). Ottawa: International Development Research Centre.

Riddle, J. M. (1992). *Contraception and abortion from the ancient world to the renaissance*. Cambridge, Massachusetts: Harvard University Press.

Ross, K. W., & Oxenham, M. F. (2016). To follow in their footsteps: An examination of the burial identity of the elderly from Non Nok Tha. In M. F. Oxenham & H. Buckley (Eds.), *The Routledge handbook of bioarchaeology in Southeast Asia and the pacific* (pp. 187–219). London: Routledge.

Scrimshaw, S. C. M. (1984). Infanticide in human populations: Societal and individual concerns. In G. Hausfater & S. B. Hrdy (Eds.), *Infanticide: Comparative and evolutionary perspectives* (pp. 439–462). New York: Aldine.

Thang, N. D., Erhart, A., Speybroeck, N., Hung, L. X., Thuan, L. K., Hung, C. T., et al. (2008). Malaria in central Vietnam: Analysis of risk factors by multivariate analysis and classification tree models. *Malaria Journal, 7*(1), 28.

Thompson, C. N., Phan, M. V. T., Hoang, N. V. M., Minh, P. V., Vinh, N. T., Thuy, C. T., et al. (2015). A prospective multi-center observational study of children hospitalized with diarrhoea in Ho Chi Minh City, Vietnam. *The American Journal of Tropical Medicine and Hygiene, 92*(5), 1045–1052.

Tilley, L. (2015). *Theory and practice in the bioarchaeology of care*. New York: Springer.

Tilley, L., & Oxenham, M. F. (2011). Survival against the odds: Modeling the social implications of care provision to seriously disabled individuals. *International Journal of Paleopathology, 1*(1), 35–42.

Trang, D. T., Mølbak, K., Cam, P. D., & Dalsgaard, A. (2007). Helminth infections among people using wastewater and human excreta in peri-urban agriculture and aquaculture in Hanoi, Vietnam. *Tropical Medicine & International Health, 12*, 82–90.

van der Hoek, W., De, N. V., Konradsen, F., Cam, P. D., Hoa, N. T. V., Toan, N. D., et al. (2003). Current status of soil-transmitted helminths in Vietnam. *The Southeast Asian Journal of Tropical Medicine and Public Health, 34*(Suppl 1), 1–11.

Verle, P., Kongs, A., De, N. V., Thieu, N. Q., Depraetere, K., Kim, H. T., et al. (2003). Prevalence of intestinal parasitic infections in northern Vietnam. *Tropical Medicine & International Health, 8*(10), 961–964.

Vlassoff, C., & Bonilla, E. (1994). Gender-related differences in the impact of tropical diseases on women: What do we know? *Journal of Biosocial Science, 26*(01), 37–53.

Webb, J. (1991). Diseases of the respiratory system. In P. Stanfield, M. Brueton, M. Chan, M. Parkin, & T. Waterston (Eds.), *Diseases of children in the subtropics and tropics* (pp. 706–724). Kent: E. Arnold.

Wilkie, L. A. (2003). *The archaeology of mothering: An African-American midwife's tale*. London: Routledge.

Willis, A. (2015). *The bioarchaeology of An Sơn and Hòa Diêm: Biosocial insights into prehistoric southern Vietnam*. Ph.D. Thesis, The Australian National University, Canberra.

Willis, A., & Oxenham, M. F. (2013). The neolithic demographic transition and oral health: The Southeast Asian experience. *American Journal of Physical Anthropology, 152*(2), 197–208.

Chapter 12
Growing Old: Biographies of Disability and Care in Later Life

Rebecca Gowland

... the contamination of life by death (Kristeva, 1982, p. 149)

Introduction

Our bodies are ever-changing entities – in childhood we undergo rapid growth and development; in adulthood we continue to renew and remodel during the process of senescence. Within the Western world, age is conceptualised chronologically, but it is experienced and lived through our bodies: the reality of time is crystallised through our own wrinkling skin, greying hair and embodied interactions with our peers and other generations. Perceptions of our corporeal selves are dictated by social mores and behaviours deemed appropriate to our life course stage: we are aged by culture as much as we are by the passing of time (Arber & Ginn, 1991; Brogden, 2001).

However, the process of senescence also introduces biological constraints of frailty and forces a tangible, embodied, confrontation with the reality of time's passing (Hockey & James, 2003). As Wendell (1996, p. 18) states '[u]nless we die suddenly ... most of us will live part of our lives with bodies that hurt, that move with difficulty or not at all, that deprive us of activities we once took for granted'. Pain and impairment are expected sequelae of old age and are the source of visceral fear concerning the ageing process in contemporary society: we are the 'impaired in waiting' (Gilleard & Higgs, 2010). For example, the BBC recently reported (3rd May 2015) the story of a nurse, Gill Pharoah, aged 75 years, who, though still healthy, travelled to Switzerland for an assisted death, because of her fear of *impending* frailty. She wrote: 'I simply do not want to follow this natural deterioration through to the last stage when I may be requiring a lot of help'. Such anxieties are not exclusive to the modern industrialised world, but are also expressed in historical

R. Gowland, Ph.D. (✉)
Department of Archaeology, Durham University, Durham, UK
e-mail: rebecca.gowland@durham.ac.uk

© Springer International Publishing Switzerland 2017

L. Tilley, A.A. Schrenk (eds.), *New Developments in the Bioarchaeology of Care*, Bioarchaeology and Social Theory, DOI 10.1007/978-3-319-39901-0_12

and ethnographic sources (see Brogden, 2001; Pelling & Smith, 1991; Thane, 2000). For example, in the first century AD in Rome, Seneca writes:

> *Just as a ship that springs a leak, you can always stop the first or the second fissure, but when many holes begin to open and let in water, the gaping hull cannot be saved; similarly, in an old man's body there is a certain limit up to which you can sustain and prop its weakness. But when it comes to resemble a decrepit building – when every joint begins to spread and whilst one is being repaired another falls apart – then it is time for a man to look about him and consider how he may get out* (Seneca *Ep. 30.1–2*, cited in Cockayne, 2003, p. 51).

Given the likelihood of impairment in older age, it is worthwhile considering past perceptions of old age and disability within the context of caregiving. Deteriorating health requires a creeping and continuous renegotiation of self and an increasing reliance on social networks to mitigate 'risk' and prevent increasing frailty from becoming disabling (Gilleard & Higgs, 2010). Kinship relationships are the primary source of informal caregiving in later life. It is therefore important to consider the changing relationships between family members over time and the shift in caregiving responsibilities and needs throughout life's unfolding (Aitkin & Griffith, 1996).

In today's ageing society, impairment has become a normalised facet of old age; one is not disabled, merely 'elderly' (Priestley, 2003). As a consequence, the elderly have largely been excluded from the disability literature, which has tended to focus on the social exclusion and experiences of young and middle-aged disabled adults (Priestley, 2003). Archaeological studies of disability have likewise rarely considered impairment in old age, though this stems from an overall neglect of this demographic in studies of the past, rather than disability politics (Gowland, 2007, 2015a).

This chapter adopts a life course approach to care in the past in order to better understand the potential impact of disability for older individuals and their caregiver(s). This is a theory-led chapter, which draws primarily upon the disability studies and sociological literature situated within present-day contexts. Whilst our contemporary demographic and social context may be far removed from many past societies, such literature still provides useful insights into the interrelationship between disability, caregiving and identity in later life. The chapter is structured around three key areas that have relevance for the theoretical development of a bioarchaeology of care and the Index of Care instrument (see Chap. 2, this volume). Firstly, it considers the importance of including a perspective on elder care in the context of the life course, senescence and the treatment of chronic disease; secondly, it emphasises the interrelationship between age identity and expectations of performance when interpreting concepts of disability; and thirdly it poses questions regarding the identity of the 'invisible' carer(s) – largely ignored in current accounts, in which the interpretive gaze is firmly directed at the sufferer, or within palaeopathology, on the *disease* process. The bioarchaeology of care approach specifically urges a focus on the implications of caregiving for gaining a greater understanding of the community in which care occurs (Tilley, Chap. 2 this volume), but has not explicitly explored the identity of specific caregiver(s). Before examining these factors, it is worth first considering concepts of 'age', 'old age' and 'embodiment' in studies of disability, both past and present.

Old Age in the Social Sciences

Age is a unique form of identity, because it is a cumulative, rather than an exclusive, identity. While we may know what it is to possess either a male or female identity, we have each experienced childhood, adolescence or any younger form of ourselves. Humans are somewhat unusual in that we 'remember our past and worry about the future' (Crews, 2003, p. 1). Further, what happens to us during these younger periods may have implications for both physical and social trajectories in later life. For example, the implications of early life adversity for chronic disease risk in adulthood (Developmental Origins of Health and Disease hypothesis) is currently subject to a great deal of medical and social health research (e.g. Barker, Eriksson, Forsén, & Osmond, 2002; Gowland, 2015a). Indeed, epidemiologists are increasingly adopting a life course approach to the study of disease prevalence and risk (Davey, 2011). Likewise, the skeleton does not represent a snapshot in time, but rather a selective accumulation of life experiences which impact upon the chemical and morphological structure of the bones. This temporal component of the skeleton is explicitly harnessed through the osteobiographical approach, which has proven to be theoretically fruitful for skeletal analyses (e.g. Robb, 2002), including studies of past care (e.g. Tilley & Oxenham, 2011). Likewise, it is useful to consider perceptions of elder impairment and care from a relational and biographical perspective, rather than as 'a moment in time'. The elderly skeleton represents a life lived, containing skeletal and biographical echoes of a person's childhood as well as later phases of their life (Gowland, 2015b).

The elderly body in the modern industrialised world is currently the preserve of medical gerontologists, concerned with biomedical interventions aimed at mitigating the natural processes of bodily decay (Pickard, 2014). Since the 1970s there has been an increasing medicalisation of age-related processes, such as the menopause, which is regarded as a 'condition' – existing outside of culture – requiring 'treatment' (Ferguson & Parry, 1998). It has been argued that the older body has been subjected to an 'othering' in biomedical models in which old age and disease may be regarded as synonymous (Pickard, 2014). By contrast, and again until recently, sociologists failed to engage with elderly bodies, instead examining old age as a culturally situated phenomenon alone (i.e. in relation to factors such as mandatory retirement) (Twigg, 2004). It has been argued that sociologists (in common with proponents of the social model of disability) have been guilty of writing the body out of their accounts of old age: fearing that to consider the ageing body would be retrogressive – returning to a/the position of biological determinism (Twigg, 2004). However, since the 1990s there has been a move to re-insert the physical body into discourses of identity, including ageing, and this has had profound implications for bioarchaeological interpretations (Gowland & Thompson, 2013; Shilling, 1993; Sofaer, 2006).

The physical reality of the ageing body is now emerging as a prominent force in accounts of elderly experiences and identities. As Twigg (2004, p. 66) argues, 'we need to give weight to the complexity and plurality of social and cultural meanings that have and do adhere to the bodily, recognizing the ways in which the body and bodily experience are constituted in and through discourses'. By considering life course stages such as old age in relation to biological remains, we are not returning to a position of biological determinism, but are instead acknowledging the 'tripartite relationship between social environment, human agency and the body' (Hockey & James, 2003, p. 135). In gender studies, a clear distinction is usually maintained between sex as a biological construct and gender as a social construct. While this separation between sex and gender has long been critiqued, it serves a useful discursive purpose and is generally maintained in bioarchaeological studies (see Sørensen, 2000 and Sofaer, 2006 for a discussion). Likewise, the influence of cultural beliefs and practices on the physical body in terms of the timing of age-related 'biological' changes, or the manifestation of symptoms of illness are potentially profound. The field of medical anthropology is producing some interesting results concerning the interrelationship between biology and culture in this respect. For example, amongst the traditional Inuit males, a hunting lifestyle necessitates a high degree of physical fitness. However, once their sons become adept hunters and they are able to reduce their own hunting activities, they experience disproportionately rapid physical deterioration (Beall, 1984, pp. 87–88). The timing of this physical degeneration can only be understood with reference to the particular cultural context (Gowland, 2006).

Senescence and decrepitude have long been important identifying features of the elderly, past and present (Brogden, 2001). In today's society, which fetishises the youthful body – the smooth, taut, unblemished skin, and the ability to engage in fluid and expansive bodily movements – this is particularly problematic. Within this context, the denigration of the elderly body appears to be inevitable, and it is often regarded as: 'not only functionally problematic but also aesthetically offensive' (Pickard, 2014, p. 1285). Negative attitudes towards the elderly within contemporary society are thought to have increased with industrialisation and modernisation (Cohen, 1984). The decline in oral tradition following modernity resulted in a replacement of the authority of the 'elders' with political and jural systems (Halperin, 1984). It would be wrong, however, to infer that the elder members of past communities were consistently treated with greater respect (Foner, 1984; Halperin, 1984; Shahar, 1997). Texts from both the ancient and medieval worlds supply negative descriptions of physiological decline in old age and expressions of repugnance towards the ageing body – often the subject of grotesque parody (Parkin, 2003, 2011; Pelling & Smith, 1991). Ethnographic studies have also highlighted examples in which the impaired ageing body comes to be regarded as problematic and burdensome (Brogden, 2001). For example, death-hastening behaviour towards elders who become impaired, including direct homicide, as well as more passive forms of euthanasia such as the withdrawal of care, or failure to provide sustenance or warmth, are well documented in many communities, even those which venerate elderly people (see De Beauvoir, 1973 and Brogden, 2001, for examples). Indeed, elderly people may be active agents in hastening their own deaths, often through refusal to eat, drink or receive medicine. Their motives are variable, but range from concern with being a burden to their loved ones to deeming their quality of life to be no longer endurable, due to either physical pain or social isolation (Simon, 1989).

Gilleard and Higgs (2011, pp. 137–138) argue that the ageing body is a source of abhorrence and fear, in part due to bodily decline, but also because of the proximity of old age to death. However, the finality of death, whilst a feature of modern secular society, is not a concept shared by all cultures in the past, for whom death may have marked a transition towards another, potentially more desirable, state of being. Within such cultures, the end stage of life may have been more greatly valued *because* of its proximity to death and spiritual transcendence (Gowland, in press). The following will examine concepts of old age and the life course in more detail before discussing the relevance for studies of disability and care in the past.

A Life Course Perspective on Care

Old Age and Identity

The application of the Index of Care to skeletal remains requires an osteobiographical approach, whereby an individual's impairment in terms of disablement is interpreted in relation to information obtained about their life history (e.g. Tilley & Oxenham, 2011). The life course can be conceptualised as a series of 'life pathways' and transitions over the trajectory of life from conception to death (Marshall, 1996; Moen, 1996, p. 181). It recognises the fluidity and intersectionality of identities throughout life; for example, gender identity is contingent upon life course stage. It is important to consider factors such as status, gender and age within 'bioarchaeology of care' discussions, because they influence the conferment of the identity 'disabled' in the presence of an impairment. In respect to older individuals, through language and imagery, the elderly have become both feminised and infantilised in the modern consciousness; transformations linked in that they serve to reinforce an illusion of weakness, dependency and low status (Arber & Ginn, 1991; Hockey & James, 1993). Feminisation occurs in part because the majority of the very old are in fact women, but primarily because those same social characteristics previously used to disparage women are ascribed to the older males as well (i.e. dependent and weak) (Ginn & Arber, 1995). It has been argued by Arber and Ginn (1991, p. 18) that parallels can be drawn between the social construction of women as the weaker sex, and the construction of negative aspects of old age.

Confinement to the domestic sphere, and the loss of rigidly defined gender roles, have contributed to the blurring of gendered identities with age (Ginn & Arber, 1995). Age frequently becomes the overriding defining characteristic of the elderly, often asserting a primacy over gender (Moen, 1996, p. 181). In fact, many anthropological accounts attest to a culturally androgynous state for older women (e.g. Cole, 1992; Coles, 1990; Rasmussen, 2000). For example, in Samoa, the strongly adhered to male/female avoidance patterns that begin at puberty between brother and sister no longer apply when women become old (Holmes & Holmes, 1995, p. 84). Such cultural androgyny does not necessarily coincide with menopausal change, but is more often connected to social factors that are only indirectly related to age, such as the marriage of a child or widowhood (Rasmussen, 1987). The same is also true for males, who in later life may assume roles more intimately connected with the domestic sphere. For example, Fijian men in the earlier part of the last century took on a range of domestic chores with old age and lavished greater time and affection on their wives (Quain, 1948). In some contexts, this loss of gender identity may lead to enhanced status and power, while in others it leads to marginalisation. It has been argued, for example, that elderly females in the ancient world were regarded as doubly disempowered, firstly because of their sex and secondly because of their age (Parkin, 2003). Similar observations regarding elder females have been made for societies across the world today (e.g. Rudkin, 1993). Of course there are no universals, and amongst the !Kung older women are granted the power to express their sexuality more overtly (Holmes & Holmes, 1995). Likewise, older woman in medieval and classical literature are often caricatured as sexually salacious. Older age can be a positive and empowering experience, freeing women from the more rigid social conformity that constrains the agency of their younger counterparts.

A life course approach also recognises the cumulative nature of individual biographies; in other words, it explicitly considers the way in which identities and experiences in early life may impact upon later stages (Hockey & Draper, 2005, p. 43). This is a departure from the earlier 'life cycle' approach to age, because one's identity and physiology at any moment in time is borne out of earlier phases, which may have diverging effects on individual trajectories. The above has highlighted the fluidity of gender and status identity throughout the life course. The relevance of this for studies of disability and care provision in the past will be explored further below.

Disability and Biography

Disabilities may be acquired at any stage in the life course, through accident or disease; symptoms may be chronic and degenerative, or transient and episodic. Our age and social identity at the time of impairment, however, is significant in terms of the impact of the illness and injury on an individual's identity and the provision of treatment (Priestley, 2003). In part, this relates to the fact that an individual's roles and 'contribution' – *expectations* of them – are contingent upon age norms. Infants and children are *expected* to be engaged to a different degree in economic activities (within the household or wider community) when compared to adults. Likewise, the roles of the elderly are *expected* to differ from younger adults. This is one of the reasons that the elderly are not considered truly disabled in current Western contexts – they are not excluded from the means of production on the basis of their impairment, they were already excluded because of their age. If we are to consider a life course interpretation with respect to the application of the Index of Care, then there are implications in terms of the category of 'essential activities of daily living', which are life course dependent. For example, an infant is not expected to wash or feed themselves, but an adult is. Care of an impaired infant may therefore be more 'acceptable' than for a similarly impaired adult. Likewise, 'instrumental activities' are contingent upon the identity and the age of the impaired individual and the social norms that pertain to these.

An impaired adult may once have been an impaired infant and child, or they may have acquired the disease later in life. The social implications of, for example, a chronic congenital disease may not be particularly significant during infancy when dependency is the norm, but may become increasingly apparent as more normative developmental milestones are missed during childhood and into adolescence. However, in such cases, caregiving decisions do not derive from societal reactions to, for example, a chronically ill adolescent, but have developed out of earlier, more *normative* caregiving of the impaired individual as an infant, which has then evolved to accommodate the increasingly *non-normative* physical state of the growing child.

Illness or frailty acquired during adulthood may 'strike down' someone who had been a physically active and vibrant member of the community. This could precipitate an altered identity, but one that is contingent upon a pre-impairment persona. High status and extensive social networks may serve to ameliorate any disablement or stigma. There is therefore a dialectic between impairment and the identity of the individual, with each influencing the impact of the other in terms of disability. Diseases themselves have a social identity: they may be perceived to reflect immorality or impurity, or be associated with activities that are regarded as either high or low status. However, a particular disease or impairment may be regarded differently depending on the social identity of the sufferer. For example, a leprosy sufferer from the high status burial ground of St Marylebone in London received a normative and inclusive burial, and was the recipient of (at that time) sophisticated and expensive medical treatment and subsequent care in the form of a successful amputation (Walker, 2009). The wealthy status of the individual prior to impairment resulted in a reduction in the social stigma of the disease. Similarly, in present-day Nepal, high status individuals suffering from leprosy have the resources of their families to draw upon in order to counteract social stigma (Hyland, 2000).

Males and females may have different experiences of disability as a consequence of societal norms regarding gendered performance and activity (Shuttleworth, Wedgewood, & Wilson, 2012). Different patterns of response by men and women with the same impairment (e.g. social withdrawal) may be due to societal perceptions regarding how well they are able to embody cultural norms of masculinity or femininity. The concept of 'performativity' has been particularly important in feminist research (Butler, 1990) and has implications for perceptions of disability (Pickard, 2014). Disabilities that impinge upon gendered or age-related activities may induce a loss of perceived femininity or masculinity. However, gendered performance is also life course specific; roles change as individuals grow up and grow old. This is important, because activities defined as 'instrumental' in the Index of Care approach (Chap. 2, this volume) are contingent upon the identity and the age of the impaired individual, and the social norms that pertain to this stage. For example, 'reproduction' may be considered an 'instrumental activity' for a young adult women. Infertility therefore may be a significant impairment for a woman of this age, but would be expected for an older woman.

In modern disability studies there has been an emphasis on the extent to which an impaired individual is able to participate in the 'economic means of production'. A young and middle-aged adult should be a 'productive' one, and this is tied to their social worth. If productivity is inhibited due to physical impairment, then 'accommodation' must be made for him/her by the other members of society if the individual's survival is to be ensured (Chap. 2, this volume). A disabled individual may, in fact, become perceived as more normative with increasing age, when societal expectations regarding 'performance' and 'abilities' may become more closely aligned. So while an impairment may remain biologically static throughout an individual's life course, the 'disability' may be more fluid in accordance with gendered and age-related societal expectations. Therefore a disabled person who becomes elderly, and an elderly person who becomes disabled, can experience very different social transitions. As Priestley points out, 'impairment characteristics regarded as aberrant in younger bodies are often viewed as 'normal' in ageing bodies' and thus disability identity is life course situated (Priestley, 2003, p. 152).

Of course, what constitutes a 'productive individual' is culture specific, and this concept is not necessarily one which would apply to all populations or periods. Indeed, it has been linked to capitalist ideas of economic participation that have burgeoned since in the Industrial Revolution in the eighteenth and nineteenth centuries. In actuality, many older people across cultures engage in vital child-rearing activities (i.e. care provision) and other roles that are confined to the domestic rather than the public sphere. In some societies these roles will be valued, whilst in others they may contribute to the liminal or marginalised status of the elder person – perhaps more so for males, as the domestic context is traditionally a feminine domain in which roles are poorly valued. This marginal status may then influence the level of caregiving that the elder person receives.

A biographical approach to the understanding of impairments has been emphasised by a number of disability studies' authors, including Bury (1982), who described the acquisition of chronic disease during adulthood as inducing a 'biographical disruption'. In other words, the sufferers conceptualise their illness as a form of interference. The sufferers also come to terms with their illness through reference to their biographies, i.e. referring to specific triggers or occupations that predisposed them to the disease – often with no medical justification (Sanders, Donovan, & Dieppe, 2002). With regard to the elderly, impairment is considered a biographical inevitability (Priestley, 2003). In relation to this, Sanders et al.'s (2002) study of older people's experience of osteoarthritis noted that the disease was normalised by the sufferers, and the debilitating effects downplayed. The authors state:

> *respondents seemed to feel doubly disadvantaged in that they felt a degree of stigma in being disabled, and at the same time they were not viewed as being legitimately disabled because they were old. In other words, disability should be expected and accepted in old age* (Sanders et al., 2002, p. 239).

A further development in life course research relates to a greater awareness of the interdependence of life course trajectories and roles. It is important to consider this interdependence with regard to the impact of disability on social relationships and caregiving.

Age and Carer Identities

Individuals are not monadic entities; strong interdependencies exist in terms of the life course trajectories of related individuals (Levy & the Pavie Team, 2005, p. 6). The inter-connectivity of age identity is often not explicitly stated in studies of age in the past, instead archaeologists tend to focus on individual life courses and life stages as discrete and separate entities. Age transitions, such as marriage or widowhood, precipitate changes in social relationships, interactions and individual identities: 'our identities, our sense of self … are all relational, reflecting a variety of social networks, social capital and the contextual circumstances in which we live' (Hendricks, 2012, p. 227).

The age of an individual at the point at which they became impaired is significant not only for the sufferer, but also in terms of care provision (see below) and sufferer/carer dynamics. Impairment precipitates a shift in power relationships and creates new interactions around dependency. It is not only the sufferer that enters the world of the impaired, with potential repercussions for social agency; so too does the carer. The act of caring and the roles and performativity surrounding care provision can have a transformative (both positive and negative) impact on the carer. For example, in the UK in 2013 the Office for National Statistics reported that there were currently a quarter of a million young carers (i.e. children caring for an adult relative), and this is thought to represent the 'tip of the iceberg'. This is worth considering for several reasons, because 'care' tends to be viewed as an adult (often female) role. But if the mother of a young child becomes disabled and is unable to dress or feed herself, then there is often a reversal in caregiving: the cared for becomes the carer. Accounts of child carers often refer to the children as having to 'grow up too quickly' or 'miss out on their childhood', suggesting that the act of provisioning care imbues the child with an adult identity. In this example, the mother's disability profoundly affects the identity of the child through his/her caring responsibilities.

The act of caring for a disabled person therefore also represents a 'biographical challenge' to the carer (Chamberlayne & King, 1997). The carer/cared for relationship is important to consider because it has implications in terms of both motives for caregiving and the efficacy of that care. In current studies of disability in the past the carer is largely invisible: all eyes are instead upon the impaired person. Historical studies of family life and household composition in the past have tended not to consider carer identities beyond roles such as motherhood. Within an archaeological context, accessing information on carer identity might be problematic, but would need to draw upon a range of evidence including settlement and household structure in addition to burial context.

Elderly individuals are more likely to be in a position of social and physiological dependency – i.e. requiring care from family, friends or neighbours. Over a person's life course the identity of the carer will change, traditionally from parent, to spouse, to adult offspring and grand-offspring, though children are often carers for younger siblings and (as discussed above) may act as carers for impaired adults in either a primary, or (more often) a supportive role. Power within families shifts and subverts throughout the life course: parents exercise power over their growing children, restricting and censoring behaviour, whilst in older age, role reversal may occur as parents then become dependent upon their adult children. It is important to consider the fact that carer/dependent relations are based on power imbalances, and have the potential to become abusive rather than supportive (Bennett, Kingston, & Penhale, 1997). Social networks are crucial to adequate elder care and, without them, the process of disablement may be accelerated (Bury, 1982). Frailty in old age is often linked to social isolation: an elderly person living alone is less likely to venture outside if they are in pain, or have mobility difficulties.

The provision of care for elder members of past societies has rarely been examined in the archaeological literature (though see Gowland, 2015b, in press). There is an inherent assumption that past societies lived in extended families and mutually supportive communities, in which ageing was a collective rather than an individualised, risk. It is likewise often assumed that elderly people in the past were universally respected and would have been afforded care. However, this is unlikely to have been true of all past populations. In Roman Britain, households consisted of the nuclear rather than the extended family. In such cases, care provision would have been most often provided by adult offspring of the elderly individual. That this form of household structure was common at this time is supported by various forms of historical texts relating to the Roman world (see Parkin, 2003). Gowland (in press) highlights a number of cases in which the bioarchaeological evidence indicates the marginalisation and even abuse of some elderly females from Roman Britain. For example, evidence of the liminal status of impaired older females was noted at the Romano-British cemetery of Watersmeet, Huntingdon, Cambridgeshire. At this site, two older females, both exhibiting severe and extensive osteoarthritis and one with an un-united fractured ulna, were buried away from the main cemetery and in non-normative burial positions (Gowland, in press). Indeed, Nicholson (2006) even implies that one of them could have been buried alive (termed a 'coerced burial'). The marginalisation of older impaired females within *Romano-British* contexts could reflect a similar 'cultural distancing' and 'structural dislocation' from other ages groups that is evident in today's society (Priestley, 2003, p. 146).

Identification of abuse in the archaeological record is problematic, but it is relevant to studies of care, because people in need of care, of whatever age, are vulnerable to abuse. As Hockey and James (2003, p. 139) observe, 'agency and choice imply an empowered or embodied individual. Yet our access to power is constrained by our physicality, our dependency and our relationships with others'. Hughes et al. (2012) demonstrated an increase in prevalence of abuse in disabled individuals compared to their non-disabled counterparts. In the context of elder abuse specifically, physical and cognitive impairments in the elderly person are likely to result in a substantial increase in the likelihood that they will be abused (Lachs & Pillemer, 1995).

Present-day categorisations of abuse include the terms 'Passive Neglect' and 'Active Neglect' by a carer. These two categories are differentiated through the intent of the perpetrator and whether pain was inflicted purposefully or not (Wolf & Pillemer, 1989). Differentiation between these two forms of carer neglect would be particularly problematic in an archaeological context. Indeed, cases of neglect per se are difficult to decipher from skeletal remains, because they are likely to lead to archaeologically invisible forms of death such as starvation, or dehydration. In an immobile elderly individual, the presence of large and severe pressure sores are regarded in present-day carer settings as an indicator of neglect and, in extreme situations, as an indicator of abuse (DiMaio & DiMaio, 2001). Severe pressure sores can affect the underlying bone, potentially resulting in periosteal new bone formation, atrophy and even osteomyelitis. In theory, pressure sores could be used as an indirect indicator of elder neglect, if not abuse, in the archaeological record (Gowland, 2015b). Conversely, Tilley and Oxenham (2011) argue that the *absence* of skeletal evidence for pressure sores in a Neolithic individual with juvenile onset quadriplegia from North Vietnam can be used to demonstrate *good* quality care in the archaeological record.

The identification of active abuse within a household, either directly inflicted by the primary carer or by other family members, would need to invoke evidence of skeletal lesions indicative of physical violence in an individual who shows evidence of frailty, or was demonstrably in need of care. Gowland (2015b) compiled a list of skeletal lesions likely to indicate such abuse and, in common with other forms of family violence, these are most diagnostic when multiple lesions are present and in various stages of healing. Evidence of likely abuse is found in a nineteenth century elderly female skeleton, currently curated at the Royal College of Surgeons, London. This individual suffered from a severe form of joint disease, resulting in proliferative new bone growth and ankyloses at a number of joints. Her skeleton exhibits evidence of rib fractures, some with new bone formation, an un-united fracture to the right clavicle, a fractured right ischial ramus, and a roughened area on the posterior aspect of the right ilium, which, according to the notes accompanying the individual, corresponded to a pressure sore during life (Gowland, in press). While fractured clavicles often occur due to a fall on an outstretched hand, the presence of a very severe pressure sore, the fractured ischium, and severe degenerative disease, suggests that this woman was likely to have been bed-ridden. Rib fractures can also occur from a fall, or even vigorous coughing, and are not definitive evidence of abuse. However, the fractures reported here represent more than one traumatic event, due to evidence of osseous response in relation to some, but not all, of the trauma. The locations of the multiple injuries in different stages of healing correspond to the clinical criteria observed in elder abuse (Gowland, 2015b). The profile of the individual as old, female, and severely impaired, also aligns with victims today (Gowland, 2015b, in press). Given what is known about perpetrators of elder abuse, it seems likely (though not of course definitive) that the carer(s) in this instance would have been the adult off-spring of the elderly woman.

Care in premodern contexts is unlikely to have been a community effort in all cases, and the burden of care will have frequently fallen on those closest to the individual. Caregiving occurs within many contexts – under the public gaze of the wider community, and in the privacy of a domestic setting. Carer/sufferer relationships have the potential to become abusive, whether involving active violence or more passive neglect. Active violence towards elder people may be culturally sanctioned and involve ceremony, or it may occur as a prohibited act (Brogden, 2001). Providing care for an impaired person is not a passive, unidirectional act. It may have a profound impact on the caregiver's own identity and habitus; it can restrict their behaviour and activities in much the same way as the sufferers. Relationships are altered by impairment and disablement, and power shifts and new relationships of dependency and constraint are forged.

Conclusions

Being elderly and frail in today's society invokes images of dependency, otherness, social isolation and a lack of autonomy and agency. There are clear parallels between discourses of old age and those concerned with disability; each of these embodied states is treated with abjection (Gilleard & Higgs, 2010). The intersectionality between age identity and disability identity is also striking – old age has the power to subsume the stigma of 'disablement', replacing it instead with the construct of 'frailty'.

Disablement is not only culturally specific, but is dependent on a number of key factors:

1. The type of disease/condition and the culturally specific construction of that disease state.
2. The identity of the sufferer, including their biography, stage of the life course, status, gender, age and religion.
3. Performance/behavioural expectations pertinent to the individual's identity/life course stage, and the degree to which an impairment impinges on these activities.
4. Social context, societal and kinship norms regarding the provision of care for individuals at different life course stages and the ability/will to accommodate impairment.

Each of these factors should be considered when interpreting bioarchaeological evidence. There is a tendency within the palaeopathological literature to consider an impairment as a fixed biological state with uniform social implications, rather than one predicated upon the interaction between the individual's identity, biography and disease process. Further, in those instances in which an impairment does remain biologically static, levels of disablement may fluctuate throughout the life course as a consequence of shifting societal expectations. Conversely, diseases that *are* progressive require the sufferer's sense of identity and embodiment to be continually renegotiated over the life course. This is also true for the degenerative physical changes that accompany ageing. It is worthwhile considering these factors more explicitly in an Index of Care approach.

This chapter has shown how older people may become socially isolated or marginalised as a consequence of their impairments. This occurs today, and there are examples of it in the archaeological record (Gowland, in press). In such instances, the level of care investment provided may be insufficient, or individuals may become victims of passive neglect, or direct physical abuse. Conversely, older people may be complicit in hastening their own deaths. Finally, it is worthwhile attempting to consider the identity of those providing the care and understanding the biographical challenge inherent in caring for a loved one. Decisions surrounding care provision are multifaceted and emotional, but the act of intensive caregiving can profoundly impact upon the identity of the carer as they too are drawn into the world of the disabled.

Acknowledgements Many thanks to Alecia A. Schrenk, Lorna Tilley and Debra Martin for inviting me to participate in the SAA session. This chapter would not exist (for better or worse!) without the encouragement of Lorna Tilley and her very generous feedback and comments on an earlier version of the manuscript. Thanks to Rebecca Redfern for drawing my attention to the old lady at the Royal College of Surgeons. Finally, thanks to Tim Thompson for his comments on a previous draft.

References

Aitkin, L., & Griffith, G. (1996). *Gender issues in elder abuse*. London: Sage Publications.

Arber, S., & Ginn, J. (1991). *Gender and later life*. London: Sage.

Barker, D. J. P., Eriksson, J. G., Forsén, T., & Osmond, C. (2002). Fetal origins of adult disease: Strength of effects and biological basis. *International Journal of Epidemiology, 31*, 1235–1239.

BBC News. (2015, August). Gill Pharoah's Decision to Attend Suicide Clinic Defended. Retrieved August 4, 2015, from http://www.bbc.co.uk/news/uk-england-london-33759490.

Beall, C. M. (1984). Theoretical dimensions of a focus on age in physical anthropology. In D. I. Kertzer & J. Keith (Eds.), *Age and anthropological theory* (pp. 82–95). Ithaca, New York: Cornell University Press.

Bennett, G., Kingston, P., & Penhale, M. B. (1997). *The dimensions of elder abuse*. London: Palgrave Macmillan.

Brogden, M. (2001). *Geronticide: Killing the elderly*. London: Jessica Kinglsey Publishers.

Bury, M. R. (1982). Chronic illness as biographical disruption. *Sociology of Health and Illness, 4*, 167–182.

Butler, J. (1990). *Gender trouble: Feminism and the subversion of identity*. London: Routledge.

Chamberlayne, P., & King, A. (1997). The biographical challenge of caring. *Sociology of Health and Illness, 19*, 601–621.

Cockayne, K. (2003). *Experiencing age in ancient Rome*. London: Routledge.

Cohen, R. (1984). Age and culture as theory. In D. I. Kertzer & J. Keith (Eds.), *Age and anthropological theory* (pp. 234–249). Ithaca, New York: Cornell University Press.

Cole, T. R. (1992). *The journey of life*. Cambridge: Cambridge University Press.

Coles, C. (1990). The older women in Hausa society. In J. Soklovsky (Ed.), *The cultural context of ageing* (pp. 57–81). London: Bergen and Garvey.

Crews, D. (2003). *Human senescence: Evolutionary and biocultural perspectives*. Cambridge: Cambridge University Press.

Davey, S. G. (2011). Epidemiology, epigenetics and the 'gloomy prospect': Embracing randomness in population health research and practice. *International Journal of Epidemiology, 40*, 537–562.

De Beauvoir, S. (1973). *The coming of age*. Harmondsworth: Penguin.

DiMaio, V. J., & DiMaio, D. (2001). *Forensic pathology* (2nd ed.). CRC Press: Boca Raton.

Ferguson, S. J., & Parry, C. (1998). Rewriting menopause: Challenging the medical paradigm to reflect menopausal women's experiences. *Frontiers A Journal of Woman Studies, 19*, 20–41.

Foner, N. (1984). Age and social change. In D. I. Kertzer & J. Keith (Eds.), *Age and anthropological theory* (pp. 195–216). Ithaca, New York: Cornell University Press.
Gilleard, C., & Higgs, P. (2010). Frailty, disability and old age: A re-appraisal. Health: An interdisciplinary.*JournalfortheStudyofHealthIllnessandMedicine*.doi:10.1177/1363459310383595.
Gilleard, C., & Higgs, P. (2011). Aging abjection and embodiment in the fourth age. *Journal of Aging Studies, 25*(2), 135–142.
Ginn, J., & Arber, S. (1995). 'Only connect': Gender relations and ageing. In S. Arber & J. Ginn (Eds.), *Connecting gender and ageing: A sociological approach* (pp. 1–14). Buckingham: Open University Press.
Gowland, R. L. (2006). Ageing the past: Examining age identity from funerary evidence. In R. L. Gowland & C. J. Knüsel (Eds.), *Social archaeology of funerary remains*. Oxford: Oxbow.
Gowland, R. L. (2007). Age, ageism and osteological bias; the evidence from late Roman Britain. *Journal of Roman Archaeology Supplementary Series, 65*, 153–169.
Gowland, R. L. (2015a). Entangled lives: Implications of the developmental origins of health and disease (DOHaD) hypothesis for bioarcheology and the life course. *American Journal of Physical Anthropology, 158*(4), 530–40.
Gowland, R. L. (2015b). Elder abuse: Evaluating the potentials and problems of diagnosis in the archaeological record. *International Journal of Osteoarchaeology*. doi:10.1002/oa.2442.
Gowland, R. L. (in press). That tattered coat upon a stick, the ageing body: Elder marginalisation and abuse in Roman Britain. In L. A. Powell, W. Southwell-Wright, R. L. Gowland (Eds.), Care in the past: Interdisciplinary perspectives. Oxford: Oxbow.
Gowland, R. L., & Thompson, T. J. U. (2013). *Human identity and identification*. Cambridge: Cambridge University Press.
Halperin, R. (1984). Age in cultural economics: An evolutionary approach. In D. I. Kertzer & J. Keith (Eds.), *Age and anthropological theory* (pp. 159–194). Ithaca, New York: Cornell University Press.
Hendricks, J. (2012). Considering life course concepts. *Journal of Gerontology B Psychological Sciences and Social Sciences, 67*, 226–231.
Hockey, J., & Draper, J. (2005). Beyond the womb and the tomb: Identity, (dis)embodiment and the life course. *Body and Society, 11*, 41–47.
Hockey, J., & James, A. (1993). *Growing up and growing old*. London: Sage.
Hockey, J., & James, A. (2003). *Social identities across the life course*. Basingstoke: Palgrave MacMillan.
Holmes, E. R., & Holmes, L. D. (1995). *Other cultures, elder years* (2nd ed.). California: Sage Publications.
Hughes, K., Bellis, M. A., Jones, L., Wood, S., Bates, G., Eckley, L., et al. (2012). Prevalence and risk of violence against adults with disabilities: A systematic review and meta-analysis of observational studies. *The Lancet, 379*(9826), 1621–1629.
Hyland, J. (2000). Leprosy and social exclusion in Nepal: The continuing conflict between medical and social-cultural beliefs and practices. In J. Hubert (Ed.), *Madness, disability and social exclusion. The archaeology and anthropology of difference* (pp. 168–179). London: Routledge.
Kristeva. (1982). *Powers of horror: An essay on abjection*. New York: Columbia Press.
Lachs, M. S., & Pillemer, K. (1995). Abuse and neglect of elderly persons. *The New England Journal of Medicine, 332*, 437–443.
Levy, R., & the Pavie Team. (2005). Why look at life courses in an inter-disciplinary perspective. *Advances in Life Course Research, 10*, 3–32.
Marshall, V. W. (1996). The state of theory in aging and the social sciences. In R. H. Binstock & L. K. George (Eds.), *Handbook of aging and the social sciences* (4th ed., pp. 12–30). New York: Academic.
Moen, P. (1996). Gender, age and the life course. In R. H. Binstock & L. K. George (Eds.), *Handbook of aging and the social sciences* (4th ed., pp. 181–187). New York: Academic.
Nicholson, K. (2006). A late roman cemetery at Watersmeet, Mill Common, Huntingdon. *Proceedings of the Cambridge Antiquarian Society, 95*, 57–89.
Parkin, T. (2003). *Old age in the Roman world*. Baltimore: John Hopkins University Press.

Parkin, T. (2011). The elderly children of Greece and Rome. In C. Krötzl & K. Mustakallio (Eds.), *On old age: Approaching death in antiquity and the middle ages*. Turnhout: Brepols.
Pelling, M., & Smith, R. M. (1991). Introduction. In M. Pelling & R. M. Smith (Eds.), *Life, death and the elderly historical perspectives* (pp. 1–38). London: Routledge.
Pickard, S. (2014). Biology as destiny? Rethinking embodiment in 'deep' old age. *Ageing and Society, 34*, 1279–1291.
Priestley, M. (2003). *Disability: A life course approach*. Oxford: Polity Press.
Quain, B. H. (1948). *Fijian village*. Chicago: Chicago University Press.
Rasmussen, S. J. (1987). Interpreting androgynous women: Female aging and personhood among the Kel Ewey Tuareg. *Ethnology, 26*, 17–30.
Rasmussen, S. J. (2000). From childbearers to culture bearers: Transition to postchildbearing among Taureg women. *Medical Anthropology, 19*, 91–116.
Robb, J. (2002). Time and biography: Osteobiography of the Italian Neolithic lifespan. In Y. Hamilakis, M. Pluciennik, & S. Tarlow (Eds.), *Thinking through the body: Archaeologies of corporeality* (pp. 153–172). New York: Kluwer Academic/Plenum Publishers.
Rudkin, L. (1993). Gender differences in economic well-being among the elderly of Java. *Demography, 30*(2), 209–226.
Sanders, C., Donovan, J., & Dieppe, P. (2002). The significance and consequences of having painful and disabled joints in old age: co-existing accounts of normal and disrupted biographies. *Sociology of Health and Illness, 24*, 227–253.
Shahar, S. (1997). *Growing old in the middle ages: 'Winter Clothes us in Shadow and Pain'*. (Trans Hebrew by Yoel Latan). London: Routledge.
Shilling, C. (1993). *The body and social theory*. London: Sage Publications.
Shuttleworth, R., Wedgewood, N., & Wilson, N. J. (2012). The dilemma of disabled masculinity. *Men and Masculinities, 15*, 174–194.
Simon, R. I. (1989). Silent suicide in the elderly. *Bulletin of the American Academy of Psychiatry Law, 17*, 83–95.
Sofaer, J. (2006). *The body as material culture*. London: Routledge.
Sørensen, M.-L. (2000). *Gender archaeology*. Oxford: John Wiley and Sons.
Thane, P. (2000). *Old age in English history*. Oxford: University Press.
Tilley, L., & Oxenham, M. (2011). Survival against the odds: Modelling the social implications of care provision to seriously disabled individuals. *International Journal of Paleopathology, 1*, 35–42.
Twigg, J. (2004). The body, gender, and age: Feminist insights in social gerontology. *Journal of Aging Studies, 18*, 59–73.
Walker, D. (2009). The treatment of leprosy in 19th century London: A case study from St Marylebone Cemetery. *International Journal of Osteoarchaeology, 19*, 364–374.
Wendell, S. (1996). *The rejected body: Feminist philosophical reflections on disability*. New York: Routledge.
Wolf, R. S., & Pillemer, K. A. (1989). *Helping elderly victims: The reality of elder abuse*. New York: Columbia University Press.

Chapter 13
Caring for Bodies or Simply Saving Souls: The Emergence of Institutional Care in Spanish Colonial America

Julie K. Wesp

Introduction

The modern healthcare industry is a multibillion dollar enterprise that has influenced the way that we think about bodily care in the present. If we have a medical emergency, one of the first things we do is go to the hospital to seek care, and if we have a chronic condition we are likely to end up seeking hospital treatment at one point or another. In Western society, if you have not already experienced a hospital visit, it is likely you will at least once in your lifetime as either a patient or a visitor. I have had the misfortune of needing to rush to the hospital a couple of times in my life already and, like most people, did so without really thinking about what people would do in the past before hospitals existed. Being a bioarchaeologist, the last time I was in a hospital bed recovering I began to wonder about the history of such institutions: When did hospitals begin to care for the sick? How did these hospitals operate? What kind of care did they provide?

This chapter explores the origins of these institutions of care that we often take for granted in our own lives today, and focuses on the last of these questions to consider the type of care that people may have received at some of the earliest hospitals. Modern medicine at hospitals concentrates on the treatment of bodily illness, and skeletal remains provide a method for bioarchaeologists to explore the implementation of bodily care in the past. The bioarchaeology of care, as outlined by Tilley in this volume and elsewhere (Tilley, 2012; Tilley & Cameron, 2014), provides a step-by-step methodology for looking at specific cases of caregiving in the past. Bioarchaeological research unavoidably focuses on bodily caregiving, although it is also important to think about and discuss what other treatments might have been

J.K. Wesp, Ph.D. (✉)
University of California Institute for Mexico and the US (UC MEXUS), Riverside, CA, USA

Mexico's Consejo Nacional de Ciencia y Tecnología (CONACYT), Mexico City, Mexico
e-mail: juliewesp@berkeley.edu

© Springer International Publishing Switzerland 2017

L. Tilley, A.A. Schrenk (eds.), *New Developments in the Bioarchaeology of Care*, Bioarchaeology and Social Theory, DOI 10.1007/978-3-319-39901-0_13

offered, such as remedies that fulfill spiritual or psychological needs in addition to bodily ones. One could certainly even argue that our understanding of the mind/body/spirit connection is still poorly understood by modern science (Dhabhar, 2009; Louveau et al., 2015), and that methods for treating one of these may have a direct impact on the others (Goyal et al., 2014; Mora-Ripoll, 2010). Healthcare today, particularly that covered by basic health insurance, has diversified to encompass a variety of different options for treating ailments of both the mind and the body, and we would be remiss to not explore the possibility of other kinds of caregiving in the past. While psychological and spiritual care practices cannot be easily verified scientifically, even using the bioarchaeology of care methodology, we can use historical, archaeological, and other forms of data to explore how these concepts may have been intertwined with bodily care at specific times and in specific places. The emergence of care institutions in Europe and later in the Americas are linked with religious institutions, but also financially supported by political institutions. These links may influence different aspects of the operational side of hospitals, which in return guide the kind of caregiving that was provided.

As a case study, I will focus on one hospital in particular, the *Hospital Real San José de los Naturales* (HSJN), founded by European missionaries in Central Mexico shortly after the conquest in the sixteenth century. In the Americas in particular, many hospitals were created to care for the local population, as many members of this population fell ill from widespread infectious diseases that were introduced along with Europeans (Larsen, 1994). The creation and sponsorship of these hospitals by both Christian missionaries and the colonial government, however, may have created a kind of treatment that included both bodily care for the primary source of labor for construction projects and a concern for the patients' spiritual well-being. Thus, at the HSJN, it is possible that evangelization and conversion to Christianity was as much a part of the hospital mission as the bodily care provided by medical professionals. A large collection of skeletal remains associated with the hospital structure provides a route to understanding bodily care through the bioarchaeology of care methodology, while archaeological evidence and historical documents pertaining to the hospital provide an avenue for exploring other possible kinds of care.

To be a Good Christian

Providing care for others in your community has an ancient history, as detailed by others in this volume, yet the emergence of institutions of care with specialized staff has a more recent history. We might think of this as a shift from providing individual care as needed to people in your community to creating a permanent care facility, or team of caregivers, that is readily available. Consequently, the way we think about care in the past must also undergo a conceptual shift. The responsibility to provide care for those in need likely expanded to include people that you may not have been socially obligated to care for. The emergence of this altruistic behavior is still debated, yet it appears as though caring expanded to include a wider range of people that extended beyond biological relationships. In the same way, people in need of care might now have been required to seek it out actively. Both the caregivers and those in need of care have different concerns in terms of the agency involved; in the case of the former, in addressing the question of whether to provide or to *not* provide care and, in the case of the latter, whether to seek or to *not* seek care. These decisions are further complicated by other aspects of institutional care, such as treatments available and cost; two key facets that continue to influence our healthcare choices in the present.

Many of the first institutions of care in Europe are associated with the rise of Christian communities. As early as the fourth century CE, there is evidence for infirmaries and other residences specifically dedicated to caring for the sick (and others in need) in large urban centers throughout the Roman empire (Risse, 1999). These institutions differ from previous models of care services that may have occurred in the home or been provided by roaming specialized practitioners. The message of Jesus Christ, which was gaining popularity during this time, focused on aiding those in need, especially the members of society that may have previously been considered unworthy of care. Charity became a key principle of good Christian behavior, which is inherently linked with the idea of caring for the poor and the sick. With this shift in religious doctrine the choice of whether or not to care for a stranger or for someone with a contagious illness, such as leprosy, became a moral dilemma. Correspondingly, this dilemma had direct spiritual consequences, since Christian belief states that a place in an eternal afterlife is guaranteed in return for service while on earth. It is no surprise, then, that most of the earliest institutions of care were created by religious organizations as a means of fulfilling this moral responsibility. This motivation to care for others out of a sense of obligation may have influenced the type of care that people received. Many early Christians rejected the idea of bodily comfort altogether, recognizing bodily desires as weaknesses that needed to be controlled through fasting, vigils, or physical labor (Risse, 1999).

Patients seeking care at a Christian healthcare institution may have been equally focused on fixing a spiritual ailment. Early Christian healthcare coexisted with secular understandings of medicine, but caring for the earthly body seems to have always been secondary to maintaining spiritual health (Ferngren, 2009). Ailments of the body were often perceived as penance for sins committed, so rather than curing the bodily problems it was more important to cure the sinful behavior in order to improve the patient's health. Some early Christians believed that faith was the only medicine necessary, therefore care at institutions that provided the minimum material necessities for survival, such as shelter and food, might ensure that a person could at least confess and repent their sins before death in order to secure an eternal afterlife (Muriel, 1956). In the same manner, the "good Christians" were ensuring their own promise of an eternal afterlife by participating in this care, whether though financial sponsorship or physical labor. This is certainly a different definition of care than today, but following Tilley's characterization of care (Chap. 2 this volume) services that may have provided spiritual comfort and survival are also worth exploring.

Institutions of care throughout the Renaissance period not only provided physical care for those suffering from disease, but were also viewed as necessary for maintaining social function, because they provided – if indirectly – a kind of psychological support. Migration to urban centers and a general increase in population had an effect on the frequency of diseases during this time period. Illnesses can easily spread within densely populated urban areas, especially without proper hygiene and sanitation. However, isolation of the sick and a timely removal of dead bodies from public areas can help to prevent epidemics. This idea of a social separation of the sick is particularly well illustrated by the formation of institutions that sequestered people suffering from leprosy at the extreme periphery of urban settlements (Flexner, 2012; Risse, 1999). The separation of the sick, however, has less to do with caring for the ill than with making the healthy population feel comfortable and safe. The rapid attack of infectious diseases can cause psychological distress among a population that feels as though there are no safe places to hide from the sickness (I have seen a single sneeze in a crowded lecture hall wreak havoc during flu season). In this way, specific social and cultural factors can influence the motivations behind providing care, and these motivations may, in fact, be concerned not only with healing the sick or caring for the dying, but also with the concerns of a "healthy" population worried about contracting disease and the desire of philanthropic Christians to boost their chances of attaining a place in Heaven.

These spiritual and psychological accommodations are difficult, if not impossible, to identify on the basis of archaeological or bioarchaeological evidence alone, but are still worth considering when discussing the creation of institutions of care. The decision-making around caring for others is continually entwined with broader decisions about personal and societal benefits. Would these institutions have been created without these other social benefits and cultural influences? The moral and psychological reasons for caregiving must have played an important part in justifying the financial and operational overhead of establishing a permanent care institution.

The personal and societal motivations behind creating an institution of care shift during the sixteenth century, when European-style hospitals begin to emerge in the Americas.

Institutions of Care in the Americas

Much of what we know about bodily health-related care practices in Pre-Hispanic societies comes from written documents created by Europeans after their arrival in the Americas, and although (as with all historical documents) it is important to remember for whom and for what purpose they were created, they are nonetheless still useful for establishing if, and how, care was administered.

By the time the Europeans arrived in Central Mexico in the early sixteenth century the Mexica empire had become the dominant political power in the region, and the contemporary conceptualization of illness and methods to cure it were based in the broader cosmological belief system of the indigenous people in the Mesoamerican region. In particular, a kind of "physical-magical" (Cárdenas de la Peña, 1976, p. 14) understanding of health existed, where life and death were simply two aspects of the same reality that followed the same cyclical destruction and renewal as the sun each day or the maize crops each year. While bodily care practices were considered specialized knowledge in Mexica society, it is more accurate to categorize bodily care as an hereditary skilled occupation passed on from parent to child within the home. Practitioners had a detailed understanding of anatomy, with specific words for anatomical elements such as heart, bone, blood, nerves, and skin in the indigenous language, Nahuatl (López Austin, 1988). Documentary and archaeological research throughout the Mesoamerican region provides evidence for dental modifications and dentistry, amputations, cranial surgery (trepanation), and detailed obstetric practices including contraception, inducing abortion, and midwifery (López Austin, 1975, 1988; Márquez Morfín & González Licón, 1992; Tiesler Blos, 2001). Additionally, other documents exist that highlight the importance of hygiene, including personal washing, washing clothing, the regulation of prostitution and drunkenness, and the maintenance of private and public space (Sahagún, 2000).

It is important to emphasize these indigenous understandings of the body, health, disease, and care because they seem to both complement and counter the European knowledge that was introduced in the sixteenth century. The entanglement of religion and bodily care within Mesoamerican societies was perceived by the colonizing missionaries as superstitious and full of erroneous calculations (Cárdenas de la Peña, 1976), while at the same time, European institutions of care were similarly tied to, or carried out in, institutions established and operated by religious organizations. Understanding these social conditions and the interaction between both of these models of care will help us to better answer the questions about the agency involved in seeking or providing care, and about the kind of care that may have been offered in early healthcare institutions in the Americas.

A key difference between the need for care in European society and the need for care in the colonial society of the Americas is the difference in the disease environment. While European traditions of care were brought to the Americas, they were coupled with the transfer of European diseases that also traveled to the Americas for the first time. During the first century after the arrival of the Spanish in Mexico it seems that each generation was afflicted by an epidemic (Table 13.1) (Cárdenas de la Peña, 1976; Lugo Olín, 2005; Márquez Morfín, 1994). These same illnesses had plagued European cities a couple centuries earlier, and prompted the creation of many of the first institutions of care in Europe. The lack of immunological defenses within the Mesoamerican indigenous population had devastating effects, especially in the capital of New Spain when coupled with close living proximity in an urban landscape. Various researchers estimate that indigenous deaths in Mexico during the sixteenth century reached nearly twenty million people, and that the Mexican population did not reach Pre-Hispanic numbers again until the early twentieth century (Acuna-Soto et al., 2002; Acuna-Soto, Romero, & Maguire, 2000; Cook & Simpson, 1948).

Table 13.1 Dates of known major infectious disease epidemics in urban New Spain during the sixteenth, seventeenth, and eighteenth centuries from historical sources (Cárdenas de la Peña, 1976; Lugo Olín, 2005; Márquez Morfín, 1994)

Dates cited	Diseases cited in historical sources
1531	Measles
1538	Smallpox
1545	Cocoliztli[a]
1564	Unknown epidemic referred to as "the great death"
1576	Cocoliztli
1595	Mixture of measles, mumps, and *tabardillo* (disease similar to typhus)
1601	Cocoliztli
1604–1605	Cocoliztli and measles (epidemic prolonged by a major earthquake in urban New Spain)
1612–1613	Cocoliztli
1615–1616	Cocoliztli, measles, and smallpox
1630	Unnamed plague
1633–1634	Cocoliztli
1639	Measles
1641	Cocoliztli
1651	Unnamed plague
1653	Smallpox
1662–1663	Smallpox and typhus
1678	Smallpox
1686	Typhus
1692	Measles
1695	Unnamed epidemic
1735	Typhus? (source is unclear regarding specific disease)
1762–1763	Smallpox
1779	Smallpox
1797	Smallpox
1813	Typhus
1833	Cholera

[a]*Cocoliztli* refers to an unknown pestilence that likely resembled hemorrhagic fever, but the use of this Nahuatl term could also simply refer to an infectious disease epidemic in a general sense

Prominent European individuals with a desire to fulfill their call to Christian charity sponsored a number of early care institutions in the Americas. In the sixteenth century alone, historical documents identify the establishment of 33 different hospitals in both urban and rural locations within the Viceroyalty of New Spain (Rodríguez-Sala, 2005). Some of these institutions were designed to care for individuals with specific ailments, such as leprosy or syphilis, while others were designated for specific portions of the population (Suarez, 1988).

The same desire for social separation that we see with the establishment of specific European hospitals occurs in the Americas, but the kind of separation needed takes on a whole new meaning. While contagious diseases had been the motivation for creating separate settlements and institutions in Europe, a new kind of "unhealthy body" emerged with the conceptual "othering" of the local population within the European mindset. Phenotypic differences created a noticeable distinction between different members of colonial society, and this was compounded by Mesoamerican cultural practices that Europeans often characterized as "savage" or "barbaric" (Ryal Miller & Orr, 2000; Sahagún, 2000). This lack of understanding about cultural differences influenced the creation of separate towns (*Repúblicas de Indios*) and laws that restricted interaction between Europeans and the local population (Cope, 1994; Gibson, 1964). This conceptual othering extended to include discussions of the very humanity of the indigenous population, and the basic rights and services that they might or might not be entitled to under colonial rule.

The issue of decisions taken regarding providing or not providing care must also be examined through this complex lens of Spanish colonial society. Many early hospitals established by religious institutions in New Spain provided care for Europeans, but separate institutions were created for the treatment of the local population. Some of the earliest institutions for the indigenous population were founded through individual sponsorship by wealthy Europeans, who felt it was their moral responsibility to help solve the problems created by their entrance to the continent (Muriel, 1956). Historical documents indicate that the infamous conquistador, Hernan Cortes, was one such sponsor who believed it was his duty to care for the sick after all the deaths caused by his conquest mission (Rodríguez-Sala, 2005).

The issue about whether this care for the local population was a societal obligation was not fully resolved, however, until nearly two decades after the conquest. In 1537, Pope Paul III issued the *sublimus dei* (a papal bull) declaring that the indigenous populations of the Americas were rational beings with souls, who had a right to liberty, and were prime subjects for evangelization (Thornberry, 2003). This proclamation transformed colonial society and the way that the colonial government operated. First, the Pope explicitly addressed the humanity of the local population and declared that they were not only capable of understanding the Christian faith, but in need of it to convert them from their pagan traditions. The manner in which this conversion should take place was linked with the idea of Christian charity and the necessity of caring for an ailing population. In fact, a 1541 law mandating the creation of hospitals for the indigenous population specifically mentions this as an act of "caridad Cristiana" (Christian charity – Zedillo Castillo, 1984, p. 127). This was a key development in the discussion of the emergence of care institutions in the Americas, because following this declaration many religious organizations began to establish hospitals throughout New Spain. In 1554, the second Archbishop of Mexico, Alonso de Montúfar, declared that more hospitals were needed in Mexico. A year later in 1555, the First Mexican Council ordered that in every town a hospital should be erected next to the church so that the priests could easily visit the sick and the poor and perform sacraments (Ricard, 1986). Furthermore, a report by Franciscan priests in the mid-sixteenth century states that hospitals were built to not only take in the sick, but to indoctrinate the healthy (García Icazbalceta, Pomar, & Zurita, 1941).

Second, and importantly, the papal bull also declared that the enslavement of indigenous populations in the Americas was forbidden, although it did not address the ongoing enslavement of Africans, which was a crucial component of colonial society. For the native population, their new status as free members of colonial society meant that they were able to take advantage of the judicial system, and often took legal action when they were denied property ownership or when services were inadequate (Kellogg, 1995). This social status also meant that the indigenous population had the option of seeking care at a hospital (albeit a segregated one) if they chose to do so.

The shifting responsibility for care institutions from individual sponsorship to religious institutions and the colonial government in New Spain influenced who provided care, who could seek care, and what kind of care they received. Changes to the operation of healthcare institutions were compounded by the specific cultural environment of colonial life, in which not every member of society was treated equally. The responsibility to care for the sick and the poor that Europeans felt was their Christian duty was entangled with changing perceptions about the indigenous population. While the indigenous population was declared worthy of care, a separation between native peoples and those of European descent was still perceived to be necessary. The indigenous hospital provided health-related care, but the association with religious institutions may have also resulted in a wide range of motivations for caregiving, such as the need to convert the indigenous population to Christianity and put a stop to their pagan traditions.

The Hospital de Indios in New Spain

In response to the increasing number of indigenous deaths from both the various disease epidemics and the hard physical demands of labor requirements, the colonial government petitioned the Spanish crown to establish a royally funded hospital that specialized in care of the indigenous population. In 1553, this petition was granted, and rather than found a new hospital, the *Hospital de Sanct Joseph* (originally founded in 1531 by the Franciscan Priest Fray Pedro de Gante) was reestablished as the *Hospital Real de Indios* (later called the *Hospital Real San José de Naturales*) (Ricard, 1986; Zedillo Castillo, 1984). As with the segregated townships established during this time, the hospital was located within the indigenous neighborhood of San Juan Moyotlán, and therefore maintained the physical separation from the European part of town (Fig. 13.1). While originally established under the traditional Christian charitable mission and administered by a religious institution, the crown sponsorship of the HSJN symbolically emphasized that the native peoples of the Americas were considered human beings worthy of care and dignity, and that these were a direct concern of the Spanish monarch. This concern was emphasized in a letter from the Spanish king to the viceroy of New Spain in 1568, in which he stated that it was of primordial importance that the hospital for the indigenous population function properly (Zedillo Castillo, 1984, p. 342).

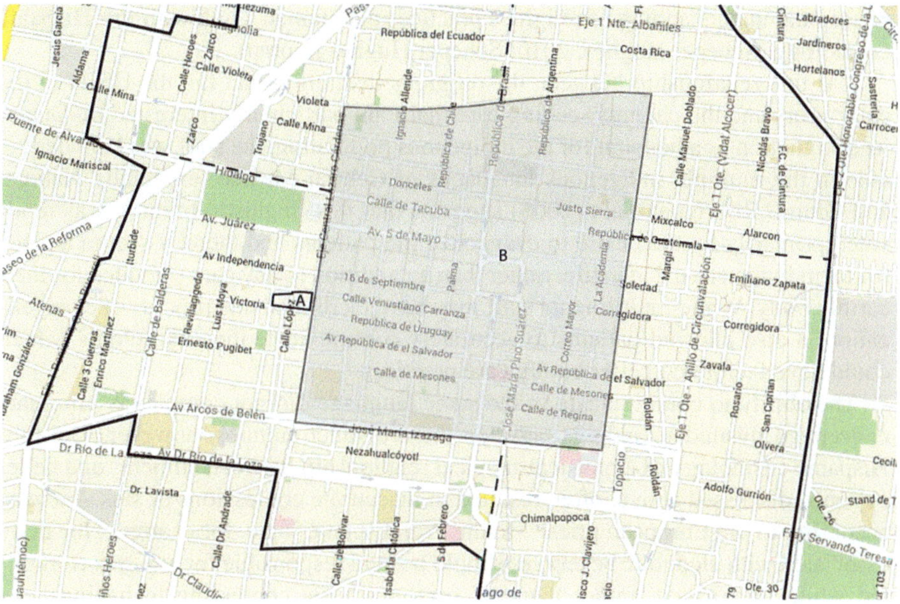

Fig. 13.1 Map of present day downtown area in Mexico City with solid black lines indicating the limits of the city in the sixteenth century. The HSJN (**a**) was located in San Juan Moyotlan, one of the four indigenous neighborhoods (*dashed lines*), and just isolated from the area designated for Spanish residences (*grey square*) and the religious and political center of town (**b**). Imagery © 2013 DigitalGlobe, Map data © 2013 Google, INEGI, Sanborn

The creation of the HSJN certainly suggests a desire to care for a population that was suffering from disease epidemics, yet given the social climate in which it was created it is important to explore the idea that bodily care may not have been the only service provided. The Codice Osuna details a lawsuit protesting a lack of proper services, brought by the indigenous population against the colonial government, which was heard during an inquiry of the Viceroy Luis de Velasco in 1563–1566. Among other services, the HSJN is specifically identified as lacking quality healthcare service because of a lack of funding. The financial support from the Spanish crown did not fully cover all of the costs associated with providing care, especially during the difficult epidemic years. During the epidemics, in particular, extra financial support was provided through alms paid as penance after members of the indigenous population came to confess their sins – sometimes as often as every Friday amidst an epidemic (Ricard, 1986).

Participation in the sacrament of confession and payment of alms by the indigenous population may indicate an acceptance of spiritual care and reflect the importance that faith can have in healing. Yet it is also possible that these payments might simply have been conceived of as a kind of offering to please a deity in order to receive a desired outcome, a practice that was common in Pre-Hispanic Mesoamerican traditions. Research in religious studies suggests that this fervent mission to convert the indigenous population may have been abandoned when it became clear that the conceptual understanding of religious practices maintained a link with Pre-Hispanic cosmology (Scheper Hughes, 2010; Scheper Hughes in prep).

It is this relationship between the religious institution that ran the HSJN in the early years and the patients seeking care that I am particularly interested in. Due to its designation as a hospital for the indigenous population, the staff was knowledgeable in the multiple indigenous languages of Central Mexico, especially Nahuatl and Otomi. Rodríguez-Sala (2005) suggests that this linguistic training was motivated primarily by the desire to evangelize the patients and thereby secure a place for them in the eternal afterlife, rather than an addition to any care provided for their earthly body. While multilingual staff may have facilitated this process of evangelization, it also allowed patients to accurately communicate their symptoms, which could have facilitated better bodily care practices.

The ability to communicate in the same language did not completely eliminate conceptual misunderstandings between these distinct cultures, however. The Pre-Hispanic cosmology of a physical-magical relationship between ailments and belief systems, discussed above, often resulted in inaccurate confessions of sins – at least according to the European priests. In the Pre-Hispanic logic, for example, the deity associated with alcoholic beverages should be held responsible for any sins committed while intoxicated, rather than the person who is confessing to having been drunk. In fact, people born on a specific day within the ritual calendar are considered destined to be imbibers, and a confession of sins will not prevent future acts committed while intoxicated or convert that person to a teetotaler. The European logic, on the other hand, holds that inebriation is in itself a sin that must be confessed and repented, along with any other acts committed while intoxicated (Ricard, 1986). This difference in logic regarding "wrongful acts" was not cured by the ability to communicate in the same language.

Since infectious disease attacks the body quickly, conversion to Christianity and the confession of sins before death needed to happen swiftly within the hospital. The design of hospital buildings was such that a small altar would be placed in an inner courtyard, enabling patients to see the priest from their hospital beds as he said mass in the central location (Muriel, 1956; Ricard, 1986). Even with a church attached to the HSJN, this design of a central courtyard around which patient rooms are located continued to be an important architectural feature at the hospital, as seen from this mid-eighteenth century plan map (Fig. 13.2). Furthermore, a number of different rooms were designated for priests to live on-site and in close proximity to the patient halls, which may have helped to facilitate impromptu confession.

Finally, the position of the indigenous population as a conceptual "other" within the European mindset provided the opportunity for some controversial practices to take place. Medical knowledge continued to advance during this time period, yet throughout the world there was a struggle to collect accurate information because of the lack of human bodies available for scientific examination. Religious beliefs against desecrating the body, even after death, meant that families often refused the consent necessary for the study of the bodies of the deceased, and grave robbing emerged as a method of sourcing cadavers for this purpose (Moores Ball, 1989). In Mexico, the overwhelming number of people who died from infectious diseases

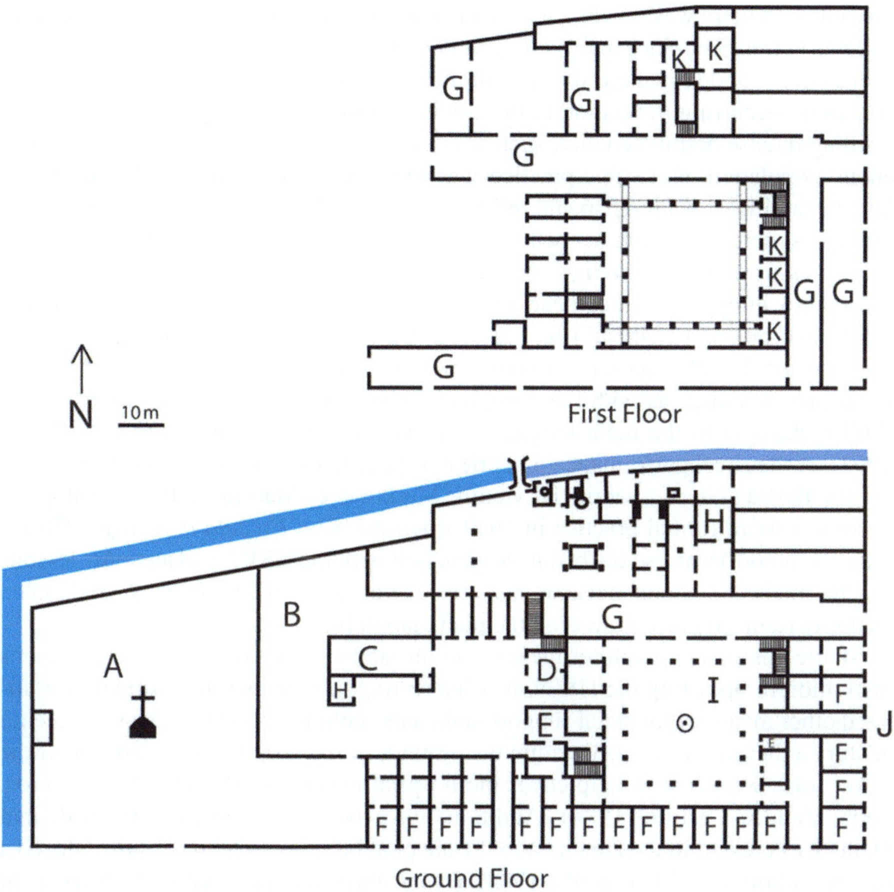

Fig. 13.2 Plan map of the ground floor and first floor of the HSJN circa 1750s, created to document renovations after a fire destroyed much of the hospital in 1722. (*A*) Cemetery (*B*) Separated section of the cemetery that was used as an infirmary during epidemics (*C*) Cemetery chapel (*D*) Anatomy room (*E*) Kitchens (*F*) Consultation rooms (*G*) Patient halls (*H*) Sacristies (*I*) Main courtyard (*J*) Main entrance, currently Eje Central Lázaro Cárdenas (*K*) Chaplain's bedrooms. Redrawn from Zedillo 1984, Original maps are located in the Archivo General de Indias in Seville, Spain

provided an ample source of cadavers for study. Conducting autopsies was valued as a way to gain more knowledge of human anatomy, and documentation suggests this practice began at the HSJN in 1576 following the great cocoliztli epidemic of that year (Rodríguez-Sala, 2005). The doctors were likely not required to give any explanation as to why they conducted autopsies, or even ask permission from family members before doing so.

Although official records state that these anatomical explorations were intended to find the cause of the disease in order to prevent further outbreaks, it is more likely that this practice was motivated by the general lack of corpses available for medical instruction. While autopsies of Europeans would not have been acceptable, it is possible that there was less of a moral quandary in utilizing the deceased indigenous patients in this way, since many still regarded the local population as being of a lower social status, or doubted the sincerity of their conversion to Christianity. As with the confusion occurring in relation to the confession of sins, many priests avoided prescribing intense bodily penance, such as auto-flagellation, for members of the indigenous population, since this practice was too closely associated with the bloody human sacrifices of Pre-Hispanic religious practice (Ricard, 1986). The emergence of these syncretized religious beliefs may have prompted doctors at the hospital to simply assume that the indigenous population would not object to such invasive procedures after death since heart extraction, among other things, was a common practice of human sacrificial ritual (Chávez Balderas, 2007). In fact, bodily dissection and display of dead human bodies was an important part of Central Mexican ritual practice, such as with the decapitated heads displayed on the *tzompantli*, or skull rack, next to the main temple of the Mexica in Tenochtitlan (López Lujan, 1994), or the ritual performance of a priest impersonating the deity *Xipe Totec* wearing the flayed skin of a sacrificial victim (Markman & Markman, 1992). Autopsies become a more formal practice in 1639 when the *Real Escuela de Cirugía* (Royal Surgery School) was established in conjunction with the HSJN, and anatomy lessons for the medical students became customary (Rodríguez-Sala, 2005). A designated anatomy room (D) can be seen on the plan map in Fig. 13.2.

While this chapter explores the motivations and methods of the original religious institution in operating the HSJN, it is interesting to note that the hospital also utilized other means of financial support in the later colonial period. In the seventeenth century a theater was created within the grounds of the hospital, and a portion of the ticket sales was used to help cover the hospital expenses (Muriel, 1956; Viveros, 2005; Zedillo Castillo, 1984). Additionally, a botanical garden with medicinal plants was created in the area next to the hospital building to help subsidize the cost of medications (Zedillo Castillo, 1984). By the early nineteenth century, the costs of repairing and maintaining the hospital became difficult to sustain. The financial state of the hospital was further exacerbated in 1814, when the crown ceased to provide a financial contribution. Attempts were made to appeal to the church as a possible financial resource, as well as charging patients for hospital care, but none of these actions provided enough money to sustain such a large hospital. Thus at the beginning of 1822, shortly after independence, the new Mexican government decided to close the HSJN, and the land and buildings were reutilized for other business ventures (Zedillo Castillo, 1984).

The HSJN provides an interesting case study for exploring the emergence of institutions of care in the Americas because, in addition to being described in contemporary historical documents, archaeological excavations accompanying an expansion of the Mexico City metro system in the early 1990s uncovered the architectural foundations of the hospital and a large associated collection of skeletal remains (Báez Molgado & Meza Peñaloza, 1995; Sánchez Vázquez et al., 1996). Utilizing the bioarchaeology of care methodology, skeletal remains provide another form of evidence to explore questions about the agency of care and kinds of care provided in the first hospitals established in the Americas.

Applying the Bioarchaeology of Care in the Americas

Bioarchaeologists have the ability to examine the actual remains of those who were likely cared for in the past, and the bioarchaeology of care approach provides a framework for interpreting the evidence gained in this process. But the bioarchaeology of care methodology has certain limitations, since we base our analysis on a need for care inferred from physical indicators of disease (Tilley, Chap. 2 this volume). Although other forms of care are also important to overall personal well-being, a need for spiritual or psychological care would not leave a discernable mark on the skeleton and is therefore unlikely to receive consideration. A bioarchaeology of care that includes a discussion of forms of care additional to physical care, however, is likely to be a purely theoretical one, and one without a method to satisfactorily verify alternative forms of care. This lack of a discernable osteological trace may lead to some dismissing these issues as purely speculative, yet I would argue that such a Cartesian division between bodily care and kinds of care necessary for mental well-being do not accurately represent the reality of how we care for others as human beings – either in the present or the past. Addressing these questions, while maybe only an exercise in educated speculation, can help to diversify our perspective on caregiving in the past. To this end, I will draw on archaeological context and historical documentation, in addition to skeletal material, to examine one case in which it is likely that physical bodily care was only one of many kinds of caregiving provided in the HSJN.

First, all bioarchaeological research on care analyzes portions of a population that died. The development of a methodology for a bioarchaeology of care, as Tilley states (Tilley, 2015), has always been limited by the knowledge that, whether or not as bioarchaeologists we can discern caregiving, the people we analyze ultimately did not survive. All of the individuals in the skeletal collection associated with the HSJN, totaling over 600 recovered individuals, represent people who died while seeking care at the hospital. At its peak in the eighteenth century, the hospital had two floors and could accommodate up to 200 patients a day, and documentary evidence indicates that between 1795 and 1799 a total of 11,490 patients entered the hospital and of those 1810 died (Zedillo Castillo, 1984). The skeletal sample recovered during archaeological excavations, then, represents a limited view of the total population of hospital patients that was cared for over the nearly 300 years of existence of the HSJN. None of the patients who came to the hospital seeking care for an ailment and ultimately survived will be represented in this skeletal population.

The fact that some people were buried within the hospital grounds may serve as evidence to indicate care – in whatever form or combination of forms – was provided for hospital patients, even if no other indicators are available. On the one hand, formal burial might be characterized as the ultimate form of care for a member of society; and one that was extended to those people who died in the hospital. On the other hand, burial might not represent this at all, but rather reflect a pragmatic removal and isolation of bodies that died from infectious disease. In other words, burials may simply have been performed to help prevent illness from spreading and served as a form of care for the "healthy" living portion of the population, rather than for the dead.

The archaeological excavations occurred along the eastern edge of the hospital, on the opposite side of where the cemetery (A) was located in the eighteenth century (Fig. 13.2). The archaeologists believe that they uncovered a small area that may correspond to an earlier cemetery. However, they also discovered a large number of bodies within the construction fill of a hospital remodeling that likely occurred in the early eighteenth century, after a fire destroyed most of the building (Sánchez Vázquez et al., 1996). Most of the skeletal remains were recovered from the area beneath the main entrance of the hospital (J) and the adjacent consultation rooms (F) and patient hall (G). This led the archaeologists to hypothesize that during epidemics the increased number of cadavers would have overwhelmed the designated cemetery areas, and that the administrators took advantage of this construction work to dispose of bodies. The dead recovered from the fill possibly pertained to the epidemic in 1735 (Cabrera Torres & García Martínez, 1998). A historical document from the eighteenth century registers a formal complaint made by one of the neighbors of the hospital who was uncomfortable with so many dead bodies close to his home, which further supports the hypothesis of an arbitrary designation of burial places throughout the entire hospital grounds (Zedillo Castillo, 1984).

In areas of burial within architectural features many of the individuals were piled on top of each other in a kind of ossuary, rather than individually placed in the rows more typical of Christian burial practices (Cabrera Torres & García Martínez, 1998; Sánchez Vázquez et al., 1996). This indiscriminate mortuary practice could indicate the large number of deaths that occurred and the speed with which the hospital needed to remove dead bodies during epidemics, but then again it may also indicate a lack of final care for these people. While these bodies were buried haphazardly, other people in the skeletal collection were buried individually, with their hands crossed on their chest, three individuals were buried in wooden coffins, and three infants were buried with crowns made of wood or flowers and a cross (Meza Peñaloza & Ortuño Cos, 1995; Pulido Méndez, 1994). Could the commingled burials represent people who were not fully evangelized before death, or even people who resisted conversion? Another possibility is that there was not enough time for anything other than palliative bodily care. The hospital may only have had the resources to make patients as comfortable as possible until they ultimately succumbed to the infection.

During the epidemics the rapid onset of disease, quickly followed by death, means that a requirement for long term care of infected patients was unlikely. It also means that the remains of people who suffered and died would appear to be those of "healthy individuals," in the sense that death would have occurred before the development of skeletal indicators of disease (Wood et al., 1992). This paradox is inherent in all skeletal research, yet for the individuals in this skeletal sample to be buried in the hospital grounds they must have died while they were patients receiving care. Burial in the hospital grounds, then, serves as a proxy indicator of experience of disease, despite absence of skeletal manifestations.

Table 13.2 Demographic information for the articulated individuals in the HSJN skeletal collection recovered from the salvage excavations. Other skeletal remains recovered consist of isolated crania or long bones and are not included in this analysis

	Male	Female	Unknown sex	Total
Subadult (0–17)	0	0	79	79
Young Adult (18–34)	75	78	12	165
Middle Adult (35–49)	104	44	0	148
Old Adult (50+)	5	10	1	16
Unknown Adult Age	7	3	19	29
Total	191	135	111	437

The bioarchaeology of care methodology focuses on studies of skeletal indicators in individual remains to build a case for the need for care. Since we may assume that anyone included in the HSJN skeletal sample died while seeking care, I instead focus on the range of skeletal indicators of bodily care discernable within the skeletal assemblage (Table 13.2). These skeletal indicators clearly suggest that, despite religious affiliation, some forms of bodily care were emphasized at the hospital, yet it is probable that this care was also integrated with alternative kinds of spiritual or psychological care.

The HSJN skeletal collection consists of 437 articulated individuals, the majority of which (82 %) are adults aged 18 or older, and of these adults there is a slightly higher percentage of males (53 %) than females (38 %). It is also important to note that only 16 adults fall within the old adult (50+ years) age group. These individuals were recovered from different areas of the excavation and therefore may represent deaths that occurred throughout the nearly 300 year existence of the hospital, but it is likely that most date to the seventeenth and eighteenth century. Other than this, the records of excavation did not provide a clear indication of when each burial area might have been used. An additional 200 individuals are represented by isolated crania or long bones from commingled mortuary contexts, and have not been included in this population level examination.

Analyses of nutritional stress indicators suggest that the establishment of the HSJN helped to fulfill the Christian charitable mission of providing food and shelter to the sick and poor. Both linear enamel hypoplasia and porotic hyperostosis have been utilized as indicators of stress, and their presence in the sample suggests that the population seeking care at the hospital may have come from a background of poor nutrition (Goodman & Armelagos, 1985; Goodman, Brooke, Swedlund, & Armelagos, 1988; Goodman & Rose, 1990; King, Humphrey, & Hillson, 2005; Stuart-Macadam, 1985). The adults in the skeletal collection showed high frequencies of nutritional deficiencies (Tables 13.3 and 13.4), with 40 % of the sample (83/208 individuals with available teeth) displaying evidence of linear enamel hypoplasia on at least one tooth and 89 % (238/266 individuals with whole or fragmented crania available) showing evidence of porotic hyperostosis (Castillo Chavez, 2000).

Table 13.3 Prevalence of linear enamel hypoplasia (LEH) on permanent teeth (Castillo Chavez, 2000)

	Absence	One line	Two or more lines	Total individuals with LEH
Canines	125/208	47/208	36/208	83/208
Central Incisors	87/108	17/108	4/108	21/108

Table 13.4 Prevalence of porotic hyperostosis (PH) for individuals ($n=266$) with a complete or mostly complete cranial vault (Castillo Chavez, 2000)

	Absent	Initial or inactive	Severe or active	Total with PH	% Total individuals with PH
Subadults	14	20	0	20/34	59
Female Adults	9	89	4	93/102	91
Male Adults	5	120	5	125/130	96
Total	28/266	229/266	9/266	238/266	89

Additionally, historical documents indicate that two of the largest cocoliztli epidemics, in 1545 and 1576, were prolonged by years of drought and famine (Acuna-Soto et al., 2002). The generalized poverty and lack of adequate nutrition among the indigenous population may have been one of the reasons that many sought care at the hospital in the first place instead of other forms of treatment for disease. During an epidemic, many factors affect whether a person survives the illness, and in addition to other treatments provided at the hospital, proper nutrition and a place to rest would have provided an added benefit to patients fighting infectious diseases.

Skeletal evidence suggests that the HSJN also provided acute care for patients with acquired traumatic injuries, some of which were probably labor related. Indigenous males were required to pay tribute under the colonial encomienda system (and then later under the repartimiento rotational labor system) during the sixteenth and seventeenth centuries by working for one week approximately three or four times each year. Urban labor projects included the construction and repairs of urban buildings, especially after extreme flood damage such as that which occurred in 1555 (Gibson, 1964) and from 1629 to 1633 (Lugo Olín, 2005). This work was extremely dangerous, since much of it occurred underwater and caused many fatalities. Indigenous labor was also utilized to construct a trench through the Northwestern wall of the Basin of Mexico, a task that was strenuous and dangerous, as it meant the building of underground channels to drain out the water from the lakes and create more usable land. This project required continuous labor, especially because of the fluctuating wet and dry seasons, from the early seventeenth century until the end of Spanish colonial rule in the early nineteenth century. There were clear dangers associated with the requirements of performing this labor, but the existence of the hospital for the indigenous population meant that workers injured in accidents could choose to seek care if necessary.

The frequency of fractures for the whole skeletal population (Table 13.5) is 16%, and of the adults in the sample 21% (64/299) display fractures (Castillo Chavez, 2000). Males ($n=43$) exhibit twice as many fractures as females ($n=21$). This difference

Table 13.5 Prevalence of fractures in the HSJN skeletal collection (Castillo Chavez, 2000)

	Subadults	Adult females	Adult males	Total fractures/ No. individuals
Cranial Vault	1	6	8	15/437
Nose	1	7	26	34/437
Other Facial Fractures	1	1	4	6/437
Upper Limb	0	2	3	5/437
Lower Limb	0	5	2	7/437
Total	3	21	43	67/437

Table 13.6 Prevalence of disease indicators in the HSJN skeletal collection (Castillo Chavez, 2000)

	Subadult	Adult females	Adult males	Total disease/ No. of individuals
Syphilis	0	10	7	17/437
Tuberculosis	6	4	5	15/437
Osteomyelitis	0	15	19	34/437

between the sexes may result from the fact that the labor requirement only applied to indigenous men. Some of these fractures, notably those on the cranial vault, are perimortem, and may be the original motivation for seeking care at the hospital.

It is also important to note that violent conflict may not have ended after the Spanish conquest. For example, Individual 150 was found with shotgun pellets in the neck and abdominal cavity, and three surgical needles were found in association with his remains. It appears that surgeons at the hospital operated on him, but he did not survive (Sánchez Vázquez et al., 1996). Similarly, the most common fracture recorded in the skeletal population was on the face, typically involving the nose. These kinds of trauma might be more indicative of interpersonal violence than work-related injuries.

In addition to the skeletal indicators that point to a need for care resulting from the impact of poverty on health status or urgent injuries, a number of other people that died at the hospital present skeletal indicators of disease that suggest some form of long-term bodily care of patients was provided at the HSJN. Other hospitals in Mexico City specialized in the treatment of specific illnesses; such as leprosy, tuberculosis, or syphilis; however, remains within the HSJN skeletal sample also present skeletal indicators of these pathologies (Table 13.6).

Seventeen people show signs of advanced treponemal disease (Fig. 13.3), such as extreme periostitis and bowing of the tibia and caries sicca, or cranial lesions on the frontal and parietal bones (Espinosa Solís, 2006; Ortner & Putschar, 1981). It is possible that during the early stages of syphilis these people did not seek care, or they may have received treatment without being admitted to the hospital, but during the advanced stages complications such as blindness or mental illness may have motivated these people to ultimately seek care at the HSJN.

Similarly, 15 people show signs of tuberculosis, such as bone remodeling on the ribs and extreme spinal kyphosis, or forward bending and fusion of the vertebrae in

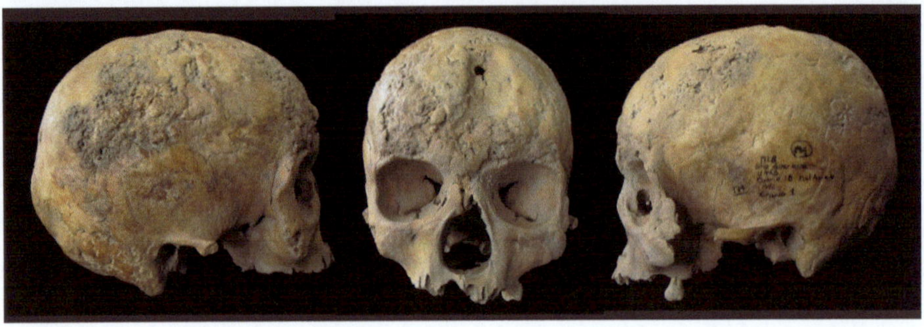

Fig. 13.3 Skeletal evidence of syphilis, indicated by caries sicca on the frontal and parietal bones on Cranium 174, skull recovered from Unit 9AB Ossuary 18 of the HSJN excavations, possibly dating to early eighteenth century

the lower spine (Castillo Chavez, 2000; Roberts & Buikstra, 2003; Santos & Roberts, 2006). Given the extensive skeletal involvement, these individuals likely would have been suffering from these ailments for a number of years. Respiratory dysfunction associated with tuberculosis may present acute complications for which a person might seek care multiple times over the course of the illness. Unlike the syphilis patients, those with tuberculosis may have sought care at an earlier stage of the disease or stayed in the hospital for a longer period of time.

A number of other patients stand out as people who likely would have had functional complications that required direct support to enable them to live their daily life. Individual 317, an old adult female, and Individual 281, a middle adult male, both have extreme osteoarthritis of the hip, with eburnation and osteophyte growth on the head of the femur and the acetabulum. The amount of osteophyte growth would have limited the mobility of these two individuals. Individual 85, an old adult female, has an extreme case of osteomyelitis that resulted in fusion of her right tibia and fibula. Individual 82, a middle adult female, presents similar osteomyelitic activity in the fibula, with the beginning of fusion between the tibia and fibula at the proximal end (Fig. 13.4). The pain and weakness associated with this kind of infection might have prompted these women to go to the hospital. Individual 386, a middle adult male, would have had his own kind of mobility problems in the upper extremity, since his left ulna and radius had become completely fused around the elbow joint, locking his forearm in a permanent state of pronation. It is difficult to know when these people might have first come to the hospital for care, the length of their visits, or even if these chronic mobility problems were their primary motivation for visiting the hospital.

Considering the age distribution of the remains studied may shed some light on the members of the indigenous population more likely to seek hospital care (Table 13.2). The majority of the skeletal sample comprises the remains of young and middle adults (77 %), while there are very few subadults (19 %) and old adults (4 %). This disparity in age groups could be the result of a number of different factors. First, since only patients who died while seeking care at the hospital were buried on hospital grounds, it could represent a heterogeneity of frailty, in which

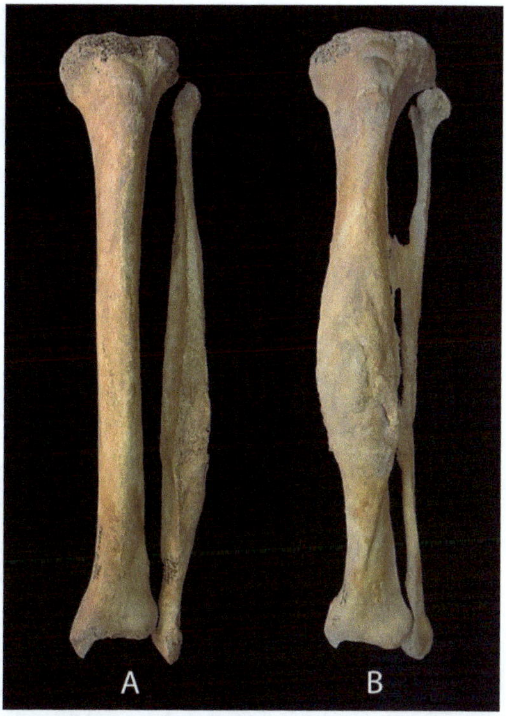

Fig. 13.4 Skeletal indicators of osteomyelitis with the beginning of fusion in Individual 82 (**a**), and fusion in Individual 85 (**b**)

infectious diseases (and traumatic injury) disproportionately affected the young and middle adult population. Alternatively, colonial period demographics may simply have been disproportionate, with fewer adults surviving to old age and fewer young people being born because of widespread fatalities from continual epidemics. Another possibility is that this difference in age groups represented in the remains reflects differential survival rates from the illness or trauma that saw the young and the old seeking care at the HSJN.

While we can never know what motivated any of these indigenous people to seek care at the hospital, it is thought provoking to speculate about what some of these motivations may have been. It is equally interesting to consider whether, in some instances, the low level of representation of particular demographic groups might indicate either a lack of motivation to seek care or even, perhaps, a motivation to *not* seek care from this particular institutional source.

The ability to make healthcare decisions for themselves would likely not have been available to children or adolescents or, alternatively, the symptoms associated with potentially serious infectious disease may not have been distinguishable from common childhood ailments, and as such not thought not to warrant hospital attention.

Adults were far more likely to have the ability to make their own healthcare decisions. The small sample of older adults may indicate that this was a group which was not motivated to seek care at the HSJN. The lack of older individuals represented in the skeletal sample may possibly be the result of sampling issues; perhaps older

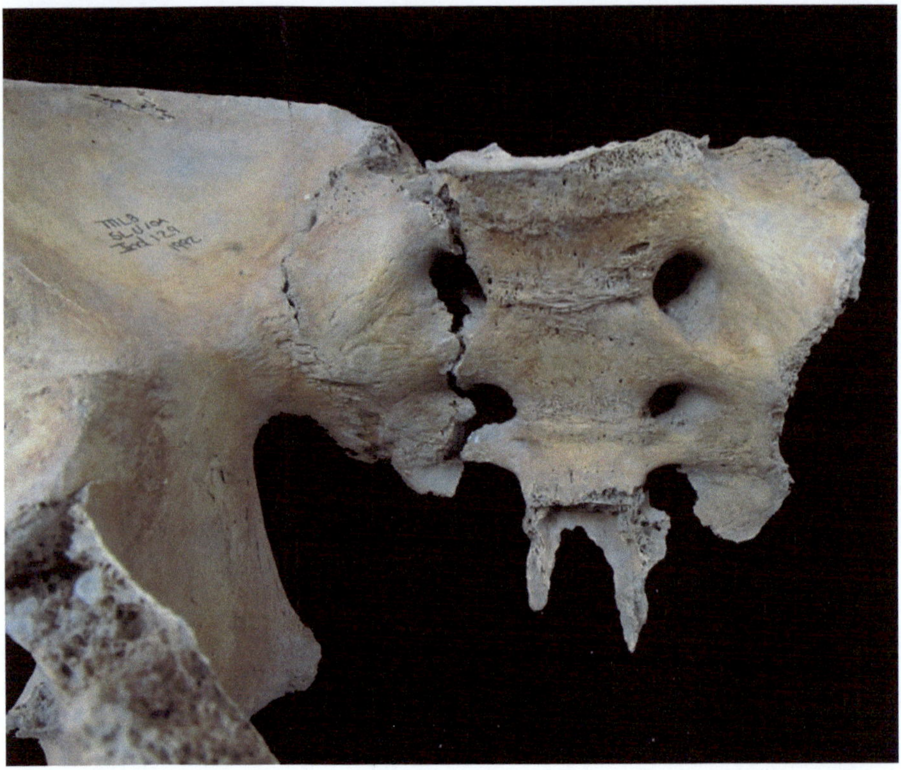

Fig. 13.5 Fusion of the os coxa and sacrum bone of Individual 129, one of the few old adult males from the HSJN skeletal collection

individuals were buried in a part of the hospital that has not yet been excavated, or perhaps poor representation is the result of poor preservation of their skeletal elements. But we should also consider the possibility that this segment of the population may have resisted seeking care at the hospital. For example, older adults may have preferred traditional methods of healthcare, and so applied to healers trained in Pre-Hispanic methods. It is possible that a lack of understanding of Christian beliefs and practice, and/or a lack of desire to have Christian spiritual care incorporated into the broader healthcare package, discouraged members of this age group from taking advantage of the services offered by the hospital.

Some older adults did avail themselves of hospital care, however. Individual 129 is one of the few old adult males in the collection; at the time of his death fusion of his right sacro-iliac joint was well underway (Fig. 13.5). Individuals 86 and 317, both old adult females, have similar osteoarthritic hip problems, with severe osteophyte growth and eburnation on the head of femur. These three conditions are likely the result of activity and aging, and without additional pathology or systemic disease complications are usually endured in a home environment. What motivated *these* people to seek care at the HSJN? Putting to one side the possibility of unrelated and archaeologically invisible pathologies requiring applied medical care, it may be that all three were pragmatically motivated by increasing challenges to their mobility – the food and shelter provided by the hospital would enable them to survive a decline in physical independence. It is also possible that the spiritual framework in which this palliative care was located offered a form of caregiving that met other kinds of needs; ones that were, perhaps, equally important to these individuals' well-being.

Conclusion

To understand care in the past we must first think about how social, political, and cultural factors influenced a person's motivation to provide care – or to seek it. With the emergence of institutions that specifically focus on providing care, there is a shift away from care as a societal obligation towards caregiving as a complex entanglement of social, political, and cultural benefits. The link between these early Christian communities and the establishment of institutions of care highlights how both the patient and the caregiver may perceive a positive benefit from their individual choices to participate in the operations of a healthcare institution. Yet this link with religious organizations prompts a discussion not only about the motivations for participation, but also about the type of care being offered. As a bioarchaeologist, it is easy to focus only on the skeletal clues that suggest someone may have needed care in the past, but bodily care is, and likely always has been, enmeshed with psychological, social and spiritual healing approaches. While "hard" evidence to support such discussion may not always be available, it is nonetheless important to contemplate how such forms of care might have been characterized.

The *Hospital Real de San José de Naturales* serves as an example for how we might incorporate skeletal remains with other forms of evidence to answer questions about care in the past. The initial motivation for establishing the hospital was likely a Christian charitable mission to provide for the poor and the sick, but the relationship between the caregiving institution and the person receiving care held a greater significance in the Americas than in the early Christian hospitals in Europe. In Mexico, hospitals became essential to survival, especially for the indigenous population who suffered greatly from widespread infectious diseases, but they also served as a way to maintain a "healthy" social distance between the distinct sections of colonial society. While the violent conquest may have occurred quickly, the conceptual one (of the Old World over the New) lasted for much of the sixteenth century, and it seems as though a secondary motivation for caring emerged when Europeans began to acknowledge the local population as peers, albeit at a slightly lower social status and in need of spiritual education. The institution of the hospital, separated from everyday life, run by religious orders, was important for responding to bodily care needs. But in a young and uneasily multicultural society facing regular outbreaks of devastating epidemic disease, the hospital also offered an important space in which to provide spiritual care, and perhaps even psychological comfort, for both caregivers and patients.

Acknowledgements I would like to thank Lorna Tilley and Alecia A. Schrenk for inviting me to participate in the conference session and for providing thoughtful critiques of this chapter. This research was supported by a UC MEXUS dissertation research grant and I was supported as a resident scholar at the institute while completing this work. I would also like to thank Dr. Lourdes Márquez Morfín for providing me with access to the HSJN skeletal collection and the academic community in the Graduate Osteology Laboratory at the Escuela Nacional de Antropología e Historía, in particular Elizabeth Hernández who served as my assistant while collecting data in Mexico.

References

Acuna-Soto, R., Romero, L. C., & Maguire, J. H. (2000). Large epidemics of hemorrhagic fevers in Mexico 1545–1815. *American Journal of Tropical Medicine and Hygiene, 62*(6), 733–739.

Acuna-Soto, R., et al. (2002). Megadrought and Megadeath in 16th Century Mexico. *Emerging Infectious Diseases, 8*(4), 360–362.

Báez Molgado, S., & Meza Peñaloza, A. (1995). Proyecto Metro Linea 8, análysis de los restos óseos del Hospital Real de San José de los Naturales. Instituto Nacional de Antropología e Historia, Dirección de Salvamento Arqueológico.

Cabrera Torres, J. J., & García Martínez, M. A. (1998). Utilización, Modificación y Reuso de los Espacios del Edificio sede del Hospital Real de San José de los Naturales, Arqueología, Escuela Nacional de Anthropología e Historia.

Cárdenas de la Peña, E. (1976). *Historia de la Medicina en la Ciudad de México*. Mexico: Tallers Gráficos de la Nación.

Castillo Chavez, O. (2000). Condiciones de Vida y Salud de una muestra poblacional de la Ciudad de Mexico en la Epoca Colonial, Antropología Física, Escuela Nacional de Antropologia e Historia.

Chávez Balderas, X. (2007). *Rituales Funerarios en el Templo Mayor de Tenochtitlan*. Mexico: Instituto Nacional de Antropología e Historia.

Cook, S. F., & Simpson, L. B. (1948). The population of central Mexico in the sixteenth century. *Ibero-Americana, 31*, 43–55.

Cope, R. D. (1994). *The limits of racial domination: Plebeian society in colonial Mexico City, 1660–1720*. Madison: University of Wisconsin Press.

Dhabhar, F. S. (2009). A hassle a day may keep the pathogens away: The fight-or-flight stress response and the augmentation of immune function. *Integrative and Comparative Biology, 49*(3), 215–236.

Espinosa Solís, E. A. (2006). Sexualidad y sífilis en la Ciudad de México en el Virreinato: Diagnóstico diferencial de enfermedad, Antropología Física, Escuela Nacional de Antropología e Historia.

Ferngren, G. B. (2009). *Medicine and health care in early Christianity*. Baltimore: The Johns Hopkins University Press.

Flexner, J. L. (2012). An Institution that was a village: Archaeology and social life in the Hansen's disease settlement at Kalawao, Moloka'i, Hawaii. *International Journal of Historical Archaeology, 16*(1), 135–163.

García Icazbalceta, J., Pomar, J. B., & Zurita, A. (1941). Códice Franciscano, Siglo XVI: Informe de la provincia del Santo Evangelio al visitador Lic. Juan de Ovando Informe de la provincina de Guadalajara al mismo Cartas de religiosos (pp. 1533–1569). Mexico: Editorial Salvador Chávez Hayhoe.

Gibson, C. (1964). *The Aztecs under Spanish rule: A history of the Indians of the valley of Mexico, 1519–1810*. Stanford: Stanford University Press.

Goodman, A. H., & Armelagos, G. J. (1985). Factors affecting the distribution of enamel hypoplasias within the human permanent dentition. *American Journal of Physical Anthropology, 68*(4), 479–493.

Goodman, A. H., Brooke, T. R., Swedlund, A. C., & Armelagos, G. J. (1988). Biocultural perspectives on stress in prehistoric, historical, and contemporary population research. *American Journal of Physical Anthropology, 31*(S9), 169–202.

Goodman, A. H., & Rose, J. C. (1990). Assessment of systemic physiological perturbations from dental enamel hypoplasias and associated histological structures. *American Journal of Physical Anthropology, 33*(S11), 59–110.

Goyal, M., et al. (2014). Meditation programs for psychological stress and well-being: A systematic review and meta-analysis. *JAMA Internal Medicine, 174*(3), 357–368.

Kellogg, S. (1995). *Law and the transformation of Aztec culture, 1500–1700*. Norman: University of Oklahoma Press.

King, T., Humphrey, L. T., & Hillson, S. (2005). Linear enamel hypoplasias as indicators of systemic physiological stress: Evidence from two known age-at-death and sex populations from postmedieval London. *American Journal of Physical Anthropology, 128*(3), 547–559.

Larsen, C. S. (1994). In the wake of Columbus: Native population biology in the postcontact Americas. *American Journal of Physical Anthropology, 37*(S19), 109–154.

López Austin, A. (1975). *Textos de Medicina Náhuatl*. Mexico: Universidad Nacional Autónoma de México/Instituto de Investigaciones Históricas.

López Austin, A. (1988). *The human body and ideology: Concepts of the Ancient Nahuas (Trans. Thelma Ortiz de Montellano & Bernard Ortiz de Montellano)*. Salt Lake City: University of Utah Press.

López Lujan, L. (1994). *The offerings of the Templo Mayor of Tenochtitlan (Trans. Bernard R. Ortiz de Montellano & Thelma Ortiz de Montellano)*. Niwot: University Press of Colorado.

Louveau, A., et al. (2015). Structural and functional features of central nervous system lymphatic vessels. *Nature, 523*, 337–341.

Lugo Olín, M. C. (2005). Enfermedad y muerte en la Nueva España. In A. Rubial García (Ed.), *Historia de la Vida Cotidiana en México: Tomo II: La Ciudad Barroca* (pp. 555–586). México: El Colegio de México, Fondo de la Cultura Económica.

Markman, R. H., & Markman, P. T. (1992). *The flayed God: The Mesoamerican mythological tradition: Sacred texts and images from pre-Colombian Mexico and Central America*. San Francisco: Harper.

Márquez Morfín, L. (1994). *La desigualdad ante la muerte en la Ciudad de México: el tifo y el cólera (1813 y 1833)*. México: Siglo Veintiuno Editores.

Márquez Morfín, L., & González Licón, E. (1992). La Trepanación Craneana entre los Antiguos Zapotecos de Monte Albán. *Cuadernos del Sur, 1*, 25–50.

Meza Peñaloza, A., & Ortuño Cos, F. (1995). De Epidemias y Muerte en la Ciudad de México. Los Enterramientos en la Unidad 12 del Hospital Real de San José. In *Presencias y Encuentros: Investigaciones Arqueológicas de Salvamento* (pp. 239–248). Mexico: Dirección de Salvamento Arqueológico.

Moores Ball, J. (1989). *The body snatchers: Doctors, grave robbers, and the law*. New York: Dorset Press.

Mora-Ripoll, R. (2010). The therapeutic value of laughter in medicine. *Alternative Therapies in Health and Medicine, 16*(6), 56–64.

Muriel, J. (1956). *Hospitales de la Nueva España: Fundaciones del Siglo XVI. Volume Tomo I*. Mexico: Instituto de Historia.

Ortner, D. J., & Putschar, W. G. J. (1981). *Identification of pathological conditions in human skeletal remains*. Washington, DC: Smithsonian Institute Press.

Pulido Méndez, S. (1994). Arqueología del Eje Central Lázaro Cárdenas de la ciudad de México: Notas de las excavaciones arqueológicas de la Línea 8 del metro. *Arqueología, 11–12*, 133–138.

Ricard, R. (1986). *La Conquista Espiritual de México: ensayo sobre el apostolado y los métodos misioneros de las órdenes mendicantes en la Nueva España de 1523–1524 a 1572*. México: Fondo de Cultura Económica.

Risse, G. B. (1999). *Mending bodies, saving souls: A history of hospitals*. New York: Oxford University Press.

Roberts, C. A., & Buikstra, J. E. (2003). *The bioarchaeology of tuberculosis: A global view on a reemerging disease*. Gainesville: University Press of Florida.

Rodríguez-Sala, M. L. (2005). *El Hospital Real de los Naturales, sus Administradores y sus Cirujanos (1531–1764), Miembros de un estamento ocupacional o de una comunidad científica?* Mexico: Universidad Nacional Autónoma de México.

Ryal Miller, R., & Orr, W. J. (2000). *Daily life in colonial Mexico: The Journey of Friar Ilarione da Bergamo, 1761–1768*. Norman: University of Oklahoma Press.

Sahagún, F. B. (2000). *Historia General de las Cosas de Nueva España. 3 vols*. México: Cien de México/CONACULTA.

Sánchez, V., & Jesús, M. et al. (1996). Proyecto Metro Línea 8, Informe Final. Instituto Nacional de Antropología e Historia, Dirección de Salvamento Arqueológico.

Santos, A. L., & Roberts, C. A. (2006). Anatomy of a serial killer: Differential diagnosis of tuberculosis based on Rib lesions of adult individuals from the Coimbra identified skeletal collection, Portugal. *American Journal of Physical Anthropology, 130*, 38–49.

Scheper Hughes, J. (2010). *Biography of a Mexican Crucifix: Lived religion and local faith from the conquest to the present*. New York: Oxford University Press. In Prep Mexican Kairos: Epidemic Disease, Indigenous Death and the Birth of New World Catholicism.

Stuart-Macadam, P. (1985). Porotic hyperostosis: Representative of a childhood condition. *American Journal of Physical Anthropology, 66*(4), 391–398.

Suarez, M. (1988). *Hospitales y Sociedad en la Ciudad de Mexico del Siglo XVI*. Mexico: Universidad Autónoma Metropolitana.

Thornberry, P. (2003). *Indigenous peoples and human rights*. Manchester: Manchester University Press.

Tiesler Blos, V. (2001). *Decoraciones Dentales entre los Antiguos Mayas*. México: Ediciones Euroamericanas INAH/CONACULTA.

Tilley, L. (2012). The bioarchaeology of care. Invited essay for special forum: New directions in bioarchaeology. *The Archaeological Record, 12*, 39–41.

Tilley, L. (2015). *Theory and practice in the bioarchaeology of care*. New York: Springer.

Tilley, L., & Cameron, T. (2014). Introducing the index of care: A web-based application supporting archaeological research into health-related care. *International Journal of Paleopathology, 6*, 5–9.

Viveros, G. (2005). El teatro y otros entretenimientos urbanos: La norma, la censura, y la práctica. In A. Rubial García (Ed.), *Historia de la Vida Cotidiana en México: Tomo II: La Ciudad Barroca* (pp. 461–487). México: El Colegio de México/Fondo de Cultura Económica.

Wood, J. W., Milner, G. R., Harpending, H. C., Weiss, K. M., Cohen, M. N., Eisenberg, L. E., et al. (1992). The osteological paradox: Problems of inferring prehistoric health from skeletal samples [and Comments and Reply]. *Current Anthropology, 33*(4), 343–370.

Zedillo Castillo, A. (1984). Historia de un Hospital: El Hospital Real de Naturales. México: Instituto Mexicano de Seguro Social.

Chapter 14
An Exploration of a Modified Bioarchaeology of Care Methodological Approach for Historic Institutionalized Populations

Lori A. Tremblay Critcher

Introduction

Lorna Tilley's bioarchaeology of care approach was designed to examine care provided to individuals in the past (Chap. 2; Tilley, 2012). While this approach provides bioarchaeologists with a framework to explore both care provision and receipt of care in prehistoric contexts, it cannot be used to examine care at the population level in prehistoric populations because we do not have evidence of either the actual disease prevalence from these time periods or the levels of care required to support those who suffered from disease and/or disability (see Tilley, Chap. 2 this volume, for further discussion on this point). However, the amount of historical documentation of medical advances and implementation during the historic period is considerable. We see the rise and growth of hospitals and various other Institutions of Care during the nineteenth century (Rosenberg, 1995). Many of the written records and accounts we have about health treatment during this period were written by, and from the perspective of, people in positions of power (e.g., medical doctors, political leaders, etc.), and a good deal of the historical scholarship written by more contemporary scholars is based on those records and accounts. As a result, we have what may be perceived as a fairly complete picture of what care provision was like at that time. But that depiction is, of course, colored by authorial and authoritative bias in those texts.

Even with sources that may provide us with information regarding past care provision, it is the human skeleton that can provide us with the most objective and empirical evidence of the human biological experience in the past (Larsen, 2002). As bioarchaeologists, our goal is both to describe and explain the lifeways and life

L.A. Tremblay Critcher, Ph.D. (✉)
Department of Anthropology, The Ohio State University, Columbus, OH, USA
e-mail: critcher.1@osu.edu

© Springer International Publishing Switzerland 2017

L. Tilley, A.A. Schrenk (eds.), *New Developments in the Bioarchaeology of Care*, Bioarchaeology and Social Theory, DOI 10.1007/978-3-319-39901-0_14

experiences of past populations and to speak for those who could not (previously) speak for themselves. We act as their voice, as their representatives, to tell others what their lives were like – what they ate, what kinds of diseases and trauma they may have suffered, whether they remained in their place of birth, or migrated to their place of death. We can use skeletal evidence to either confirm or contradict the information about care provision that we obtain from those textual sources. This then raises an interesting question: can we use a new, modified bioarchaeology of care method to consider not simply whether care (and if so, what *kind* of care) occurred in the historic period, but the extent to which such care was effective?

This chapter examines this question. It does not provide a definitive answer; rather, it is a preliminary exploration to look at whether a modified bioarchaeology of care method may be used to assess the efficacy of care at both the individual and population levels at the Oneida State Custodial Asylum in upstate New York, a late nineteenth–early twentieth centuries Institution of Care. This pilot study offers the beginnings of an approach that I hope to build upon in future research into historic-era Institutions of Care.

Institutions of Care

I define an Institution of Care as any institution, whether funded governmentally or privately, which is specifically designed to provide long-term care for those in society who cannot provide it for themselves.

Early in the nineteenth century mental illness was believed to be a moral failing, but later during that century a new way of thinking started to emerge – one that emphasized that 'insanity' was an illness that required medical treatment, just like any physical ailment. Up until that point most people who were labeled as 'insane' or as 'lunatics' were hidden at home if their families had the means to care for them, or, if they had no such support, they lived on the streets or were put in prison. Once mental illness, or insanity, was recognized as a medical condition, the ways in which the mentally ill were treated changed (Grob, 1994).

It was after this paradigm shift that we see the emergence of the insane asylums (or mental institutions) in the United States. Dorothea Dix was influential in the movement that resulted in the establishment of insane asylums across the United States, arguing for the creation of state sanctioned hospitals or institutions to care for the mentally ill as well as to serve as cultural buffers protecting them from the starvation, the dangers of disease, and the risk of injury and abuse they typically suffered in prisons and on the streets (Grob, 1994). The ultimate goal of these institutions of mental health treatment, in addition to serving as a cultural buffer, was to rehabilitate those afflicted by mental illness (Phillips, 2001), as it was believed that most could be cured if they were treated in large institutional settings specifically designed for that purpose (Grob, 1994; Yanni, 2003).

Examining Efficacy of Care

The Oxford English Dictionary (2015) defines efficacy as the "power or capacity to produce effects; the power to effect the object intended."

If the intended effect of institutional care was not only to cure mental illness, but to act as a cultural buffer against the risk of starvation, trauma, and disease that the mentally ill would have been subjected to on the streets, in almshouses, or in prisons, then we may be able to use skeletal evidence to attempt to determine whether, and to what extent, these institutions may have met that latter goal. We cannot, of course, measure the efficacy of the former goal (i.e., recovery from mental illness) using skeletal evidence because mental illness does not manifest in any way on the human skeleton. We can, however, attempt to evaluate institutional performance in terms of evaluating how well it met its goal of providing a cultural buffer.

The bioarchaeology of care approach defines care along a continuum of direct support to accommodation (Tilley, Chap. 2 this volume), and we might approach assessment of *efficacy of care* based not only on what is recorded about the type and amount of direct support and accommodation provided, but also on what we may be able to tell about the *impact* of that caregiving through its expression and/or reflection in individual and collective indicators of physiological stress in the form of lesions associated with pathological conditions or trauma. (While the term pathological condition refers to any abnormality, for purposes of clarity and distinguishing between the etiologies of lesions associated with disease from those associated with injury, I am using the term pathological condition in this chapter to refer solely to the skeletal indicators associated with any disease process, be they infectious or metabolic.) We know that in institutions basic direct support was provided in terms of housing, food, etc., and that in most institutions some level of accommodation, in terms of providing opportunities for inmates/patients to participate in social activities, was likely practiced. Opportunities to participate in economic activity (such as maintaining the facility), if these were available, would have varied at an individual level as well as within and between institutions.

Modified Method

In attempting to modify the bioarchaeology of care approach for examining the efficacy of historic institutions of care, I created two variants of an experimental method: one that could be used at the individual level, and one that could be used at the population level. This was an exercise in trial and error. While these modified approaches may work successfully in some instances, there are a number of limitations that may prevent them from working as well as I had originally hoped. I attempted, and not entirely successfully, to test these two variants of the modified method in examining efficacy of care in the Oneida State Custodial Asylum. Below is a description of the proposed new method, followed by an account of its attempted application to one individual from that sample and to the population as a whole. While this new method is not yet sufficiently evolved to produce results that have a high degree of accuracy, it serves as a starting point for thinking about how we might begin to assess 'effective treatment' in historic era institutions.

Tilley's original bioarchaeology of care method is composed of four stages of analysis (Chap. 2 this volume). These four stages are the basis for the four stages of analysis in this modified method, with its two variants for assessing efficacy of care at individual and population levels, respectively. In the discussion that follows, these four stages are described in relation to their application at the individual level specifically, although the many of the same processes are followed in assessing care outcomes at a collective, or population, level. Indeed, when working at the population level, analyses in stages one, two and, to some extent, three, must be carried out at the level of the individual remains although information gathered on lifeways context will be equally relevant to all subjects. The results of these analyses are then collated in order to provide a general picture of risk for physiological stress within the institution, allowing an estimate of healthcare efficacy.

Efficacy of Care at the Individual Level

As in the standard bioarchaeology of care approach, the first stage of the modified approach requires a description of the skeletal evidence indicating that an individual lived with a debilitating or potentially incapacitating condition, as well as a diagnosis of that condition (if possible).

Importantly, the 'modified method' Stage 1 analysis varies from the original in pursuing a focus on differentiating between the presence, prevalence, and distribution of active pathological lesions and evidence for perimortem trauma. The reason for the focus on active lesions and perimortem trauma, and for distinguishing such indicators within a more general 'presence of lesions' category (which combines healed and active lesions together in one count), is because although asylums were long-term institutions of care, in most cases we cannot know with certainty how long a particular individual was under the state's care and control. While many inmates lived in institutions for years, unless we have personal medical records that we can associate with an individual set of remains – and these are rare – we cannot ascertain exactly how long an individual resided in the institution or, using anthroposcopic methods alone, how long prior to their death a healed pathological lesion or fracture may have occurred. Emphasizing active lesions and perimortem trauma allows bioarchaeologists to say with more certainty that particular pathological condition or traumatic injury likely occurred and/or was experienced while the individual was institutionalized. At the level of population analysis, a number of individuals displaying a particular type of indicator may allow identification of a pattern of occurrence of a specific pathological condition or traumatic injury.

Stage 1 also includes a thorough description of lifeways context, but the search for information about the subject's environment needs to focus particularly on features of the institutional context and the place of the institution in the community, which can often be obtained via contemporary historical documentation.

The second stage requires consideration of the clinical and functional impacts of any identified conditions for each individual in question. Information about clinical effects can be obtained from modern medical literature, and the functional impacts can be inferred based on how those clinical impacts may have interfered with an individual's ability to engage in the activities of everyday living; again, in applying this new method, information allowing analysis of functional impact is likely to draw on historical sources. While mental illness certainly has clinical impacts, because there is no evidence of this kind of condition on the skeleton we cannot, without individual identification, attempt to ascertain what those impacts were. There is no need at this point to determine whether direct support was needed for this individual because, as an institutionalized person, the existence of direct support and accommodation are a given rather than a question. However, in this context Stage 2 does allow for the estimation of type of care required in broad terms of 'direct support' and 'accommodation.'

The third stage comprises consideration of the detail of care likely required by the individual examined in the first two stages, and then constructs a model of the care that may have been provided *within the corresponding institutional setting*, taking into account what is known about the institution and its practices from historical sources, as well as information about its goals, available resources, and the treatments available at the time. The range of material available should allow the researcher to develop a relatively detailed picture of what care may have been available on paper and (not necessarily the same thing) what care may have actually been offered to patients.

The fourth and final stage of this new approach is completely different from the original bioarchaeology of care Stage 4. It requires the researcher to focus exclusively on what the information acquired to this point may reveal about the outcomes of institutional care for the subject of their study. In other words, can the care provided be assessed as having been effective in meeting institutional healthcare goals of protecting vulnerable inmates from disease and injury and, where possible, providing treatment adequate for inmates' immediate health needs (according to the standards of the time)? If the care provided does not appear to have been effective in meeting institutional goals then, dependent upon the extent and reliability of information available, the researcher may also able to consider what care, available in theory, was lacking in practice (e.g., dental care, fracture alignment), and why this may have been the case.

Efficacy of Care at the Population Level

This second variant of this modified method examines of the efficacy of the institution in meeting its goal of providing a cultural buffer *for the sample as a whole*, as well as assisting the researcher to compare and contrast level of treatment efficacy (i) between different institutions and (ii) between male and female inmates within and across institutions.

The first stage in this variant requires a description of the *patterns and distribution* of all pathological and traumatic lesions present either on individual skeletal elements or systemically, noting which of these lesions are active, and whether these are well established or the result of perimortem activity. Disease diagnosis and descriptions of patterns of nonspecific pathological lesions and trauma should be included where possible. Additionally, at this stage, all information on disease and causes of death available from historical and/or medical records associated with the institution should be recorded.

The second stage requires a general overview of the clinical and functional impacts of any emergent patterns of prevalent pathological conditions and/or traumatic injuries elicited from the Stage 1 analysis. Stage 2 analysis is only relevant *if* clear patterns of disease emerge; if there are no such patterns, then in this variant of the bioarchaeology of care methodology, Stage 2 becomes redundant and the researcher proceeds directly to Stage 3.

In the third stage, the 'model of care' of the institution should be described. This will be based on data obtained from available historical and medical records that provide general information about what kinds of treatments were provided by the particular institution to the inmate population during the relevant time period.

In the fourth and final stage, the institutional program of care is analyzed to evaluate the efficacy of the institution's performance. In Stage 4, the focus is on the care choices that were made – on the impact of the care provided as well as, on occasion, the care *not* provided (e.g., failure to provide dental care). Where skeletal data, historical documents and/or medical records permit, it might be prudent to attempt comparison between the patterns and distributions of pathology and causes of death within the institutional population with those of the general population and/or those of other contemporary and vulnerable populations in the same locality (such as the population of a pauper's cemetery, an almshouse, or a prison). Taking due account of caveats arising from consideration of the characteristics of the population serviced by an 'Institution of Care' (by definition, residents are more likely to be in need of caregiving), this comparison might provide insights into the ability of a particular institution to meet its health-related goals. This exercise might also allow cautious comparison between the performance of different institutions with similar aims and mandates.

Although an unknown length of time spent in the institutional setting is a constraint in the individual model, it is less so in this collective model variant, because these kinds of institutions were long-term care facilities. As such, most of the inmates who resided there had done so for at least one, if not many, years. Other constraints may include difficulty in accessing comparative data, because there may not always be contemporary skeletal collections or documentary information available for comparative purposes. Without these data, it will be difficult to assess whether patterns of disease or trauma, active or healed, were unique to the institutionalized population or whether they were ubiquitous in the wider community. Another limitation can lie within the sample itself; if there are many burials with differential preservation or completeness, obtaining accurate data in relation to the number of active and healed pathological lesions is potentially problematic.

Application of the New Method

Oneida State Custodial Asylum

For the initial application of the new method, I chose the Oneida State Custodial Asylum, known later as the Rome State Custodial Asylum, in upstate New York. This was a long-term Institution of Care for the mentally ill that was deemed state of the art for its time (Phillips, 2001).

The Oneida State Custodial Asylum was originally established as almshouse in 1825, but was, by the late 1860s, used primarily as an asylum for the 'incurably insane' (Carlisle, 1918, p. 41; Phillips, 2001). While it served as both a poorhouse and an asylum until 1894, the human skeletal remains recovered have been associated with the asylum population for a number of reasons. First, the burials recovered were believed to have been interred in the 1880s (when the asylum housed almost 300 inmates) and at this time the poor did not reside in the institution, but instead received outdoor relief. Second, the records from both the asylum and the New York State legislature indicate that during the latter part of the nineteenth century the institution served primarily as an asylum for the mentally ill, as well as for some who were physically disabled. Third, the demographics of the sample are not in line with those expected of a poorhouse. Poorhouse cemeteries typically contain high numbers of infants and children, and the sample from this institution contains only one infant (Phillips, 2001).

The Oneida State Custodial Asylum was considered state of the art in the late nineteenth century because it used the most up-to-date psychiatric treatment (Phillips, 2001). At the end of the nineteenth century it was believed that physical labor could cure mental illness and mental disability, so the Oneida State Custodial Asylum used labor therapy for approximately 95 % of its inmates as a means both of keeping the asylum functional and treating the inmates by helping them to achieve a sense of normality (Grob, 1994; Phillips, 2001). The labor therapy used at the Oneida State Custodial Asylum was divided on gender lines, with men responsible for farm work and women responsible for household maintenance (Phillips, 2001). While the primary goal of the institution may have been to 'cure' its inmates of their mental illness, it also served to protect these vulnerable people from the risks they would have faced on the streets or in prisons.

Materials

The remains of more than 80 individuals who were associated with the Oneida State Custodial Asylum have been recovered. However, preservation and completeness varied throughout the sample. I analyzed the remains of 46 adult individuals (see Table 14.1) assessed as being in a condition allowing description for demographic and/or diagnostic purposes. The remainder of the burials were either incomplete (some contained only a single element) or the preservation was too poor to allow analysis. The entire original sample is composed of adults (with the exception of one neonate subadult).

Table 14.1 Sex and age composition of study sample

Sex	N.	<30	30–45	45–60	60+	Adult (unknown age)
Male	32	4	10	5	4	9
Female	10	3	3	2	0	2
Indeterminate	4	0	0	0	1	3
Total	46	7	13	7	5	14

Individual Level Analysis

I chose to use an individual labeled as Burial 29 for the application of the new model at the individual level. This individual is a 35–50-year-old male who exhibits multiple potentially debilitating antemortem injuries to his vertebral column, left arm, and left ribs. He does not exhibit any perimortem trauma or active lesions, with the exception of one small carious lesion on his lower right second molar. While this individual does not exhibit active lesions, I chose him as a case study because he clearly required both direct support and accommodation due to the debilitating nature of his injuries.

The remains of Burial 29 exhibit (Stage 1) a healed complete antemortem fracture that separated the dens from the second cervical vertebra, both DISH and Schmorl's nodes in the thoracic and lumbar vertebrae, and severe trauma to the left elbow, with what appears to be concurrent trauma to his left ninth and tenth ribs. Together, the traumatic lesions would have (Stage 2) constricted the movement of his elbow joint and spine, in addition to causing potential pain and stiffness associated with Schmorl's nodes and DISH (Mayo Clinic Staff, 2012; Takatalo et al., 2012).

Stages 3 and 4 are where the limitations of this new method emerge. In relation to Stage 3, we know that the model of care at the Oneida State Custodial Asylum involved labor therapy, but because of Burial 29's physical limitations it is difficult to assess whether this standard treatment, which applied to most inmates, was used with this individual. There are no signs of atrophy of either his upper or lower limbs, so we can assume that his gross movement was not restricted. Unfortunately, we are missing one very crucial piece of information about this individual – his name. Because he is unidentified, we cannot know whether he resided in the institution for one month or for years, and not knowing this means that it is not possible to determine whether he sustained his injuries before or after admittance to the asylum.

Not having this information makes Stage 4, assessing the efficacy of care of the institution for Burial 29, very problematic. This is one of the biggest limitations of this variant of the proposed new method. If his injuries occurred prior to his admittance, then his admittance to the asylum could have been, in part, because of the physical limitations resulting from those injuries. If this were the case, then the efficacy of institutional care could be rated as 'high' for this individual, because he does not exhibit either active pathological lesions or the same extensive patterns of dental disease that his contemporaries in this asylum do (see discussion in the following section on this latter point).

Alternatively, if Burial 29 had resided in the asylum for a number of years, and had sustained his injuries in a labor-therapy related context, the efficacy of the institutional care for this individual would be low – because it did not protect him from the risk of injury equivalent to that which he would likely have faced in the streets or in an almshouse.

Population-Level Analysis

In applying the population-level variant of the model, in Stage 1, I found a high prevalence of Schmorl's nodes, dental caries, and antemortem tooth loss (AMTL) (see Table 14.2 for the numbers of individuals who exhibit dental caries, antemortem tooth loss, and Schmorl's Nodes). In Stage 2, where in the clinical and functional impacts are examined, it can be argued that the Schmorl's nodes likely caused a moderate-to-severe amount of back pain (Takatalo et al., 2012). Ongoing back pain may have made engagement in daily tasks difficult, but whether it would have prevented individuals from engaging in those tasks, be they self-care tasks or labor therapy tasks, is unknown. The clinical impacts of Schmorl's nodes and poor dental health can be painful, but are not necessarily permanently debilitating. However, advanced dental disease can have larger systemic effects that we are unlikely to see on the skeleton, but which could well have had an impact on overall health and quality of life (Garcia, Henshaw, & Krall, 2001).

In considering the 'model of care' (Stage 3), historical records indicate that labor therapy was employed in the asylum. As previously noted, there was a sexual division of labor, with men typically undertaking outdoor and agricultural work (clearing fields, planting and maintaining crops, chopping wood, tending animals, etc.) and women typically working indoors, undertaking more domestic tasks such as cooking, cleaning, and sewing. One would expect this kind of treatment may have put individuals at risk for work-related accidents. However, the range of assigned tasks would have put different individuals at risk for different kinds of occupational injury. This means that although there was a very general prescribed category of treatment – 'labor therapy' – variations in the nature of this treatment make it impossible to generalize about the impacts of labor therapy practices across the asylum population.

In the fourth stage, I compared the demographic and pathology data I had to data from the Albany Almshouse (in Phillips, 2001). While dental health care was available to the public at this time, it may not have been provided to the inmates at this institution. The overall dental health of the Oneida State Custodial Asylum population was significantly poorer (58 % exhibited caries) than that of their contemporaries (16.94 % of the Albany Almshouse sample exhibited caries noted in [Phillips, 2001]). Additionally, while there is no consensus on the etiology of Schmorl's nodes (Dar et al., 2010), it has been found that populations that engage in heavy labor tend to exhibit higher rates of Schmorl's nodes than occur in other populations (e.g., Lai & Lovell,

Table 14.2 Frequencies of individuals who exhibit dental pathologies and Schmorl's nodes

Sex	Caries	AMTL	Schmorl's Nodes
Male	21/32	25/32	8/32
Female	5/10	8/10	3/10
Indeterminate	4/4	3/4	1/4
Total	30/46	36/46	12/46

1992), thus the high prevalence of Schmorl's nodes in this institutional population might be associated with engagement in physically demanding forms of labor therapy.

'Exhaustion,' a nonspecific term that simply means 'to be drained,' was noted as the most frequent cause of death in the Oneida State Custodial Asylum, equivalent to all deaths from all the 'infectious respiratory diseases combined' (Phillips, 2001, p. 43) at a time when respiratory disease and accidents were the most common causes of death in the nineteenth-century United States. There were few deaths attributed to accidents at the Oneida State Custodial Asylum. How does this pattern of mortality reflect on the question of efficacy? Was this institution, based on these data, effective in serving as a cultural buffer to protect its charges from the risks they would have encountered on the streets or in prisons?

The limitations of available data, as well as the limitations of this newly conceptualized model, make such a determination problematic. On one hand, based on the historical records, the Oneida State Custodial Asylum did protect its inmates from death due to accidental injuries and from the infectious respiratory diseases that plagued the general population, yet on the other hand, based on both the skeletal data and contemporary documentation, it put the inmates at risk of Schmorl's nodes and death by 'exhaustion' by virtue of the labor therapy employed by the asylum caregivers. So the answer to the question of whether this institution was effective in meeting its goal of serving as a cultural buffer is both yes and no.

While the strength of this population-level analysis is that it has the potential to let us identify patterns of disease and injury within institutions, giving us a more realistic picture of the lived experiences of their inmates, it is not yet at a point where it can be used to give a reliable assessment of the efficacy of an institution for the inmate population as a whole. The design of care programs is complex, with many factors that need to be accounted for. There are possible trade-offs for protection from certain health risks that may ultimately lead to other kinds of health challenges. For example, while inmates may not have been as exposed to the respiratory diseases rife among the general population, at the Oneida State Custodial Asylum they suffered from poor dental health, which may have ultimately led to health conditions as serious as the respiratory diseases they were protected from.

Furthermore, although analyzing the prevalence of pathological lesions may allow us to see patterns of disease and trauma, when we include healed lesions this can potentially be misleading, because unless detailed patient case histories are available we have no way of knowing when each individual developed a particular disease or sustained a particular injury. Therefore, while lesion patterns may suggest that a relationship between activities in the asylum and certain forms of acquired disease or trauma is possible or even probable, such hypotheses must always be conservative.

Conclusions and Future Directions

This chapter has presented a possible method for examining and assessing the efficacy of caregiving in late nineteenth and early twentieth-century institutions of care that is based on an adaptation of the bioarchaeology of care methodology. Whether, and to what extent, we can apply either the individual or the population-level variant of the proposed new approach successfully remains an open question; this new approach suggests intriguing possibilities, but it is in its infancy and requires further testing and refinement. However, combining evidence from skeletal and documentary sources to focus on the effectiveness of institutional care provision may, at the very least, encourage us to think about the lifeways of institutionalized people in the historic-period United States in a new light. It may also provide a foundation for exploring the impact of caregiving (or lack of caregiving) experienced by those belonging to some of the most vulnerable and marginalized groups of people in the historic period, such as the inmates of mental asylums – as illustrated in this study.

Many of the practical limitations of this new, and still experimental, method have already been canvassed. These include, for example, those problems that impact all bioarchaeological analysis, such as poor skeletal preservation compromising the description and diagnosis of pathological conditions. A problem more specific to research into efficacy of care is difficulty in ascertaining whether pathological lesions and/or healing occurred before or after patient admittance to the care institution. There are a number of other constraints that need acknowledgement. First, this method can only work with skeletal samples that come from known institutional burial grounds, as it relies on the knowledge that the remains examined are associated with residence in a long-term care facility. Second, both historical records, and histories produced by modern scholars, often contain bias (as do all texts, to some extent) and/or inaccuracies in descriptions of treatments and conditions of care institutions. Last, working with skeletal remains is inherently limited, in that information about diseases experienced during care that manifest only in soft tissue will be unavailable to us unless case histories exist and, more cogently, we are able to match individual skeletal remains to these. This factor, perhaps more than any other, will prohibit us from achieving a truly robust and comprehensive understanding of whether an institution met their healthcare goal of protecting their charges from infectious diseases or physical harm.

This pilot study has been a first step at looking at the question of efficacy of care in a systematic manner, and lays the groundwork for future, more extensive research. To give just one example, stable isotope analysis has the potential to address whether local and nonlocal residents differed in terms of risk for disease or trauma within an institution – and therefore, perhaps, whether they differed in terms of effectiveness of the care received. Despite its limitations, this new approach offers a valuable perspective for those investigating aspects of past care provision.

Acknowledgements I owe a great debt of gratitude to Lorna Tilley for not only inspiring the ideas put forth in this chapter, but for her unwavering support and insightful and thought-provoking feedback.

References

Carlisle, C. L. (1918). 'The Causes of Dependency based on a survey of Oneida County' State of NY State Board of Charities, Division of Mental Defect and Delinquency. Eugenics and Social Welfare Bulletin No. XV The Capitol, Albany NY.

Dar, G., Masharawi, Y., Peleg, S., Steinberg, N., May, H., Medlej, N. P., et al. (2010). Schmorl's nodes distribution in the human spine and its possible etiology. *European Spine Journal, 19*, 670–675.

Garcia, R. I., Henshaw, M. M., & Krall, E. A. (2001). Relationship between periodontal disease and systemic health. *Periodontology, 2000*(25), 21–36.

Grob, G. N. (1994). *Mad among us: A history of the care of America's mentally ill*. New York, NY: The Free Press (Simon & Schuster Inc).

Lai, P., & Lovell, N. (1992). Skeletal markers of occupational stress in the Fur trade: A case study from Hudson's Bay company Fur trade post. *International Journal of Osteoarchaeology, 2*, 221–234.

Larsen, C. S. (2002). Bioarchaeology: The lives and lifestyles of past people. *Journal of Archaeological Research, 10*(2), 119–166.

Mayo Clinic Staff. (2012). Diseases and conditions: diffuse idiopathic skeletal hyperostosis. Mayo Clinic. Retrieved from http://www.mayoclinic.org/diseases-conditions/diffuse-idiopathic-skeletal-hyperostosis/basics/symptoms/con-20024713.

Oxford English Dictionary. (2015). Oxford: Oxford University Press.

Phillips, S. M. (2001). *Inmate life in the Oneida County Asylum, 1860–1895: A biocultural study of the skeletal and documentary records*. Dissertation. The University at Albany.

Rosenberg, C. E. (1995). *The care of strangers: The rise of America's hospital system*. Baltimore, MD: Johns Hopkins University Press.

Takatalo, J., et al. (2012). Association of modic changes, Schmorl's nodes, spondylolytic defects, high-intensity zone lesions, disc herniations, and radial tears with low back symptom severity among young Finnish adults. *Spine, 37*(4), 1231–1239.

Tilley, L. (2012). The bioarchaeology of care. New directions in bioarchaeology, part II. *The SAA Archaeological Record, 12*(3), 39–41.

Yanni, C. (2003). The linear plan for insane asylums before 1866. *Journal of the Society of Architectural Historians, 62*(1), 24–49.

Chapter 15
Subadult Mortality Among Hunter-Gatherers: Implications for the Reconstruction of Care During Prehistory

Marco Milella

Introduction

The presence of social support to disabled individuals during prehistory (defined here as the late Pleistocene – i.e., up to ca. 11.0000 years BP) has been debated in the archaeological and anthropological community (Degusta, 2002; Dettwyler, 1991; see also Hublin, 2009). Theories on health-related caring behavior during prehistory are typically developed on the basis of fossil findings that exhibit traces of pathological conditions inconsistent with self-subsistence of the individual. In such cases, external support from other members of the group is invoked as an explanation for the survival of the subject. Among such paleopathological cases we can cite an adult Neanderthal male from Shanidar, Iraq (Solecki, 1971; Trinkaus, 1983; Trinkaus & Zimmerman, 1982) exhibiting various traumas and degenerative joint diseases, an edentulous subject from Dmanisi, Georgia, who survived despite evident masticatory impairments (Lordkipanidze et al., 2005), a mandible from Aubesier, France exhibiting marked tooth loss (Lebel et al., 2001), a case of craniosynostosis from the site of Atapuerca (Middle Pleistocene, Spain) (Gracia et al., 2009), and an Upper Paleolithic dwarf from the site of Romito, Italy (Frayer, Macchiarelli, & Mussi, 1988; Tilley, 2015) which likely necessitated social support for his survival. The link between the fossil evidence and caring behavior has been questioned on the basis of too simplistic assumptions about degrees of disability, reactions from the group toward disabled subjects, lack of ethnological and contemporary comparisons, and lack of comparative studies on non-human primates (Degusta, 2002; Dettwyler, 1991). Such pessimistic views have been recently opposed by the introduction of the Index of Care, a methodological framework allowing a critical evaluation of possible healthcare behavior on the basis of the paleopathological evidence (Tilley & Cameron, 2014; see also Chap. 2 this volume).

M. Milella, Ph.D. (✉)
Department of Anthropology, University of Zurich, Zurich, Switzerland
e-mail: marco.milella@aim.uzh.ch

© Springer International Publishing Switzerland 2017

L. Tilley, A.A. Schrenk (eds.), *New Developments in the Bioarchaeology of Care*, Bioarchaeology and Social Theory, DOI 10.1007/978-3-319-39901-0_15

It is interesting to note the paucity of discussion based on ethnological data in the biocultural interpretation of paleopathological cases. In particular, no attempt has been made to systematically compare these with what is known for modern hunter-gatherer societies when analyzing prehistoric case studies. The advantages of an approach based on the analysis of data from hunter-gatherers are manifold: (1) modern hunter-gatherer societies can be (cautiously) used as proxy of prehistoric human communities; (2) the ethnological literature provides a good amount of data on several aspects (e.g., ecology, demography, life history variables) of hunter-gatherers, which can be used to test working hypotheses; (3) analyses of data on hunter-gatherers allow comparisons with more structured, sedentary human communities.

Attitudes toward disabled subjects among hunter-gatherers have been poorly investigated, with references in the literature amounting mostly to sporadic mentions of specific behaviors in certain societies. Examples include the support provided to disabled elderly subjects among the !Kung (Daly & Wilson, 1980) or, on the other hand, the lack of care toward incapacitated individuals observed in some Arctic societies (see Dunn, 1968). The lack of systematic data strongly hampers a survey of such behaviors among hunter-gatherers. On the other hand, more systematic attention has been paid to childhood, subadult mortality (see below), and attitudes (including care) toward children in these type of societies (e.g., Hill & Hurtado, 1996, pp. 423–425; Hewlett & Lamb, 2005). Accordingly, in this work I decided to focus on behaviors related to parental (or alloparental) investments (food provision, custodial care – admittedly a rather coarse and indirect definition of care, but, I believe, justified by the quantity and quality of available data) and to discuss these in the more general perspective of healthcare behaviors.

From a general point of view, in order to investigate care in hunter-gatherers one can first try to deconstruct healthcare behaviors (or any other behavior) into their major components. If considered from a biocultural perspective, these will include the **causes** leading to these behaviors, the **factors** influencing such behaviors, and the **dynamics** characterizing the behaviors.

In relation to 'causes,' we can distinguish between biological and cultural causes. For biological causes, I refer here to biologically driven behaviors (i.e., kin selection, the process by which specific traits are favored due to their positive effects on descendant or nondescendant offspring [Griffin & West, 2002]). For cultural causes, I refer to the case of behaviors mediated by cultural factors such as social norms and taboos (see, for example, the taboo among the Ngandu concerning the supposedly poisonous nature of breast milk provided to infants by women other than the mother [Hewlett & Winn, 2014]).

As far as 'factors' are concerned, environmental factors include those aspects such as geological or climatic variables possibly influencing the expression of a certain behavior. On the other hand, demographic factors include the possible role played by features of the population (e.g., population size and density, mobility, mortality – see for example the relationship between demographic changes and disease emergence among modern humans [Jones et al., 2008]).

Finally, in considering the 'dynamics' of a behavior, we can distinguish between singular versus collective dynamics, as when we have a single versus multiple social actors enacting a specific behavior (in the present work I will focus especially on collective dynamics).

Altogether, causes, factors, and dynamics combine to express a behavioral model. Behavioral models can then be used for comparing different social units and may represent a complementary tool of analysis when posing hypotheses concerning behavioral patterns in prehistory.

Here, I explore the possible causes, factors, and dynamics of healthcare behaviors in modern hunter-gatherers using a large ethnographic dataset taken from published data. In particular, I try to isolate variables likely to be correlated with caring behavior and explore their relationship with other variables describing demographic or environmental contexts. Due to the limits of the available data (see later), I focus my attention on subadult (infant – first year of life, and juvenile – to the age of 15 years) individuals, used in this study as proxy of subjects needing care and, in their mortality percentages, assumed to indirectly express levels of healthcare.

The choice to focus on subadult mortality results from the discriminant variables considered designing my study, which are survival odds and relative exposure to health-related risks. Lacking more specific information, I adopted a probabilistic approach, i.e., assuming the youngest age classes as a subsample of a population to be particularly vulnerable from this point of view. Note that I am not proposing an equation between childhood and sickness, but merely focusing on a section of the population more likely to be the recipient of health-related (parental or alloparental) caring behaviors. On the other hand, I recognize the limitations of this approach. Among these, the main issues are the risk of ethnocentrism in viewing children as passive entities lacking of agency, and the difficulty in adopting a univocal concept of childhood, given the cultural characterization of age distinctions (see Baxter, 2008; Bugarin, 2005; Kamp, 2001). Moreover, one should also consider the fact that among hunter-gatherers children usually start to be relatively independent after a certain age (e.g., after 3–4 years old – see Bird-David, 2005). Finally, because of the nature of the data to hand, sex is not considered as variable in the present study (for the relevance of considering gender in any archaeological discussion on childhood see Kamp, 2005). These considerations demonstrate the difficulty in approaching the present work in a simplistic way, especially when dealing with data on juveniles, given the relatively wide age interval included in this class (in several societies older children not only contribute to the economy of the social group, but may also provide care for their siblings – see Bugarin, 2005). However, fine-grained (in terms of age classes) systematic data on childhood mortality among hunter-gatherers are not available. I therefore decided to approach this study in a cautious way, by conducting separate analyses on infants and juveniles and by taking into consideration the aforementioned issues in the discussion on my results.

It should also be noted that I chose to consider specific variables that I assessed as likely to be linked to the question at hand, which is the development of health-related caring behavior in hunter-gatherer societies. The lack of explicit information on these behaviors in the source material led to an indirect approach; in other words, a focus on a variable (infant and juvenile mortality) possibly linked to costs (in terms of time and energy spent by the provider) and expression of caring behaviors.

The experience of mortality, and the factors surrounding mortality, are indeed expected to be relevant from a behavioral point of view and to trigger healthcare behavioral responses. In relation to demographic and environmental variables, I decided to focus on population density, population mobility, and environmental productivity in relation to care. These variables were chosen in order to outline, at least in general terms, a demographic and environmental background for the observed mortality values and specific types of stress acting on the population as a whole.

Material and Methods

The Binford dataset (http://intersci.ss.uci.edu/wiki/index.php/Binford_hunter-gatherer_data#Spreadsheets; Binford, 2001) consists of data from 390 hunter-gatherer societies covering a wide geographic area. For each society, a large number of variables describing different features of the population are listed. These range from environmental data (e.g., type of vegetation, rain fall, etc.) to more demographic information (e.g., population size, population density, etc.).

The Marlowe forager dataset (http://intersci.ss.uci.edu/wiki/index.php/Binford_hunter-gatherer_data#Spreadsheets; see also Kramer, 2011) contains data from 479 societies. In this dataset, too, each society is described by a list of variables, some of them (e.g., infant and juvenile mortality) not present in the Binford dataset. The existence of this additional information led me to merge these two partially overlapping datasets when trying to explore specific relationship between variables, with the view to increasing the power of my analyses.

Relationships between variables were investigated by means of linear regression analyses and correlation tests (Spearman's rho test). All analyses were conducted in JMP 11.0 (SAS Institute), setting alpha at 0.05.

Results

In Figs. 15.1 and 15.2 I plot infant and juvenile mortality against, respectively, yearly average number of movements by the local group and yearly average distances walked by the local group. Results show overall negative, although not significant, correlations (Table 15.1). It must be noted that data on mortality are taken from Marlowe and are available only for a small subset of societies (14). Moreover, in this and the following analyses, one should take into consideration the relatively large variance characterizing each subset, and the influence exercised by outliers in such small samples.

On the other hand, when plotting infant and juvenile mortality against population density (Fig. 15.3) a positive (although not significant) correlation between these two variables is evident (Table 15.1).

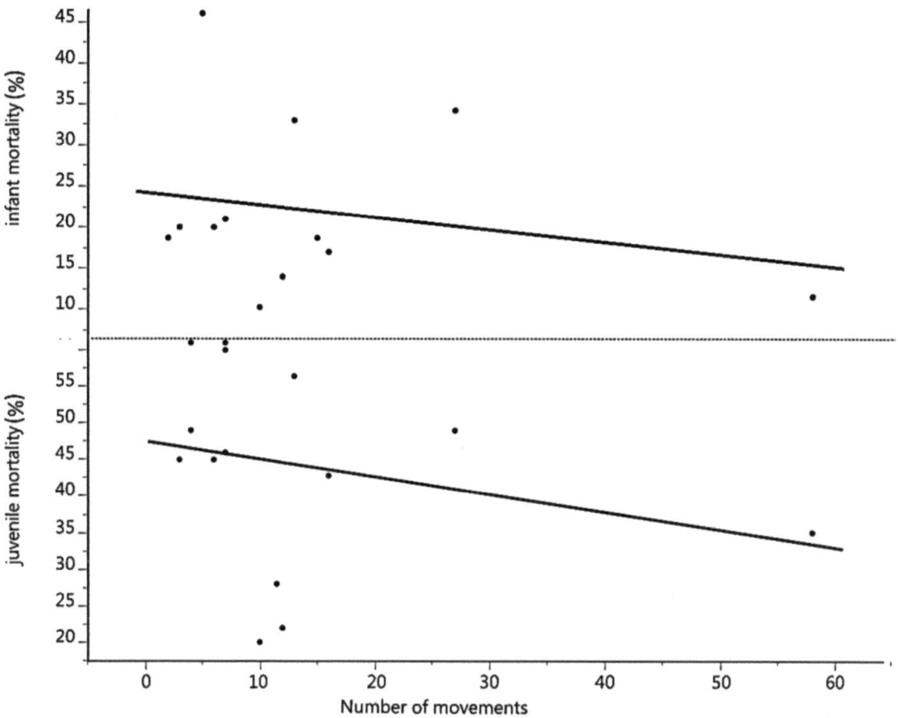

Fig. 15.1 Plots of infant and juvenile mortality vs. number of yearly movements

I then calculated a proxy of mean environmental productivity by subdividing net primary productivity (NPP) by population density and checked for the correlation between this new variable and mortality values.

Interestingly, while no significant correlation was found for infants, I obtained a strong and significant negative correlation between these variables for juvenile mortality (Fig. 15.4, Table 15.1).

Discussion

In relation to the specific trends highlighted by my analyses, it is interesting to note the lack of correlation between subadult mortality and group density. This suggests that the likely greater availability of alloparental care in more dense societies, as opposed to that available in more sparse groups, does not play a relevant role in terms of subadult survival. It also seems that higher population density does not influence mortality, as would be expected due to the relevance of the former variable in the emergence and diffusion of diseases (note, however, that in this case even relatively dense populations would be composed of few members in comparison with agricultural or industrial societies).

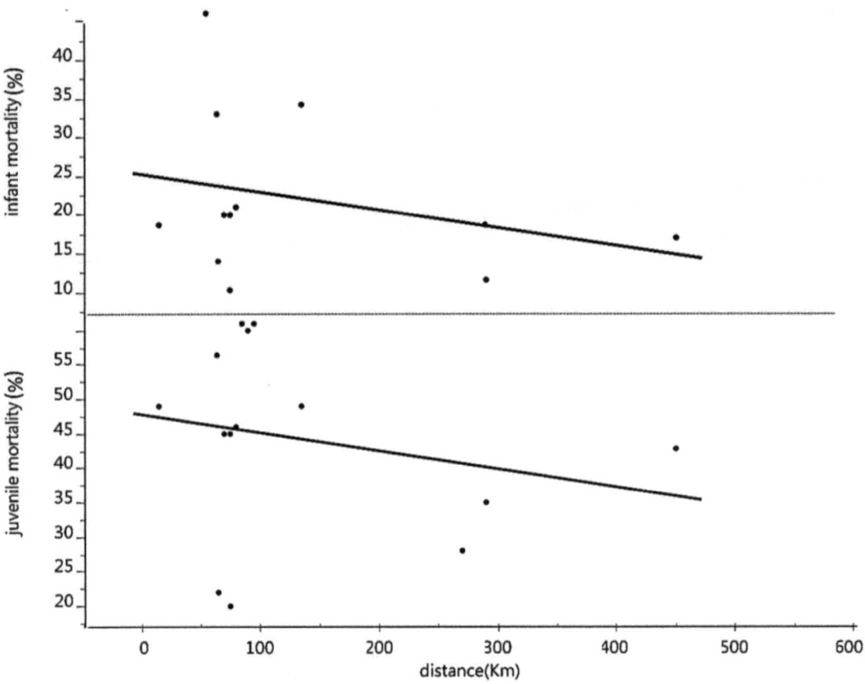

Fig. 15.2 Plots of infant and juvenile mortality vs. distance walked yearly

Table 15.1 Spearman's correlation values between variables

		Spearman's rho	*p*
Pop. Density	Infant mortality	0.3263	0.3006
Pop. Density	Juvenile mortality	0.4961	0.0712
N. of movements	Infant mortality	−0.2386	0.4552
N. of movements	Juvenile mortality	−0.3592	0.2072
Distance walked	Infant mortality	−0.3286	0.2969
Distance walked	Juvenile mortality	−0.0585	0.8425
Net Primary Productivity/Pop. density	Infant mortality	−0.2947	0.3524
Net Primary Productivity/Pop. density	Juvenile mortality	−0.8159	0.0004

However, the inverse correlation observed between number of movements and walked distances on one hand and, on the other, subadult mortality, is of special interest, since it suggests (with the caution necessary due to the inherent biases of my data) that an increase in mobility, together with associated physical tasks, do not expose a group to an increase in subadult mortality. A possible relevant factor in this case could be the care offered by parents and other members of the group as a buffer against the risks linked to a high mobility. In addition, a higher level of mobility would result in an overall 'healthier' living environment, which would mitigate against the development of disease-related conditions associated with more sedentary populations.

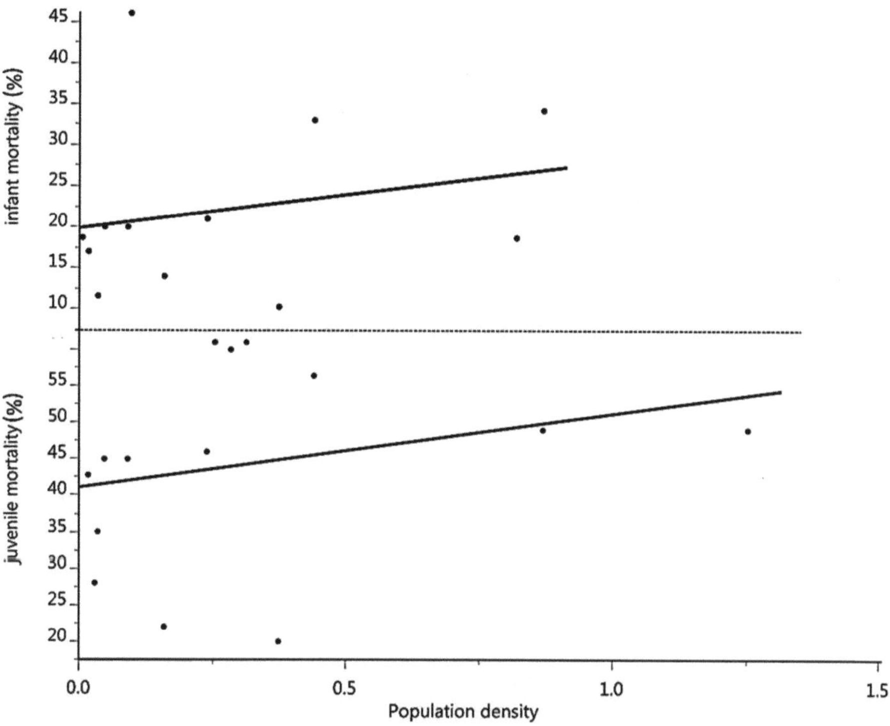

Fig. 15.3 Plots of infant and juvenile mortality vs. population density

In the results of analyses of the relationship between mortality and environmental productivity, the presence of a strong negative correlation between this variable and juvenile mortality only is of interest, since it is consistent with a differential parental investment for different classes of subadults (cf. Daly & Wilson, 1980). In particular, it seems that older children will be advantaged compared with infants when there is an increase of food availability, a pattern that is possibly related to the higher social and productive value of older subjects (cf. Kramer, 2011), to strategies of population control (Hayden, 1972), and to the fact that healthy older children would have higher chances of survival and attaining adulthood compared with the higher risks and exposure to diseases of infants. In the case of infants, however, the possible role of breastfeeding as a buffer against environmental variability needs to be stressed. This point is important, since it would contribute to explaining the lack of correlation with environmental productivity in this age class.

Discussions about behaviors in the past are often affected by a certain lack of contextualization with regard to their biological, environmental, and social correlates. Such issues have been already highlighted by other authors. De Gusta (2002) stressed the lack of comparative data on caring behavior in nonhuman primate communities when discussing similar behaviors and attitudes in hominids (for a review of nonhuman primate behaviors see Fashing & Nguyen, 2011). Dettwyler (1991),

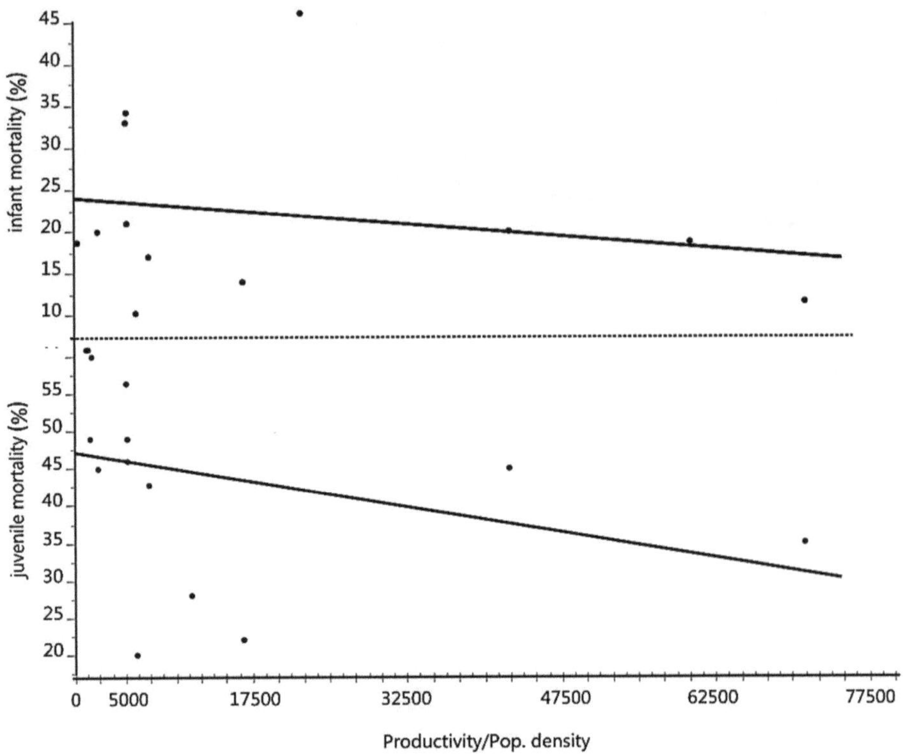

Fig. 15.4 Plots of infant and juvenile mortality vs. net primary productivity/population density

on the other hand, expressed a more general criticism to positing hypotheses about caring behavior in the past on the basis of paleopathological data. Variability in the context of disability, reaction to disability by the social group, relative contribution of the apparently sick to the economy of the group should all be considered when postulating hypotheses on supposed caring behaviors (Dettwyler, 1991; for further discussion of Dettwyler's views, see Doat, Chap. 17 this volume).

A renewed attention to the possibility of reconstructing caring behavior in the past has recently been stimulated by the introduction of a bioarchaeology of care approach (Tilley, 2015; Tilley & Cameron, 2014; Tilley & Oxenham, 2011; Chap. 2 this volume). The associated instrument, the Index of Care, aims to assist the researcher in testing hypotheses on the possible presence of caring behaviors, starting from a critical evaluation of the paleopathological evidence. In particular, the differential diagnosis of each case is followed by an estimate of the degree of disability of the subject, which allows inferences on possible support provided by other subjects.

Of particular interest is the set of factors (environmental and social) driving specific behaviors, such as the ones which are the target of this study. This is particularly relevant since, without a contextualization of each case or cases, the presence and meaning of determinate behaviors risk being disconnected from their biological and social components, which are the basis of any biocultural hypothesis. This is especially true for studies focused on prehistory, a time period for which we do not have access to direct information on the sociocultural dimension of a specific society, but must infer it from indirect data (geological, paleoenvironmental, archaeological, and anthropological).

In this context, the results from the present study are relevant for the discussion about the possibilities and limits of reconstructing caring behaviors in the past. As already mentioned, the major limit of this study is the lack of explicit data on caring behaviors, which are typically underrepresented in the ethnological literature. Furthermore, the available studies reveal contrasting attitudes toward disabled subjects in different social groups, a fact likely linked to divergent cultural factors (cf. Fabrega, 1999; Marlowe, 2010). The choice to use subadult mortalities as a way to evaluate the possible costs involved in caring behaviors, though justified by the available data, is not immune from specific issues, as already mentioned earlier. Given their relative independence, this is especially true when considering data on juveniles, a fact that is likely to influence my analyses. The paucity and ambiguity of the available data suggest that my results, rather than describing specific behaviors, are useful for a reflection on their possible (biological and social) background.

I note, moreover, that by using a dataset including a heterogeneous sample of societies, my results represent only general tendencies and cannot be extended to specific social contexts.

My results, even if not directly involving care behaviors, are nonetheless interesting since they *do* provide a useful background for posing biocultural hypotheses. The experience of death and the perceived associated risks of death (for a given environment) must indeed influence the type and amount of support provided by the social group. Accordingly, I postulate that a behavioral response in terms of caring attitudes will be directly linked to the risks and costs specific to a given environment and to previous experiences in terms of illness and mortality for a specific human group in a specific environment.

In this work, I focused my attention on environmental and demographic factors which might be included in a model of caring behaviors among hunter-gatherers societies. We should, however, take into consideration also the possible role played by cultural causes. A good example is represented by the attitudes toward elderly subjects, who in some societies like the !Kung are highly valued and routinely given care to (though with a variability associated with the presence or absence of next of kin) (Daly & Wilson, 1980; see also Marlowe, 2010, pp. 160–161). This emphasizes the obvious qualification that, in reconstructing a behavioral model for hunter-gatherers (and by proxy prehistoric human communities), one must consider not only the available environmental and demographic data possibly influencing such behaviors, but also the role played by cultural variables on the expression of these behaviors. Clearly, one may object to such a discrimination between natural vs. cultural causes, given their possible overlap (e.g., biological vs. affective value of offspring) (but see Hayden, 1972). I nonetheless believe in the usefulness of maintaining the two dimensions separated, at least initially, in order to test working hypotheses.

Finally, considering the possible dynamics characterizing caring behavior in prehistory, it is interesting to note the general lack of care provided by single individuals in hunter-gatherer societies. Rather, support (e.g., in case of illness) is usually provided by the family or social group, or by a certain number of specialists (Fabrega, 1999; Hayden, 1972). This is of relevance in positing archaeological research questions, since it is consistent with the presence, also during prehistory, of complex social networks (cf. Apicella, Marlowe, Fowler, & Christakis, 2012) regulating interindividual relationships and behaviors.

Conclusion

In the present study, I explored the possible usefulness of data on modern hunter-gatherers as a tool to model caring behaviors in prehistory. Systematic reviews on caring behaviors in hunter-gatherers are absent from the literature. However, a study of the relationship between mortality in infants and juveniles (used here as classes of subjects needing care) and variables such as group density, group mobility (translated in yearly average movements and walked distances), and environment productivity provides interesting results. In particular, it highlights the complex nature of care among hunter-gatherers, which seems independent from both group density and mobility but is, instead, consistent with biological and cultural responses to specific environmental stimuli. It appears that, in order to investigate conspecific care in prehistory, we need to adopt multifaceted models which take into consideration both a biological and cultural component. The present study represents the first attempt to discuss the bioarchaeology of care from a perspective that is not based on isolated case studies, but rather considers data from a multi-population perspective. I believe this approach to be of potential value, especially due to the possibility of its use in predicting specific behavioral responses to specific environmental and sociocultural stimuli.

On the other hand, it is obvious that what has been applied in this study is a preliminary version of a model that must be further refined and tested in order to be of direct use. In particular, one of its shortcomings is that due to the limits of available information I was forced to address the issue of healthcare indirectly, focusing on subadult mortalities and their possible relevance for the problem at hand. Besides the limitations arising both from using subadults (especially older ones) as proxies for subjects needing care and from the small number of societies considered, it must be emphasized that in this work I focused on a specific type of care (parental or alloparental). Accordingly, it is not possible to simply extend the specific results from this study to more general health-related caring behaviors (e.g., toward the sick). In order to do this, more specific ethnological data are needed. These would allow an increased number of variables to be studied and compared, and possibly the extension of this research approach to several age classes (e.g., including also elderly subjects, another population segment which would be interesting to study from a healthcare point of view). Systematic medical studies of modern hunter-gatherer populations would, moreover, allow a better definition of the type of epidemiological risks these populations are exposed to, allowing a more precise contextualization of the studied behaviors. Finally, the availability of data at an individual level (i.e., raw data from all – or at least a representative number of – members of a population rather than population means as the ones used here) would allow the exploitation of complementary statistical tools (e.g., social network analysis), leading to more fine-grained and focused analyses.

Despite the caveats acknowledged earlier, I believe that the methodology described in this chapter helps to address and refine research questions on both subadult mortality and healthcare during prehistory. It does this by providing an alternative framework for examining these topics, by shifting the perspective from an individual to a population level, and by stressing the relevance of social and environmental variables when studying caring behaviors.

Acknowledgements I am grateful to Alecia A. Schrenk, Lorna Tilley, and Debra Martin for inviting me to the session 'Building a Bioarchaeology of Care' at the 80th Annual meeting of the Society for American Archaeology. Thanks to Alecia A. Schrenk, Lorna Tilley, and to the two anonymous reviewers whose comments greatly improved the present contribution. Many thanks to Ruth Haegi for the support provided during the bibliographic research and to Simone Callegari for the useful comments to this manuscript.

References

Apicella, C. L., Marlowe, F. W., Fowler, J. H., & Christakis, N. A. (2012). Social networks and cooperation in hunter-gatherers. *Nature, 481*(7382), 497–501.

Baxter, J. E. (2008). The archaeology of childhood. *Annual Review of Anthropology, 37*, 159–175.

Binford, L. R. (2001). *Constructing frames of reference: An analytical method for archaeological theory building using hunter-gatherer and environmental data sets*. Berkeley, CA: University of California Press.

Bird-David, N. (2005). Studying children in 'hunter-gatherer' societies. In B. S. Hewlett & M. E. Lamb (Eds.), *Hunter-gatherer childhoods: Evolutionary, developmental, and cultural perspectives* (pp. 92–101). New Brunswick, NJ: Transaction publishers.

Bugarin, F. T. (2005). Constructing an archaeology of children: Studying children and child material culture from the African past. In J. E. Baxter (Ed.), *Children in action: Perspectives on the archaeology of childhood* (Archeological Papers of the American Anthropological Association, Vol. 15.1, pp. 13–26).

Daly, M., & Wilson, M. (1980). Discriminative parental solicitude: A biological perspective. *Journal of Marriage and the Family, 42*(2), 277–288.

Degusta, D. (2002). Comparative skeletal pathology and the case for conspecific care in Middle Pleistocene hominids. *Journal of Archaeological Science, 29*(12), 1435–1438.

Dettwyler, K. A. (1991). Can paleopathology provide evidence for 'compassion'? *American Journal of Physical Anthropology, 84*(4), 375–384.

Dunn, F. L. (1968). Epidemiological factors: Health and disease in hunter-gatherers. In R. B. Lee & I. Devore (Eds.), *Man the hunter* (pp. 221–228). New York: Aldine publishing company.

Fabrega, J. H. (1999). *Evolution of sickness and healing*. Berkeley, CA: University of California Press.

Fashing, P. J., & Nguyen, N. (2011). Behavior toward the dying, diseased, or disabled among animals and its relevance to paleopathology. *International Journal of Paleopathology, 1*(3), 128–129.

Frayer, D. W., Macchiarelli, R., & Mussi, M. (1988). A case of chondrodystrophic dwarfism in the Italian Late Upper Paleolithic. *American Journal of Physical Anthropology, 75*(4), 549–565.

Gracia, A., Arsuaga, J. L., Martínez, I., Lorenzo, C., Carretero, J. M., de Castro, J. M. B., et al. (2009). Craniosynostosis in the Middle Pleistocene human cranium 14 from the Sima de los Huesos, Atapuerca, Spain. *Proceedings of the National Academy of Sciences, 106*(16), 6573–6578.

Griffin, A. S., & West, S. A. (2002). Kin selection: Fact and fiction. *Trends in Ecology and Evolution, 17*(1), 15–21.

Hayden, B. (1972). Population control among hunter/gatherers. *World Archaeology, 4*(2), 205–221.

Hewlett, B. S., & Lamb, M. E. (Eds.). (2005). *Hunter-gatherer childhoods: Evolutionary, developmental, and cultural perspectives*. New Brunswick, New Jersey: Transaction publishers.

Hewlett, B. S., & Winn, S. (2014). Allomaternal nursing in humans. *Current Anthropology, 55*(2), 200–229.

Hill, K., & Hurtado, A. M. (1996). *Ache life history. The ecology and demography of a foraging people*. New York: Aldine de Gruyter.

Hublin, J.-J. (2009). The prehistory of compassion. *Proceedings of the National Academy of Sciences, 106*(16), 6429–6430.

Jones, K. E., Patel, N. G., Levy, M. A., Storeygard, A., Balk, D., Gittleman, J. L., et al. (2008). Global trends in emerging infectious diseases. *Nature, 451*(7181), 990–994.

Kamp, K. A. (2001). Where have all the children gone?: The archaeology of childhood. *Journal of Archaeological Method and Theory, 8*(1), 1–34.

Kamp, K. A. (2005). Dominant discourses; lived experiences: Studying the archaeology of children and childhood. In J. E. Baxter (Ed.), *Children in action: Perspectives on the archaeology of childhood* (Archeological Papers of the American Anthropological Association, Vol. 15.1, pp. 115–122).

Kramer, K. L. (2011). The evolution of human parental care and recruitment of juvenile help. *Trends in Ecology and evolution, 26*(10), 533–540.

Lebel, S., Trinkaus, E., Faure, M., Fernandez, P., Guérin, C., Richter, D., et al. (2001). Comparative morphology and paleobiology of Middle Pleistocene human remains from the Bau de l'Aubesier, Vaucluse, France. *Proceedings of the National Academy of Sciences, 98*(20), 11097–11102.

Lordkipanidze, D., Vekua, A., Ferring, R., Rightmire, G. P., Agusti, J., Kiladze, G., et al. (2005). Anthropology: The earliest toothless hominin skull. *Nature, 434*(7034), 717–718.

Marlowe, F. (2010). *The Hadza: Hunter-gatherers of Tanzania*. Berkeley, CA: University of California Press.

Solecki, R. S. (1971). *Shanidar, the first flower people*. New York: Knopf.

Tilley, L. (2015). Accommodating difference in the prehistoric past: Revisiting the case of Romito 2 from a bioarchaeology of care perspective. *International Journal of Paleopathology, 8*, 64–74.

Tilley, L., & Cameron, T. (2014). Introducing the index of care: A web-based application supporting archaeological research into health-related care. *International Journal of Paleopathology, 6*, 5–9.

Tilley, L., & Oxenham, M. F. (2011). Survival against the odds: Modeling the social implications of care provision to seriously disabled individuals. *International Journal of Paleopathology, 1*(1), 35–42.

Trinkaus, E. (1983). *The Shanidar Neandertals*. New York: Academic.

Trinkaus, E., & Zimmerman, M. (1982). Trauma among the Shanidar Neandertals. *American Journal of Physical Anthropology, 57*(1), 61–76.

Chapter 16
Digitised Diseases: Seeing Beyond the Specimen to Understand Disease and Disability in the Past

Andrew S. Wilson, Keith Manchester, Jo Buckberry, Rebecca Storm, and Karina Croucher

Introduction

Digitised Diseases is a major web-based 3D resource of chronic disease conditions that manifest in changes to the human skeleton. The resource was established through funds from Jisc[1], the University of Bradford and Bradford Visualisation. The multidisciplinary team involves project partners MOLA (formerly Museum of London Archaeology) and the Royal College of Surgeons of England (RCS), together with associate partners in London and York. The project has undertaken a programme of mass digitisation of pathological type specimens from world-renowned archaeological, historic and medical collections represented across the partner institutions.

We continue to augment this resource through insertion of new content. The resource was always envisaged as needing to appeal to a diverse user community, having an impact not just among academic and clinical beneficiaries, but also enriching the wider understanding of public health in the past. From the outset, our focus was on making sure that the digitised palaeopathological exemplars were represented and understood within a broader clinical context. In essence, we wanted to emphasise the impact of living with disease and disability in an era before modern therapies were available and the significance of the care provision that would have been required at a societal level, given the longevity of many of these conditions.

This chapter discusses how the web-based resource Digitised Diseases (www.digitiseddiseases.org) might be used in conjunction with the Index of Care (Tilley,

[1] Jisc (formerly the Joint Information Systems Committee) is a publicly funded body in the United Kingdom that supports higher education and research by providing digital resources, network and technology advice and services.

A.S. Wilson, Ph.D. (✉) • K. Manchester, D.Sc. (Hon.), M.B.B.S. • J. Buckberry, Ph.D.
R. Storm, Ph.D. • K. Croucher, Ph.D.
School of Archaeological Sciences, University of Bradford, Bradford, UK
e-mail: A.S.Wilson2@bradford.ac.uk

© Springer International Publishing Switzerland 2017
L. Tilley, A.A. Schrenk (eds.), *New Developments in the Bioarchaeology of Care*, Bioarchaeology and Social Theory, DOI 10.1007/978-3-319-39901-0_16

Chap. 2 this volume; Tilley & Cameron, 2014) to look beyond the simple quantification of disease. It presents the rationale for Digitised Diseases and describes the way in which it operates through specimen-level description and clinical synopses of corresponding disease. We are keen to see Digitised Diseases used in research into past caregiving. With this in mind, we also consider some limitations currently faced as we attempt to achieve a greater emphasis on the person who lived with disease, as opposed to focusing solely on the disease itself – as past palaeopathology studies have tended to do.

Digitised Diseases is a large multidisciplinary study, funded predominantly through taxpayer money in the UK (it has received almost £1 million). The mission statement focuses on the digital documentation of specimens to inform clinical understanding of chronic conditions affecting the skeleton, with a further aim of safeguarding fragile and often unique specimens (Wilson, 2014). We have now digitised over 1600 specimens using 3D laser scanning, complemented by descriptions, radiographs and CT images that accompany the specimens. In view of the emphasis on documenting type specimens we have had to target our approach in working with different institutions and collections because of the low prevalence of many of these specific diseases, and the fragmentary nature of archaeological skeletons and the often small size of some of the skeletal assemblages available have also posed problems. Fortunately, partner organisations such as the RCS and MOLA hold diverse collections, varying from separate bone elements to whole assemblages of skeletal individuals. Many of the elements scanned at the RCS, for example, originate from anatomy and pathology collections and reflect an historic practice of specimen collection.

Without such practices we would now have a far more limited comparative set of examples of bone change that pre-dates the advent of modern medical intervention, particularly for those diseases that result in very fragile bone change (e.g. neoplastic change and those conditions affecting bone mineralisation, such as osteomalacia), which for obvious reasons survive less well in the archaeological record. Whilst we use the word 'specimen' within Digitised Diseases, we recognise that this contradicts the 'personhood' approach aspired to when using a bioarchaeology of care approach. We selected this term to emphasise the educational value of being able to show type examples of pathological conditions, whilst acknowledging the lack of a suitable, more inclusive word to describe individual bone elements succinctly and without negative connotations. Whether working with Digitised Diseases or the Index of Care, the focus should always be on how the evidence can be used to inform health impact and care needs at the individual level, and this is reflected in the Digitised Diseases clinical synopses.

In creating an online open access resource available to the wider public, the need for high-level explanatory documents that described these chronic conditions and contextualised our understanding of health and caregiving in the past was seen as important. We have included two documents for this wider user base that introduce 'living with disease and disability in the past' and 'dental health and disease in the past'.

For those specifically researching healthcare in the past, we recognised the importance of clear descriptions of pathological change to accompany each 3D model. Not only do these guide the user through the appearance of possibly unfamiliar diseases,

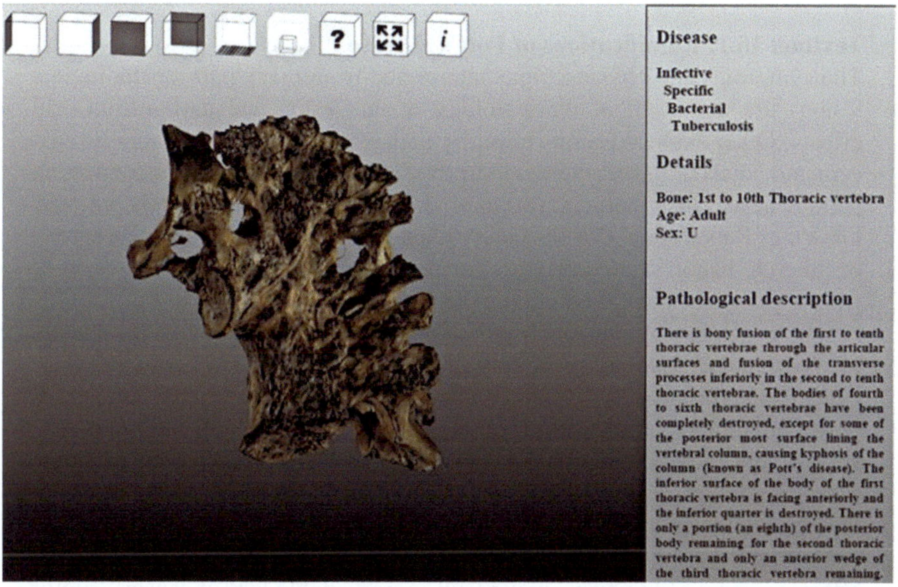

Fig. 16.1 Thoracic angular kyphosis – an example of Pott's disease (screen shot from Digitised Diseases http://www.digitiseddiseases.org/mrn.php?mrn=B0036)

but they also record changes that may not be immediately evident on photographs or scans. In addition, some of the 3D models have supplementary content, such as radiographs and CT scans, in order to help the user more fully appreciate the extent of the boney reaction in each disease. These internal images are important, as they help us understand the progressive nature of many of the diseases in a holistic sense, and provide a fuller picture of lesions that are not always visible on the bone's surface.

From the outset of the project individual 'type specimens' invariably had to be placed within their context, and for many diseases it was not possible to consider elements in isolation. Looking at an individual bone element or series of elements, we almost always found we needed to emphasise the distribution of lesions across the skeleton, along with any co-existing pathology, in order to understand both the expression of the disease in a particular area of the body and how this disease would relate to the overall health of the individual (Fig. 16.1 and Textbox 16.1 illustrate this point); in particular, this was an important aspect of the pilot project *From Cemetery to Clinic*, which focused on leprosy (http://www.barc.brad.ac.uk/FromCemeterytoClinic/). These two key issues interplay – for some pathological conditions, the distribution of lesions across the body is as important as lesion appearance for diagnosis. Furthermore, the overall distribution and interaction of the target disease with other pathological conditions, together with the clinical description of each individual, is also important when considering how individuals lived with chronic disease. Based on this information we can seek insight into how an individual living with a particular chronic disease interacted with their environment, and how, in turn, society viewed and treated them.

Textbox 16.1: Ramifications of Pott's Disease

The symptoms and physical signs interpreted from many palaeopathological lesions are the result of the aetiology of the lesion and its constitutional effects. Other skeletal lesions have, by their corporeal site in relation to viscera and adjacent tissue, more widespread systemic effects due to continuing pathogenesis. The thoracic vertebral destructive collapse of tuberculosis, known as Pott's spine, is a secondary phenomenon of haematogenous spread of tubercle bacilli from a primary (or post-primary) pulmonary infection or from a gastrointestinal tuberculous focus.

The general symptoms of shortness of breath, persistent cough productive of blood stained sputum or bloody diarrhoea, accompanied by weight loss, anaemia, night sweats and malaise, are joined by the secondary effects of progressive tuberculous osteomyelitis of the spine, with deep chronic boring spinal pain, increasing kyphosis and circum-chest pain due to costal nerve entrapment. A more serious consequence of this kyphosis, not apparent from the skeletal lesion itself, is the likely entrapment, compression and functional compromise of the spinal cord at the level of thoracic spine collapse. This effect, a sequel of kyphosis, may result in irreversible loss of sensory, motor and autonomic nerve function below the level of collapse.

The individual to whom the thoracic vertebrae in Fig. 16.1 belong may have had paresis or paralysis of both lower limbs, loss of bladder and bowel control and, if male, impotence. Such profound disablement required major care and support for long-term survival, for mobility, and for attention to bodily functions. The management and means for urinary and faecal retention are unknown in the absence of catheterisation and enema. But the problems do not stop at this gross disablement. The neuropathic limb may ulcerate with the development of a chronic infected suppurating skin ulcer of the lower leg, with the ultimate risk of marginal cancerous change.

It is necessary to look beyond the lesion itself. Thus, interpretation of such complex skeletal lesions must be undertaken with reference to regional anatomy and an understanding of the physiology of related structures and the dysfunction thereof. When the implications of disease sequelae are proposed, a suggestion can be made regarding the emotional, psychological and physical care (including equipment) necessary for the patient.

A Complementary Tool to the Bioarchaeology of Care

As a research and teaching resource, Digitised Diseases has three main intentions: (a) to illustrate and explain the impacts and implications of disease indicators manifest on bone; (b) to support (through [a]) consideration of clinical and social implications of evidence for the lived experience of disease in the past – in relation both to the individual affected and to their kin and/or wider community; and (c) to help enable (through [a] and [b]) a deeper understanding of what constituted health and disease in the past and community views, values and behaviours in relation to these.

With that first aim of providing clear evidence for interpreting bone change, our 3D viewer enables the user to manipulate and understand comparative evidence from a library of specimens, and can perhaps be seen as a prequel to using the Index of Care by helping confirm the extent of bone change relative to reference material. Seeing these bone changes in their context helps with differential diagnosis, but also through examination of comparative cases helps to emphasise the relative advancement of chronic conditions at the end-stage of life. This evidentiary foundation allows for inferences to be drawn in relation both to past need for care and to past care provision in response to this need.

At present, Digitised Diseases can provide valuable input to the Index of Care Step 1, in which researchers are focused on disease indicators and the location and description of these in relation to an individual. Our specimen-level descriptions and overarching clinical synopses provide a further linkage between Digitised Diseases and the Index of Care Step 2, in which the functional aspect of disease impact is considered within a lifeways context. The clinical synopses, important in recognising the limitations of a solely pathological description in isolation, were crafted to accompany each class of disease. They range from overarching summaries to more detailed clinical interpretations. These combined approaches give linkage between the physical manifestation of bone change as seen in individual elements across the skeleton and the extent to which these impacted on function, and help us consider how lesions relate to pain and other symptoms, moving towards a full body approach.

By coupling the Digitised Diseases resource with further observations from clinical practice we hope to extend the reach of this resource to complement the Index of Care Step 3, in which a 'model of care' is developed. The remainder of this chapter considers this aspiration, which considers aspects of clinical and functional impacts to identify likely care needs and care responses to these needs, whilst exploring some of the challenges facing this approach.

Case Reviews Informed by New Approaches

Leprosy

Both the Index of Care and Digitised Diseases offer potential for providing new insights into existing collections. During initial pilot work for Digitised Diseases, the 3D scanning of skeletal elements from the Medieval leprosarium of St James and St Mary Magdalene at Chichester [see also Roberts, Chap. 6] highlighted the opportunity for obtaining new information made possible by this initiative. This structured approach has helped in the reanalysis of a number of individuals, revealing further examples of leprous skeletal change not recorded in original monographs, and it also offered the chance to reexamine the diagnoses made in some of the original cases (Magilton, Lee, & Boylston, 2008).

Of course, limitations in reporting on leprosy cases can be due to many factors, including the possibility of an early or latent stage of infection prior to osseous involvement, the state of preservation and completeness of the skeleton, and/or whether or not enough features of leprosy are found in the skeleton to enable a diagnosis of this disease. With the skeletons from St James and St Mary Magdalene, many of the individuals had manifest non-specific inflammatory changes in the lower limbs, which (erroneously) were not considered to be among the diverse characteristics of leprosy. The exact number of individuals who lived with leprosy and were buried at this site was therefore likely much higher than has been documented.

Modern records help us to consider the personal symptoms of pain, of fever, the immediate disabilities of specific diseases, and their physical manifestations in living individuals. The understanding of disease and disability in antiquity therefore has a wide remit, incorporating the effect on the individual, on their immediate companions and on wider society – as we see in other chapters in this volume. The experience of disease involves a complex mixture of physical, psychological and emotional impacts and their social and economic ramifications. The focus of this chapter, and of the symposium in which it was originally presented, in on re-fleshing skeletal remains – stressing the importance of seeing not simply the localised picture, but the widespread change and the context of how it affects the individual.

Looking at the concept of 'illness' (an individual's experience of disease) versus 'disease' (a pathophysiological process in body structure, chemistry or function) requires us to examine how, traditionally, we view disease in palaeopathology. In fact, we employ a scientific, 'objective' approach, which in some cases provides a somewhat limited insight into the life and morbidity of the individual. The inference and understanding of the subjective effects of disease in an individual from the past can only be attempted by reference to clinical experience and to recorded clinical descriptions in more recent contexts.

Chronic Infection: Osteomyelitis

In the Index of Care Step 1 we can diagnose a non-specific osteomyelitis from the osseous lesions, such as those seen in Fig. 16.2, but we must deduce the pathogenesis and the clinical sequelae from the specific pathological characteristics.

From palaeopathological lesions it is possible, in many diseases, to predict the nature of the symptoms which were presented in antiquity, although not their severity because this was, and is today, not constant between individuals. It is possible to predict the outward signs that individuals presented with greater certainty, because these are the product of physical variables and not influenced by emotive and psychological factors in the patient. As such, signs are dependent on the site of the pathological lesion, the severity of the disease and its rate of progression. The severity and

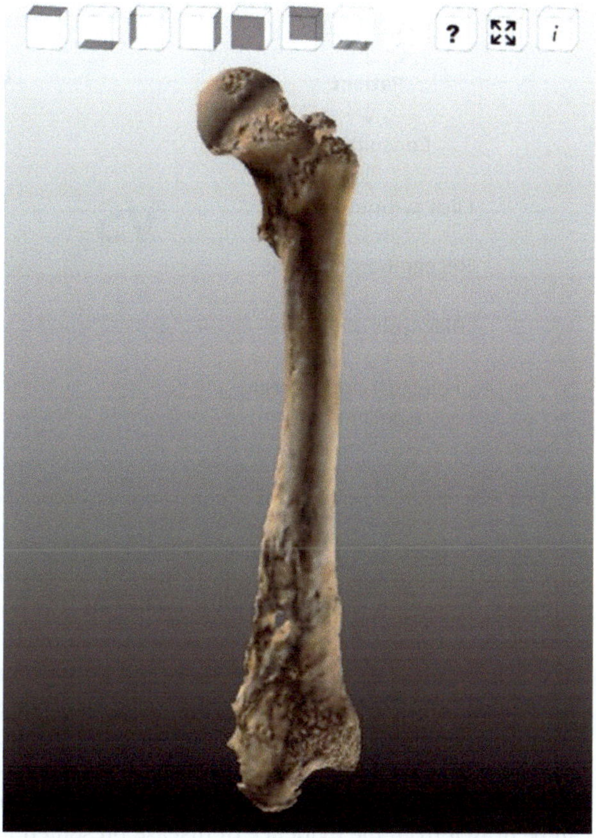

Fig. 16.2 Left femur displaying non-specific osteomyelitis (screen shot from Digitised Diseases http://www.digitiseddiseases.org/viewer/viewer_overlay.php?MRN=0080)

progression of a disease (particularly infectious disease) is determined by the general health status of the individual, co-morbidity and the immune status of the "patient".

It is interesting for us to reflect on the different perspectives of the clinician and palaeopathologist, outlined in Fig. 16.3. The patient presents to the clinician with the symptoms of disease which will, in many cases, point to the nature of the disease (e.g. infection, neoplasm, metabolic or rheumatic disease). Verification of the diagnosis may be achieved by subsequent clinical physical examination and ancillary imaging and pathological investigations.

As palaeopathologists, however, we are often limited in our interpretation by our level of knowledge of the cause and the extent of an injury and the effect it had on the individual, although we can use contextual information to infer both the pathogenesis and course of some diseases. Taking the case of the individual who experienced the pathology responsible for the lesions in the femur shown in Fig. 16.2, we have no direct access to the almost certainly associated symptoms of fever; the chronic boring bone pain; the swelling; the tenderness of the leg; the inability to weight bear; and the hot, red, tender subcutaneous abscess at the site of the cloaca. Observed in isolation and in the absence of direct bone trauma, a case of osteomy-

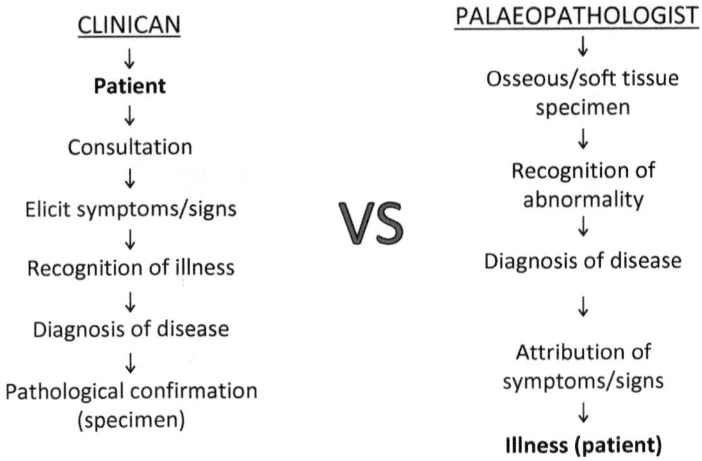

Fig. 16.3 The different perspectives of clinician and palaeopathologist

elitis does not allow us to examine further the haematogenous spread of pyogenic pathogens from some distant bodily infection. Although we can make inferences between cases with associated trauma such as an open fracture, versus cases where there is no evidence of trauma, with more likely haemotogenous spread, fractures can remodel and be hard to identify if very well aligned. Furthermore, the actual pathogen cannot be identified without use of biomolecular methods. However, by extrapolating from the pattern of infections today we can argue certain bacteria are the most likely cause. Textbox 16.2 describes in further detail the inferences that can be drawn from the evidence of disease presented in Fig. 16.2.

Textbox 16.2: Progress of Disease

There may be a significant, sometimes long, period of time between onset of disease and skeletal change, the pathogenesis of which may itself be slow. During this prodromal phase there may be profound incapacitating symptoms for which there can be no palaeopathological evidence. In the case of this femur with a distal osteomyelitic lesion associated with local trauma, we can infer a compound fracture with direct spread of pathogens from the skin surface.

Superimposed on the femoral fracture - which in itself was a cause of acute intense pain and immobility - there was the more long standing chronic osteomyelitis with the intractable deep boring bone pain, and associated local inflammatory signs of soft tissue inflammation, relieved only by the bone cortical perforation of cloaca, and discharge of pus into the adjacent soft tissue. In the absence of antibiotics or surgical drainage, this became a chronic condition with the constitutional symptoms of ill health. In antiquity, just as today, such ill health requires emotional support. But, unless death super

(continued)

(continued)
vened, this infection resolved and the osseous lesion became quiescent, maybe with intermittent discharge of pus. The individual is likely to have been able to walk, although not perform heavy manual work. Therefore, continued physical support and care was not necessary.

Final long-term sequelae of this chronic infective process may have been the development of amyloid change in vital body organs such as liver and kidneys, with resultant hepatic and renal failure and death. Thus, a consideration and interpretation of the care needed in antiquity, based solely upon the palaeopathological manifestation of disease without reference to modern clinical data, falls short of the holistic implications of the illness for the individual.

Tuberculosis

In the modern consulting room, the patient presents the subjective symptoms of disease; for example, constitutional symptoms include pain, fever, limitation of movement, lethargy and weight loss. These are not pathognomonic of a specific disease, but indicate the class of disease (for example infection, neoplasia, metabolic). These symptoms can be organ specific; for example, in pulmonary TB these might include a persistent cough and bloodstained sputum, with physical signs such as red, swollen, tender cervical lymph nodes.

As previously noted, the scope and potential to postulate the overall disease presence and impact (physical, psychological or social) in the past is limited by the nature of palaeopathological evidence. Primary soft tissue disease, which encompasses the vast majority of diseases affecting humans today and throughout history, is undetectable in the palaeopathological record, other than where there is secondary osseous involvement. In palaeopathology we are denied the benefit of symptom presentation and, usually, soft tissue or physical signs. We therefore have to provide an objective description of pathological lesions looking at generalised or localised effects, and using context to infer the course of some diseases. For example, pulmonary TB can be inferred from skeletal lesions of rib erosion and new bone formation secondary to peripheral lung lesions and pleural inflammation.

Complementary historic resources, such as radiographs, add further value in understanding disease in antiquity and, in particular, the pathogenesis and course of disease. These historic radiographs are of particular value in the context of infectious disease since they pre-date effective treatment using antibiotics. Two major radiographic archives complement Digitised Diseases. These are (1) the BARC Andersen collection of leprous x-radiographs from India, Nepal and Ethiopia, and (2) the radiographs and clinical records from the Stannington Children's TB Sanatorium in Northumberland. The radiographs of leprous patients collected by Clinical Leprologist Dr Johs Anderson are curated in the Biological Anthropology Research Centre at the University of Bradford, and were digitised as part of the Jisc-funded project 'From Cemetery to Clinic'; they date largely from the era before the introduction of anti-leprous triple therapy. A major proportion of the Stannington archive also dates from before the introduction of anti-tuberculous antibiotics. Through the joint efforts of the University of Bradford and the Northumberland Archive Service, the unstable nitrocellulose Stannington radiographs were saved from destruction in the 1980s and converted to microfilm. These have since been digitised by Northumberland Archive Service with funding from The Wellcome Trust, and examples are shown in Fig. 16.4. The x-radiographs in these two archives parallel the findings in palaeopathological specimens of leprosy and TB.

An Integrated Discipline

The essence of palaeopathology is to enhance knowledge and understanding of the pathological processes and pathogenesis of disease in the past. This understanding is informed by the subjective symptoms and objective physical signs of disease. A corollary of this is an understanding of the consequent effects and sequelae of disease and illness upon the individual, family and immediate society, and the significance of the disease within the wider population.

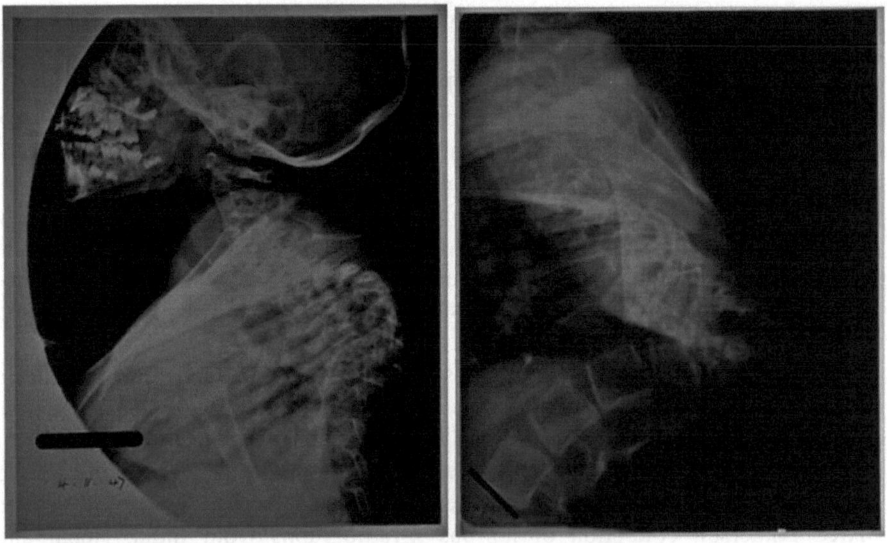

Fig. 16.4 Radiographs from the Stannington archive HOSP/STAN/7/1/2/2157_39 (lateral view of upper spine and skull); HOSP/STAN/7/1/2/494_02 (extreme deformity in spine). With permission from Northumberland Archives, Woodhorn and the Caldicott Guardian

Whilst the fundamental sources are the observations and investigations of palaeopathology, the validity of diagnosis of pathological changes and lesions in archaeological human remains is dependent upon the knowledge and understanding of such lesions in diagnosed diseases in current clinical practice, verified by available ancillary investigations. This integrated approach in the diagnosis and interpretation of palaeopathological lesions has been central to the Digitised Diseases project and facilitates a 3D study of skeletal lesions in antiquity.

The significant difference with palaeopathological study is that these archaeological lesions exhibit pathological processes that were not influenced by effective therapy, particularly antibiotics in infectious diseases. The end of the disease progression in the past was, in many cases, death. The end of the disease progression in many cases in current practice is resolution following therapeutic intervention.

There are, however, interesting parallels between (i) the transformative approach offered by the Index of Care and the introduction of new information and digital datasets, as with Digitised Diseases, and (ii) the revolutionary new approaches in modern healthcare delivery, with their increasing emphasis on targeted therapy and personalised medicine. Central to both is the idea of the patient/skeleton as an individual – someone who perceives pain and may experience change of mood – although there is consensus that individual response to disease is highly variable and hard to predict.

What cannot be predicted from skeletal remains, nor, indeed, from living patients, are the psychological effects of the disease on the afflicted person. The psychological sequelae of physical disease are varied and multiple in their presentation and severity in different patients. What may be accepted and tolerated in one person may be overwhelmingly distressing in another. One person may have a resigned acceptance of therapeutic failure and inevitable death, whilst these may be a source of great anguish in another. The degree of pain associated with a specific disease is variable between people, dependent to some extent on the pain threshold of the person. The psychological effects of disease in an individual determine the degree and extent of kindred physical and emotional support required. Conversely the emotional and physical support given will affect the psychological adaptation of the patient to his or her illness. Whilst this is unlikely to influence the outcome of the disease, it will alter its tolerable course.

In bioarchaeology we have increased access to markers and tools for assembling information on physiological stress and the diachronic picture for our health experience. Drawing on a life course/life history approach, we can similarly tailor information using a bioarchaeology of care approach to reach a better understanding of health and wellness at the individual level, reflective of a lifetime of interaction with the world (Buzon, 2012). It is also important to expand interactions between palaeopathologists and archaeologists, using approaches such as archaeothanatology (Duday, Cipriani, & Pearce, 2009; Willis and Tayles 2009) and new understanding from taphonomy (Wilhelmson & Dell'Unto, 2015) to explore the context of deposition. Of course for some diseases the staging of disease may present more challenges, and following a bioarchaeological approach can certainly add investigative procedures to help, in some cases, to see the invisible – the use of radiography/computed tomography (CT) [see Conlogue et al., Chap. 8 this volume), histopathology, DNA and proteomics, stable light isotope analysis and other markers of physiological stress, palaeoparasitology and analysis of biomarkers of medicinal plants.

Disease Management

Modern surgery and chemotherapy make a difference to individual lives and to the survival of individuals, but not to the overall pattern of disease. The development of antibiotics has made a difference to the global picture of disease, with many diseases once fatal, now controlled and in some cases eradicated. Whilst patients in antiquity were denied effective therapy capable of altering the course of disease (the modern context), medical management in antiquity was not absent or universally ineffective. Heuristic approaches led to practical solutions to problems, as with the use of bespoke spinal braces to correct for kyphotic change to the spine resulting from tuberculous infection (see Fig. 16.5). Active therapeutic reduction of fractures may not have been attempted because of the associated risks of haemorrhage, infection and/or shock induced by the actions involved in setting a broken limb; in the case of a break to the upper leg these risks would be coupled with the difficulty in reducing femoral shaft fractures, where powerful thigh muscles pull the fracture out of alignment. In the modern context, the management of disease at the individual level and the control of disease at the population level have been influenced by increased public health measures, access to better food, improved housing and living conditions and harnessing epidemiology to limit causal agents.

The pathological specimens represented in Digitised Diseases belonged to people suffering illnesses with recognisable symptoms and presenting physical signs of disease. These people may not have had formal medical treatment but may have received emotional support. From the Medieval period onwards we see varied practices of care, with the role of hospitals encompassing spiritual care as well as treatment (see Wesp, Chap. 13 this volume); the concept of the four humors; the emergence of skilled personnel, as in the barber-surgeon in the later Medieval period; and increased evidence of autopsy, anatomy training and amputation in eighteenth/nineteenth centuries. While it is evident in the cases discussed earlier that a certain level of care would have been necessary to ensure survival, care does not necessarily mean that it involved compassion. Although the study of emotion in archaeology has been debated (see Harris & Sørensen, 2010; Tarlow, 2000), and emotions can be argued to be rooted in their material contexts (Hodder, 2000, p. 734), particular types of emotive response cannot be assumed to be universal (Tarlow, 2000), even when care was clearly present. There are many different and contrasting motivations for substantive human behaviour, ranging from fear and other irrational responses (e.g. in response to risk of contagion) to compassion, respect and affection.

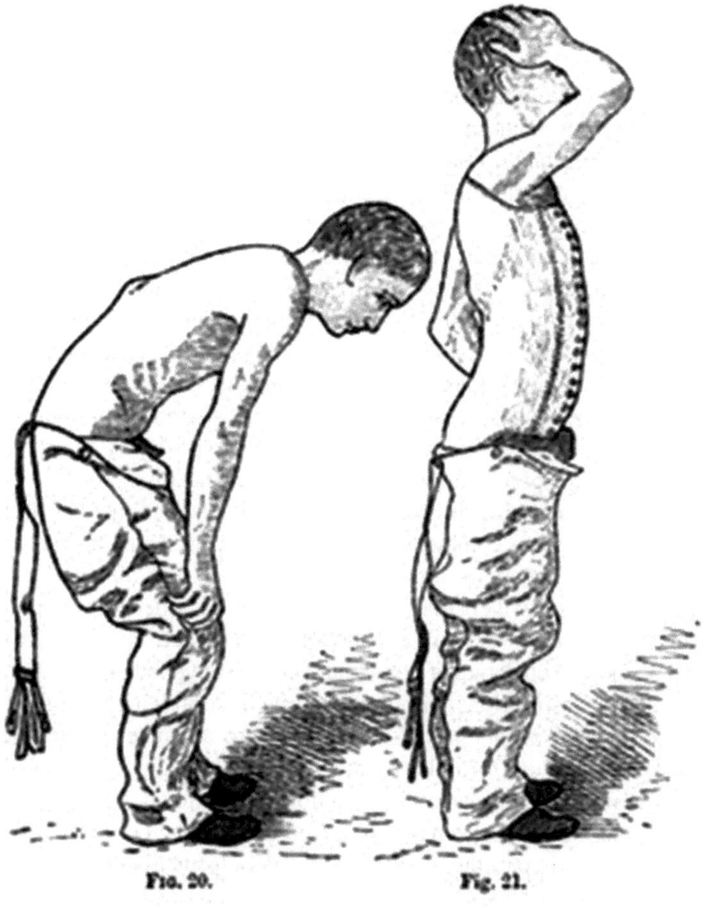

Fig. 16.5 Spinal brace to correct for kyphosis. Courtesy of the Thackray Medical Museum

The subjective effects of the disease process upon the individual should also be highlighted, since there can be considerable variance in the severity of symptoms and patient needs arising from a given disease. This variability affects the social and physical care and support required by individuals. Whilst the physical signs may be pathognomonic of specific disease, these signs will vary with the advancing course of the disease, with co-morbidity and with the immunological and nutritional status of the patient. The symptoms experienced will be influenced by the psychological well-being of the patient, by coexisting socioeconomic factors within the patient's life and by the patient's perception of the seriousness of the illness and their tolerance to pain. We hope to supplement the Digitised Diseases resource with contextual information wherever possible, to make users more aware of these intangible aspects of disease symptoms and treatment.

Summary

The Index of Care is transformative in the way in which it helps us to approach the bioarchaeological examination of individuals, and this chapter shows how Digitised Diseases may be used in conjunction with this instrument. There remain gaps in the ability to consider the emotional and personal features of disease that cannot be determined solely from physical evidence of pathology, and instead require the context that the Index of Care encourages in Step 4, in drawing on further clinico-social experience and knowledge, specific to different groups, of the individual's community and of this community's cultural norms. In consultation with modern clinicians, and by reference to older (pre-antibiotic era) medical texts, palaeopathologists can interpret the physical consequences and symptoms of disease in antiquity. Calling on personal life experiences, it is both valuable and justifiable to consider the psychological impacts of disease in individuals from the past. By so doing, we give life to the skeletal remains of antiquity with which we are dealing.

Digitised Diseases remains an evolving picture – a resource that is still in development – which we hope can complement themes relating to the bioarchaeology of care approach. We continue to augment this with new content, including CT and micro-CT data, and are in discussion with partner organisations to look at defining data and metadata standards that would allow us to absorb further content, including descriptive requirements based on the nomenclature of disease and the use of varied 3D data formats.

We have various aspirations with the resource in complementing the bioarchaeology of care – using a contextualised approach to advance our perspective and understanding. Taking us from element to individual (ongoing work is helping to re-associate elements); from lesion to symptoms (additional descriptive content of clinical symptoms); and from clinical to social (reattribute context, using archaeological data and historic parallels). Ultimately this helps to provide a more complete picture of the circumstances – the social, demographic and economic – that enable us to create more detailed interpretations concerning care and quality of life.

Acknowledgements With thanks to the entire Digitised Diseases team (http://www.digitiseddiseases.org/meettheteam.php), our project partners (http://www.digitiseddiseases.org/projectpartners.php) and associate partners (http://www.digitiseddiseases.org/acknowledgements.php). Thanks also to Sue Wood (Head of Collections) and Karen Rushton (project archivist), Woodhorn Museum and Northumberland Archives, for permission to use historic radiographs of a child with collapsed spine from Stannington Sanatorium, digitised as part of a Wellcome Trust-funded project.

References

Buzon, M. R. (2012). The bioarchaeology approach to palaeopathology. In A. L. Grauer (Ed.), *A companion to paleopathology* (pp. 58–75). Oxford: Blackwell.

Duday, H., Cipriani, A. M., & Pearce, J. (2009). *The archaeology of the dead: Lectures in archaeothanatology*. Oxford: Oxbow books.

Harris, O. J. T., & Sørensen, T. F. (2010). Rethinking emotion and material culture. *Archaeological Dialogues, 17*(02), 145–163.

Hodder, I. (2000). Response to Tarlow. *Current Anthropology, 41*(5), 733–734.

Magilton, J., Lee, F., & Boylston, A. (Eds.). (2008). *Lepers outside the gate: Excavations at the cemetery of the hospital of St James and St Mary Magdalene, Chichester, 1986–87 and 1993*. York: CBA.

Tarlow, S. (2000). Emotion in archaeology. *Current Anthropology, 41*(5), 713–746.

Tilley, L., & Cameron, T. (2014). Introducing the index of care: A web-based application supporting archaeological research into health-related care. *International Journal of Paleopathology, 6*, 5–9.

Wilhelmson, H., & Dell'Unto, N. (2015). Virtual taphonomy: A new method integrating excavation and post-processing of human remains. *American Journal of Physical Anthropology, 157*(2), 305–321.

Willis, A., & Tayles, N. (2009). Field anthropology: Application to burial contexts in prehistoric Southeast Asia. *Journal of Archaeological Sciences, 36*(2), 547–554.

Wilson, A. S. (2014). Digitised diseases: Preserving precious remains. *British Archaeology, 136*, 36–41.

Part III
Ethics and Accountability in the Bioarchaeology of Care

Chapter 17
What Ethical Considerations Should Inform Bioarchaeology of Care Analysis?

David Doat

Introduction

From the second half of the twentieth century, archaeological discoveries of fossilised skeletons of individuals with physical disabilities have prompted some archaeologists (Dickel & Doran, 1989; Frayer, Horton, Macchiarelli, & Mussi, 1987; Hublin, 1985; Solecki, 1971; Trinkaus, 1983) to suggest that the survival of these individuals (as demonstrated through palaeopathological investigation) provides evidence that prehistoric hominin communities showed caregiving behaviours towards their disabled members. Lordkipanidze et al. (2005) and Walker, Zimmerman, and Leakey (1982) even suggest that there are archaeological grounds for claiming that caregiving behaviours already existed within the human line around 1.5–1.77 million BP.

However, direct inference of health-related caregiving from the archaeological record alone can be problematic, and there is very limited empirical evidence for attitudes of social care and support for people with disabilities in prehistoric times. Interpretations of care provision were considered controversial by some, and this critique was most strongly expressed in the publication of a contentious article by K.A. Dettwyler (1991), *Can Paleopathology Provide Evidence for 'Compassion'?*. In this study, the anthropologist developed a set of arguments critical of the interpretations of compassionate caregiving for disabled persons in prehistory that had appeared in the palaeopathological literature until that point.

Though I am well informed of the very real technical challenges involved in the scientific debate on the topic, I am not, in this chapter, going to embrace the manner of thinking of an archaeologist. Given my own disciplinary background as an ethicist and philosopher of science, my work does not consist of excavating, protecting,

D. Doat, Ph.D. (✉)
Department of Ethics and Philosophy, Catholic University of Lille, Lille 59800, France

Centre for the Study of Science and Philosophy, University of Namur, Namur 5000, Belgium
e-mail: david.doat@univ-catholille.fr

© Springer International Publishing Switzerland 2017

L. Tilley, A.A. Schrenk (eds.), *New Developments in the Bioarchaeology of Care*, Bioarchaeology and Social Theory, DOI 10.1007/978-3-319-39901-0_17

analysing and interpreting archaeological remains in order to reconstruct the history of prehistoric populations. Rather, it consists of bringing to light the ethical and philosophical issues which appear to be related to the emerging field of bioarchaeology of care and the academic debate preceding it for the last decades. Indeed, many ethical and philosophical beliefs, goals and values are buried beneath the surface of the explicit arguments that shape academic discourse in the field. As a philosopher, it is my job both to analyse such arguments and excavate the presuppositions on which they are based. From an interdisciplinary perspective this is of importance, as philosophical and ethical beliefs underlying the work of archaeologists in the field influence the way they position themselves with regard to the development of new methodologies, narratives and theoretical models in bioarchaeology of care. Metaphorically, my work is in some ways an archaeological one.

Within the parameters outlined earlier, I would like to discuss the following questions:

1. What were the main reactions in the archaeological literature to discussion of past caregiving?
2. What beliefs and values were the first objections to inferences of care based on?
3. Are the beliefs and values informing the recently developed bioarchaeology of care model of analysis sufficiently robust to overcome past criticism?

What Were the Main Reactions in the Archaeological Literature to Discussion of Past Caregiving?

According to William James, one of the founders of American pragmatism, the history of knowledge is to some extent that of a certain clash of human values and beliefs. Whatever personal convictions a scientist shares, when practicing science he or she tries, of course, to 'sink the fact of his temperament' (James, 1984, p. 488). Scientists claim objectivity in their conclusions, as beliefs and values are not conventionally recognised in science. Yet in uncertainty and in the absence of irrefutable proofs, James claims that personal convictions and affects often underlie so-called *impersonal reasons* for choosing one direction rather than another, and, to some significant degree, science itself relies on specific beliefs and values. Undignified as such a position may seem to some 'objective' scholars, as a philosopher and ethicist I have to take account of differences in human beliefs and values as these sometimes explain some divergences in scientific debates – especially those regarding human affairs.

I observe two major contrasting rational and psychological reactions within the scientific community regarding attempts to infer the types of relationship prehistoric communities had with their disabled members. Between these two reactions I presume there is, of course, a whole set of logical, possible intermediary positions that will not be further elaborated within this chapter.

Following a first *prudent (if not sceptical) critical stance*, a number of authors (e.g. DeGusta, 2003; Dettwyler, 1991; Boyd, 1996 ; Metzler, 1999; Roca, Jiménez-Brobeil, Oumaoui, Tiristán, & Fernando, 2012; Tarlow, 2000) argue that, faced with the challenges raised by the obstacles that researchers are confronted by in interpreting palaeopathological data, only an approach of strict restraint would be reasonable from a scientific standpoint.

It is true that any effort to understand disability and care practices in prehistory is potentially exposed to many obstacles. In the skeletal record, assessing which 'abnormalities' may be defined as disabling to the individual or to the group in which he or she lived is difficult (Roberts, 1999, p. 81). As archaeologist C. J. Knüsel writes (1999, p. 32), 'we must be aware that definitions of disability and reactions to disability very likely differed in the past, as well as among different groups in the present'. It is unlikely, for example, that dyslexia would have been a disability in prehistoric societies. Moreover, because behaviours do not fossilise, there is little empirical data to assess how prehistoric societies behaved towards disability (Southwell-Wright, 2013a, 2013b). For instance, caring for disabled people with love or preventing them from dying in order to treat them as 'scapegoats' is an alternative that palaeopathological data cannot systematically help clarify (Dettwyler, 1991, p. 382). If material evidence can 'show the effects of disease or trauma a person experienced [...] on its own it cannot show the cultural or social aspects of that person's life conclusively' (Metzler, 1999, p. 64). Finally, while considering the present may sometimes be useful, contemporary researchers may 'impose their ideas upon the past, without considering that concepts and perceptions may have changed considerably through time' (Roberts, 1999, p. 81).

Given the many obstacles archaeologists face in interpreting palaeopathological data, a number of them both adopt a defensive *prudent critical stance* and are led to think that any interpretation based on empirical evidence in support of compassionate and/or inclusive attitudes of care towards disabled individuals in prehistoric times would be objectively unverifiable. Such interpretations would be, if not perhaps arbitrary, then at least revealing of the (moral, ideological and anachronic) intentions of the researchers who propose them. From an epistemological point of view, the cognitive and logical leaning of this first stance can lead to scepticism displayed by challenging the very possibility of there being any prospects for advancing research into past caregiving

Following a second *bolder (but more risky) critical stance*, some of the obstacles archaeologists face in interpreting palaeopathological data can be overcome. In philosophy, one says that such a position is a more rationalistic one than a sceptical one, since it places faith in the power of reason to further our limits of knowledge. Contrary to the conclusions of the sceptic, rationalism calls for a more comprehensive deepening of interdisciplinary dialogue between scientific disciplines. In some cases, because of lack of caution and scientific rigor, enthusiasm which characterises the first developments of such an approach leads to failure. But in many other cases it provides the necessary energy and strength for the development of innovative scientific methods and practices. Such new contributions enrich the scientific community and contribute to its progress. In archaeology, in the last 6 years, such enthusiasm has led to the development of a specific method for bioarchaeological analysis of care to help test, at a case-study level, how reasonable the inferences of caregiving may be.

Among findings from recent years, the case of a young adult male (Man Bac Burial 9) living with quadriplegia in Neolithic Vietnam (Tilley & Oxenham, 2011), and the methodology used in that study's diagnostic analysis (Tilley, 2012), reflected for the first time in bioarchaeology this bolder critical stance. In a recent article, Tilley and Cameron (2014a) highlight the value of their (perfectible) method for bioarchaeological analysis of care:

> *When health-related care provision can be inferred from evidence in human remains it offers a valuable window into the past – yet this is rarely exploited […]. Few studies engage in in-depth consideration of the functional disability for which care was required, the nature of care required and provided, and/or what this care may reveal about the cultural context in which it occurred […]. Archaeology's failure to address the subject of care in a systematic manner has had negative consequences. Lack of detailed argument has rendered claims of caregiving vulnerable to criticism […], and neglect of care provision as a focus of archaeological research has resulted in a source of rich insights into prehistoric lifeways and individuals being overlooked […]. The 'bioarchaeology of care' [has been] developed to address this problem. First employed in the study of Man Bac Burial 9 […], it asserts that it is possible, where sufficient evidence exists, to establish the presence of disability requiring support, to posit some of the more straightforward components of the care likely provided in response, and to deduce aspects of social relations and social practice of those involved in caregiving. It also offers a fully theorised, practical framework for addressing these issues* (Tilley & Cameron, 2014a, p. 5).

Most of the chapters in the current volume adopt a similar perspective. They express the willingness of a new generation of researchers to go beyond, at a case-study level, the existing pitfalls and past prejudicial scepticism in interpreting empirical evidence from the past.

The two contrasting attitudes I have painted earlier are the extremes, shaping a field which is polarised by sometimes very different attitudes with regard to scientific research. Such attitudes suggest that, faced with the same epistemological, methodological or ideological issues typical of their discipline, reactions of scholars in archaeology may be diametrically opposed, without there being any obvious 'scientific' justification for such a polarisation. This is because, for scholars, the differences between a *conservative prudent (if not sceptical) stance* or *a bolder (but more risky) critical stance* may rely less on scientific reasoning than on differences of beliefs or normative engagements, which often animate invisibly, *through affect*, the *visible* part of scientific debate.

In extending this assumption over the next sections of this chapter, I will first focus on the content of beliefs underlying the early arguments against archaeological inferences of health-related care, in particular concentrating on the objections raised by Dettwyler (1991). This is a good point of entry into discussion, as Dettwyler's article has had a chilling effect on archaeological research into caregiving behaviours in prehistory over the last decades, and many archaeologists (e.g. Berkson, 2004; DeGusta, 2003; DiGangi, Bethard, & Sullivan, 2009; Gargett, 1999; Knudson & Stojanowski, 2008; Metzler, 1999; Roca et al., 2012; Tarlow, 2000; Toyne, 2015) have, and still do, implicitly or explicitly refer to her statements to justify a conservative critical stance. After this first analysis I will present the answers to Dettwyler's objections, which, I think, are presupposed in the emerging field of bioarchaeology of care.

What Beliefs and Values Were the First Objections to Inferences of Care Based on?

The first inferences of prehistoric attitudes of care towards disabled individuals in the palaeopathological literature in the second half of the twentieth century have given birth to three kinds of objections. The first range of objections is highly motivated by the defence of the 'moral economy' of science, that is the set of values and affects which are both required by the epistemology and the methodology of any *scientific* research. A second field of criticism is semantic and conceptual, and relates to the issues arising from the reference to 'disability' in the archaeological literature. A last field of objections relates to the interpretations of the moral signification of the contents and outcomes of archaeology of care analysis. Such objections, which often reflect ethical relativism opposed to ethical universalism – both being classical widespread stances in academic fields such as anthropology and ethnology – rely on the researcher's political and moral personal position.

Objection 1: A Moral Economy of Science

The first range of objections made by Dettwyler to early claims for provision of health-related care in the past appears *at a first sight* as a purely epistemological and methodological commentary. This may be summarised like this: if one draws attention to the types of inferences made by archaeologists from palaeopathological diagnosis, one must admit that the exact nature of support benefiting disabled individuals cannot be *directly* deduced from skeletal analysis. Osteological data are *brute physical facts*. They do not give any information concerning *institutional facts* such as social status, collective behaviours and shared intentionality, symbolic functions or cultural norms which do not fossilise. Nor do they deliver any indication concerning emotions in prehistory.

But yet, if we take a closer look, this epistemological statement depends more deeply on a specific field of norms and values, on the basis of which a scientific community defines its rules of rational acceptability (Putnam, 1979) – that is, those rules in relation to inference, models, criteria and theories which it is rational to acknowledge and apply when we wish to attain some knowledge about 'reality'. In other words, epistemology and methodology in science cannot be separated from the field of human values, beliefs and affects from which communities of scholars select and shape most of their principles. As Didier Fassin and Samuel Lézé (2013, p. 343) emphasise, scientists share 'a moral vision of their activity which relies on values (…) which are inseparable from the affects which accompany them'.

The existence of an intrinsic relation between the area of science and that of morality is a well-known topic in philosophy of science, which has been studied in depth by philosophers such as Robert Merton (1942), Hilary Putnam (1979) and Lorraine Daston (1995) within the last century. The latter, especially, observed that scientific attachment to empirical evidence, precision measurement and objectivity relies on the existence of what she calls a 'moral economy' that, in one form or another, underlies the operation of scientific communities.

What is a 'moral economy'? Daston employs this term 'to denote a community of scientists governed by norms of professional integrity' (Edelman, 2012, p. 62). A moral economy is a web of affect-saturated values, virtues and rules that

> *stand and function in well-defined relationship to one another. In this usage, 'moral' [...] refers at once to the psychological and the normative. [...] [Here economy refers] to an organized system that displays certain regularities. [...] A moral economy is a balanced system of emotional forces, with equilibrium points and constraints...* (Daston, 1995, p. 4)

which influence the production of socially recognised scientific material. For instance, good scientific practice requires specific virtues of 'diligence, fastidiousness, thoroughness, and caution' (Daston, 1995, p. 11). Science itself is premised on a rich system of rules, covering both compliance with methodology, empirical verifications and obligations to justify inferences, and requirements for cognitive performance reflecting certain values, such as coherence (rather than incoherence), simplicity (rather than confusion), transparency (rather than obscurity) and related matters.

One finds, then, in connections between the moral, epistemological and methodological, the source of a first range of objections raised against attempts to infer from skeletal pathology prehistoric attitudes towards care for disabled persons. These attempts were interpreted by Dettwyler as overstepping the limits of moral decency *in* archaeology. It is precisely from this background that one can understand the origin of one of the most powerful criticisms of an archaeological focus on caregiving. Both behaviours and emotions accompanying care practices have been considered as 'immorally' inferred (with regard to moral economy of science in archaeology) at the expense of

> *the normally self-imposed constraints on archaeological interpretation. [Such constraints] have been disregarded and otherwise careful scholars have overstepped the boundaries of reasonable inference. Unfortunately, these interpretations are often accepted uncritically by others and are widely disseminated because they find their way into introductory textbooks, popular scientific writings, and even 'prehistorical' novels. These views gain the status of 'accepted wisdom' within the discipline and are perpetuated until someone steps in and critically questions their validity* (Dettwyler, 1991, p. 376).

Objection 2: Cognitive Relativism

A second range of objections comes from a specific theory that is called 'cognitive relativism', which was developed in the wave of both the 'linguistic turn' in analytical philosophy in the early to mid-twentieth century and the rise of constructionism in the humanities more generally following on from this.

According to Wittgenstein (1969), one of the most influential theorists of the linguistic turn, any worldview or account of a phenomenon – whether it be historical, sociological or scientific – is fundamentally shaped by the words we use for its description. According to 'cognitive relativism', the real world we experience is completely dependent on our concepts, the latter being themselves totally built up on the language habits – that is, the 'language games' in respect of Wittgenstein's terms – of a social group. Tell me what your language is, and I will tell you which world you think and live in! Different societies in space and time thus imply different languages, which lead to different worldviews. Consequently, we have no access at all to any 'independent' reality in itself. We have no access to an 'objective' world of brute physical and human facts, nor do we have access to the worldviews of societies other than our own, since we do not share their language. Comprehension between, and the making of inferences concerning, worlds other than our own is fundamentally impossible.

In the field of disability studies, one finds many scholars who adhere to such postmodern cognitive relativism when considering disability. If one asks what a disability is, a cognitive relativist will answer: 'Well, disability is not a brute physical fact – as, for example, 'there is snow on the Everest' – distinct from social or institutional facts; it depends upon the structure and the field of concepts of the language which is used for the description'. Is your language, as an archaeologist, dependent on your education in osteology and palaeopathology? If so, the cognitive relativist will argue that your views on disability won't be those of a prehistoric society, but a projection onto the past of a modern medical conception of disability – that is, a conception of disability as a pathology that exists in *deviant bodies* rather than something varying in time and social spaces.

Following this argument, a 'strong' version of cognitive relativism will claim that, like disability, medical classifications of pathologies and impairments are also relative from one society to another (Mallet & Runswick-Cole, 2014; Oliver, 1996; Thomas, 1999; Tremain, 1998). To the radical relativist, an impairment is not a loss or abnormality of physiological or psychological structure or function (that is a 'pathology'), nor is disability a functional difficulty (resulting from an impairment) encountered by an individual in executing a task or action. Disability is socially constructed through linguistic, representational, attitudinal, organisational and environmental processes. Furthermore, impairments are not engraved in individual bodies; they are relative[1] because on the one hand they depend on culturally shaped physiological norms of health and validity, and because, on the other hand, the

[1] Lennard Davis, one of the most important scholars in the disability studies, states that 'impairment is not a neutral and easily understood term. It relies heavily on a medical model for the diagnosis of the impairment. [...] Particularly with illnesses that did not exist in the past, the plethora of syndromes and conditions that have sprouted in the hearts and minds of physicians and patients [...] we have to question the clear line drawn between the socially constructed 'disability' and the preexistent and somatic 'impairment.' Davis finally asks: 'Is the impairment bred into the bone, or can it be a creation of a medical-technological-pharmaceutical complex?" (Davis, 2006, pp. 237–238).

content of human experience itself is completely informed by various contextually dependent cognitive systems of beliefs and values.

> *Strong constructionism as it may be implied in disability social theories, posits that the body [as in the case of impairment, for instance] does not determine its own representation in any way because the sign precedes the body in the hierarchy of signification. In fact, political ideologies and cultural mores exert the greatest power, social constructionists claim, when they anchor their authority in natural objects such as the body. (...) Bodies are linguistic effects driven, first, by the order of representation itself and, second, by the entire array of social ideologies dependent on this order* (Siebers, 2006, p. 174).

From this perspective, one can interpret the strategic use an anthropologist makes of ethnographic data as an attempt to justify a 'cognitive relativistic' philosophical position on a specific topic. The use of empirical data to argue that there are bases for comparison across different societies is well illustrated in Dettwyler's article. Her relativistic stance appears when she writes, for instance, that

> *[t]he ethnographic record tells us that societies sometimes take extreme positions with respect to people who are different (...) In some groups, individuals with abnormalities are feared or hated, and they may even be killed at birth. (...) In other groups, such individuals are revered. (...) In a discussion of Mary Douglas' work on pollution, Buckley and Gottlieb (*1988, p. 27*) note that 'anomalies are simply 'powerful'...their power being granted a negative or positive valence to be determined through specific cultural analysis rather than being attributed cross-culturally. An entity deemed polluting in one culture might, for example, be deemed holy in another.' The archeological record does not allow us to distinguish between these two alternative possibilities* (Dettwyler, 1991, p. 381).

Here one finds the source of a second range of objections to attempts to infer the provision of care to disabled person in prehistory on the basis of skeletal pathology. According to these objections, disability in the palaeopathological literature is classically identified as a functional limitation due to impairment rather than a cultural product of social reactions to corporeal differences. The argument consists in claiming that even *before* inferring social behaviours, determining a disability or an impairment from skeletal remains is simply modernising the past through current medical knowledge. As a consequence of this, archaeologists examining care would have been led into the position of interpreting prehistoric social attitudes towards persons with disabilities from the modern post-industrial, paternalistic framework (Shakespeare, 1999) of the medical relationship between a patient who has a physiological problem and a set of carers put in the position of 'being compassionate'. However, according to Dettwyler (1991) and disability scholars who adhere to cognitive relativism, the logic of such interpretation would be simply a piece of fallacious reasoning. We cannot capture what disabilities and impairments were from the point of view of our prehistoric ancestors, as both their subjective experience of their real world and the language which gave form to it cannot fossilise. As a consequence, early attempts to infer prehistoric practices of compassionate care from skeletal pathology in the archaeological literature of the second half of the twentieth century are rationally illegitimate from a cognitive relativistic perspective.

Objection 3: Moral Universalism, Moral Relativism, Moral Pessimism

Finally, the last range of objections that a philosopher is tempted to categorise relate to interpretations of the moral signification of the contents and outcomes of a bioarchaeology of care analysis. Dettwyler (1991) makes her objections clear; when she wonders why some archaeologists infringe the rules and values of the moral economy of the scientific community to which they belong, she proposes an undeclared 'moral' purpose.

According to Dettwyler, some scholars have both a political and moral hidden agenda – that is, an *un*scientific will to change cultural representations of the past in a way which might demonstrate that core human values such as compassion and respect for the most vulnerable in society are strongly inscribed in our 'noble (prehistoric)' origins (Dettwyler, 1991, p. 383). Such a critique applies, for example, to the implicit normative presupposition of archaeologist J. Renfrew, when she writes in 2009 at the very beginning of her archaeological study:

> *Caring for severely disabled members of the community must be one of the indicators of respect for the individual and for the human life. It is clear that Neanderthals fed and looked after severely [disabled*[2]*] members of their communities who were too disabled to contribute to the food quest* (Renfrew, 2009, p. 51).

Renfrew's (2009) views are not an exception. Observations such as this one underlining the normative nature of caregiving are often found in the literature (e.g. Gould, 1988; Green, 2003; Le Pichon, 2009; Solecki, 1971; Spikins, Rutherford, & Needham, 2010), implying some attachment to what one calls 'moral universalism' in philosophy. In terms of this normative view, there exist certain cross-cultural and trans-historical human values, according to which caring for disabled persons may always be intuited in human experience – in any historical and cultural situation – as being the *moral* thing that *must* be done (whether it is *in fact* done is another question).

But doesn't the ethnographic record '[tell] us that societies sometimes take extreme positions with respect to people who are different' (Dettwyler, 1991, p. 381)? Don't anthropological data show us that behaviours towards persons with disabilities fluctuate from one society to one another – sometimes in huge, contradictory ways? As a cultural anthropologist, Dettwyler completely disagrees with universalistic moral claims by opposing them with moral relativistic statements. For instance, this appears clearly to be Dettwyler's position when she writes:

---

[2] Renfrew uses in her original chapter the term 'handicapped' to designate the disabled members of a prehistoric hominid community. In the context of the quotation, the term is inappropriate. I have replaced 'handicapped' with 'disabled', since the latter is the descriptor used (at the time of Refrew's publication) by the *WHO International Classification of Functioning, Disability and Health (ICF)* (2001). Regarding differences on terminologies between English-speaking countries, I have used both the terms 'disabled persons' (GB) and 'persons with disabilities' (USA, Australia) in the chapter. I have avoided the term 'the disabled' which is sometimes regarded as pejorative.

The question of which is the compassionate choice – to expend effort to keep nonnormal individuals alive or to kill them (or, the genteel version, 'allow them to die') is far from being answered [...]. In many societies, infants who are obviously impaired or deformed at birth may either be killed outright or 'allowed to die' through the deliberate withholding of food, water, medical care. In a study of the Tarahumara of northern Mexico, Dorothy Mull and Denis Mull (1987) report several cases of infanticide involving disabled infants or toddlers. Although this may seem cruel to some people, the parents explained that life was very difficult even for 'normal' individuals and would be unbearably difficult for disabled children. For them, the 'compassionate' choice for their children was death. Even in the United States, some parents make similar choices for their disabled children. [...] To claim that facilitating the survival of a disabled person necessarily indicates compassion and moral decency [...] suggests a certainty about the moral issues in these situations, which, as 'objective' scientists, we are not justified in claiming. Speculation about the moral qualities of people who lived thousands years ago, based on paleopathological analyses of archeological remains, is particularly inappropriate (Dettwyler, 1991, p. 381).

By moral relativism, I mean a general normative position (which covers several forms in moral philosophy) according to which the content of what is right and wrong does not depend on a universal human nature, but rather relies on contextual beliefs, factors and situations that may be ecological, social, cultural and personal. As a consequence, a 'moral relativistic perspective' implies, when applied to care, that assisting, caregiving and making life possible for physically impaired individuals is not always what must be done – that is, what is 'good' – in all human societies and in all circumstances. The nature of right and wrong, good and bad, is *always* determined by highly contingent and malleable factors which do not allow the characterisation of human *agency* as motivated by universal human moral values.

However, Dettwyler's moral position is much more complex than it may appear at a first sight. On one hand, she adheres to a relativistic perspective, according to which the achievement what is 'good' or 'desirable' sometimes involves actions intended to assist or care for another and sometimes requires the exact opposite of this, with all behaviours adapting to the immediate ecological, social, cultural and other factors constraining the operation of human agency. On the other hand, some of Dettwyler's claims seem to take precedence over her moral relativistic perspective by pretending to universality.

This normative paradox appears, for instance, when Dettwyler (1991, p. 382) suggests that, like disabled people met in her field research in Mali who were kept alive, but who were 'hardly treated with compassion', Shanidar I, Romito 2 and the Windover Boy had survived, but they may have been poorly treated. By assuming ethnographic comparisons, she writes:

[f]or all we know, these individuals were ridiculed, teased, taunted, beaten, treated as slaves, physically and emotionally abused, constantly reminded of their differences and shortcomings, and threatened with bodily harm or abandonment (Dettwyler, 1991, p. 382).

Dettwyler then adds:

I am not suggesting that we ought to take a pessimistic view of earlier human societies or that we know with any certainty that disabled individuals were treated poorly. Unfortunately, the ethnographic record, including that of our own society, supports [a] dismal view of human nature more often than it supports a view of society as compassionate (Dettwyler, 1991, p. 382).

Thus along with tendency to moral relativism, Dettwyler paradoxically suggests there seems to exist – as supported by the ethnographic record – some kind of general tendency in human nature to exclude and mistreat disabled individuals rather than to care for them.

Though this universalistic normative assumption regarding human nature is contradictory with regard to moral relativism and the logical coherence it requires, I suspect that Dettwyler's moral pessimism is fully consistent with a prevailing belief in the contemporary public sphere and among many postmodern disability scholars and activists. The pessimism concerns the nature of relationships between disabled persons and non-disabled persons in human societies, according to which exclusionary practices and mistreatment of people with disabilities are both the cross-culturally and trans-historically indisputable fate that has awaited disabled people in most human societies up to the present day (Goodley, 2010; Hubert, 2000; Oliver, 1996; Shakespeare, 2006a, 2006b). This postmodern normative belief emerged in the twentieth century as a premise for political and academic engagement with disability prejudices, and clearly had an impact on Dettwyler's article. In disability studies, it may lead to thinking that it is a priori unrealistic – and just another paternalistic denial of the universal experience of persons with disabilities – to interpret evidence of survival of disabled persons in prehistory in terms of benevolent (i.e. compassionate, decent, inclusive) caregiving behaviours.

One finds here the source of a third range of objections which have been addressed within the last decades to the inference of care (and perhaps compassion) for disabled individuals from skeletal evidence alone. Both relativistic and pessimistic moral outlooks on human relationships between disabled persons and non-disabled persons have categorised such attempts as politically and morally unacceptable, as well as romantic and naïve.

Given this last objection, along with the two others I have summarised earlier, one now has to ask the following crucial question:

Are the Beliefs and Values Informing the Recently Developed Bioarchaeology of Care Model of Analysis Sufficiently Robust to Overcome Past Criticism?

As a philosopher of science and an ethicist, my answer to this question is yes. But this simple affirmative is, *of course*, not convincing on its own. It is therefore time to present the arguments that can be addressed to the three points of criticism I have presented earlier, and which underlie contemporary developments in the bioarchaeology of care. Let's take one by one the objections I have just classified. My aim is to show why basic beliefs and values in the bioarchaeology of care model seem to me to answer past criticism.

Answer to Objection 1: A Moral Economy of Science

Regarding the first category of objections that have been addressed, the *Index of Care*, introduced in 2014 as a methodological instrument for use in bioarchaeology of care research, is an adequate answer to any scholar who fears that the 'moral economy' of scientific research might not be honoured in the field.

It is true that many past reports where provision of care was inferred did not dedicate enough effort to justifying this conclusion (e.g. Dickel & Doran, 1989; Solecki, 1971; Trinkaus, 1983), meaning that a basic requirement of scientific research was not met. Comments relating to the likelihood of caregiving behaviours were often limited to almost conversational reflections in concluding paragraphs of palaeopathological studies. One can imagine how shocking the disparity between the detail of palaeopathological analysis and the general observations on the possibility of care could appear to readers, and how suspicious they might be of what could appear as 'much too-easy-to-make' speculation or poetic conclusions! Basically, what was lacking from earlier archaeological studies was, first, an operational protocol situating the individual and their experience of disease within their wider archaeological context, thereby helping to explain what disability may have meant in practice. Second, there was no rigorous framework for helping to build or select appropriate models of care on the basis of information collected from the bioarchaeological context. Third, interpretations were not constrained in respect of the order of inferences that should have been controlled – from the most irrefutable to the most probable ones (Hawkes, 1954) – by the whole process of inquiry and a dedicated methodology.

By contrast, the bioarchaeological framework presented by Tilley and Cameron (2014a) for identifying and interpreting past health-related care provision at a case study level, really does respect moral economy of contemporary archaeological practice. Its rigorous step-by-step approach does not confuse core differences, which must remain transparent, between evidence, inference and interpretation. In addition, its framework as well as its results is fully perfectible, that is, it is open to critical evaluation and ongoing development. Finally, as *fallibilism and antiscepticism often go hand in hand in the history of science*, Tilley's model for a bioarchaeology of care analysis fully admits there is no absolute guarantee that such and such a statement will never need revision. The framework and its fully accessible methodology (Tilley & Cameron, 2014b) opens the door to bioarchaeological reassessment of archaeological literature on past caregiving behaviours.

Bioarchaeology of care also opens the path to critical reading of Dettwyler's own respect or disrespect of moral economy of archaeological practice. Let's give an example: in her 1991 article, Dettwyler explains that one cannot know the detail of the 'emotional motivations' behind past behaviours of care. She is right, but she goes even further. She not only criticises inference of emotions and values, but she tends to condemn any attempt to infer behaviour from the archaeological record (Mennear, 2013): 'We can observe how disabled people are treated today, cross-culturally (…) but we cannot know with any certainty how disabled individuals were treated from archeological remains' (Dettwyler, 1991, p. 382). Elsewhere, she writes: '[…] the archaeological record does not provide answers to the question of how individuals were treated or what other people thought of them' (1991, p. 383), and equates such attempts at inference with more general tendencies to characterise past populations as 'noble savages' (Dettwyler, 1991, p. 383).

If Dettwyler were right, and inferences of 'care and compassion' always went hand in hand in the early archaeological studies, then obviously conclusions of caregiving could be regarded as dubious and should be revised. But on one point, she is not right. First, Dettwyler only focuses on three 'primary research' case studies (Dickel & Doran, 1989; Frayer et al., 1987; Solecki, 1971); in fact, not all archaeological studies pre-Dettwyler *do* explicitly interpret care as evidence for compassion. As a consequence, the small sample upon which Dettwyler relies to support her general comment renders much of her argument generalised hyperbole. Second, though Solecki (1971) briefly discusses compassion, none of the three scientific studies to which she refers explicitly conflate care and compassion. And in any case, why should archaeologists be forbidden to make interpretations? Is 'interdiction of interpretation' part of the *moral economy* of archaeology? To my knowledge, the moral economy of archaeology does not prohibit interpretation during the archaeological reconstruction of the past – in fact, attempting interpretation is a precondition for theoretical progress and underlies further discoveries in the field. In other words, Dettwyler relies on a non-existent taboo in the moral economy of archaeology.

Contrary to Dettwyler's conceptual imprecisions, the recent bioarchaeology of care rigorously makes the methodological distinction between 'caregiving behaviours' and the several possible underlying 'motivations' for these (including compassion, but also rational interest, reciprocal altruism, social rules or positions, search for social recognition, moral and religious beliefs, etc.). It clearly proposes (Tilley & Cameron, 2014b) a thorough methodological approach to caregiving analysis in the past, putting inferences of behaviours and interpretation of 'hypothetical' underlying motivations (values, beliefs, emotions, etc.) at different stages of the methodology to avoid any confusion. A step-by-step methodology is thus proposed at a case study level, using palaeopathological analysis, bioarchaeological and clinical criteria to evaluate the possibility to make (or not) inferences of caregiving behaviours. At a well-signposted step, the methodology is also opened to cautious interpretation regarding identity, motivations, values and beliefs that existed in a particular context, assuming that

> *[a] community's response to the health care requirements of its members is shaped by a combination of cultural beliefs and values; collective knowledge, skills and experience; social and economic organisation; and access to resources* (Tilley & Oxenham, 2011, p. 35).

This last level of bioarchaeology of care analysis is of course the most speculative, and this is quite recognised in bioarchaeology of care methodology (Tilley, 2015b; Tilley & Cameron, 2014a).

I will not undertake any further discussion on the points earlier as the readers may consult the previous chapters of this book, which demonstrate how much things have changed in relation to our approach to questions of care provision in the past. Let's have a look now at the class of objections coming from what I have called 'cognitive relativism'.

Answer to Objection 2: Cognitive Relativism (Medical, Social)

In Dettwyler's paper, the term 'disability' is an ambiguous one. First, though she explicitly admits that disability includes the physiological dimension of *impairment* as defined by the World Health Organization definition of 1980 (Dettwyler, 1991, p. 377), she does not focus on the pragmatic relationship that exists between the level of severity of an impairment diagnosed at an osteological level, and the clinical, psychological and contextual specificities of the social response that an individual with such impairment may have required in the past as a necessary condition for survival. Second, Dettwyler prefers to systematically refer to disability in terms of what was called in the 1990s a 'handicap' (World Health Organization, 1980), defined as *social* disadvantage which results from an impairment and its functional consequences (Dettwyler, 1991, p. 376). In other words, despite Dettwyler's claims to rely on the full WHO definition of disability (Dettwyler, 1991, p. 376), which covers impairment, functional limitation and handicap (World Health Organization, 1980), she mainly interprets disability as a *handicap* – that is the product of a cognitive construct shaped by negative social reactions to physical and cognitive difference. Third, and final, Dettwyler relies on ethnographic data to suggest that a disability is a purely linguistic phenomenon, varying from one social group to one another and, as a consequence, archaeologically unmanageable, since the prehistoric social beliefs and values that shaped behaviours towards persons with disabilities do not fossilise.

It is worth noting that Dettwyler's interpretation of disability in terms of 'handicap' has been prevalent in the field of disability studies and among disability rights concerns over the past decades. It is possible then that Dettwyler (1991), who has a personal stake in disability matters (Bower, 2002), was strongly influenced by theories and ideas common in disability rights movements in the second half of the 20th century. Among disability activists, one finds indeed both 'cognitive relativism' and a strong tendency within the 'social model of disability' (Union of the Physically Impaired Against Segregation (UPIAS), 1976; Shakespeare, 2006b) to identify disability as a form of exclusion, in which disability and also impairment (if one considers the most extreme tenets of a socio-constructivist perspective on disability) are mostly the product of prejudicial beliefs and values whose content may fluctuate from one society to one another (Shakespeare, 2006a, p. 29). Such understanding of disability as a discriminatory social construct is classically opposed to the medical model of disability (Smith, 2009; Vehmas & Mäkelä, 2009), which relies on what one might call a 'cognitive universalism'. According to the medical model, activity limitations and participation restrictions in daily life are not due to social organisation and cultural beliefs, but rather to individual problems in body function or structure.

When the medical and the social models are compared from a political and moral perspective, one can understand the a priori preference of many disability activists for a social model of disability. Indeed, such an intellectual stance offers the best insights into the experience of discrimination, as well as the most powerful motivation for combating exclusion and demanding core political and moral changes in postmodern society. If people are not disabled by their body but *by society*, the issue immediately becomes a question of *justice,* and the right to *compensation.* First, it provides a strong position in a democratic society from which to ask for the dismantlement of disabling barriers (Shakespeare, 2006a, p. 30). Second, 'replacing a traditional [medical] deficit approach with a social oppression understanding [...] [is] very liberating for disabled individuals' (Shakespeare, 2006a, p. 30). Nevertheless, though *of course* I personally do not deny the highly moral and political value of disability rights concerns, as well as the idea that disability is partly a consequence of unfair and discriminatory social barriers that *must* be withdrawn (this is part of my own personal and professional engagement), the prevalence of the social model of disability risks sometimes leading to major theoretical bias in scientific research.

As disability scholar Tom Shakespeare (2006b) points out, by systematically equating disability with stigmatisation, the perspective on disability is not any longer whether disabled people are either oppressed *or* cared for and included in a particular situation, but only the extent to which they are oppressed. 'A circularity[3] enters into disability research: it [becomes] logically impossible [...] to find disabled people who are not oppressed' (Shakespeare, 2006b, p. 201). Even caregiving behaviours (whether compassionate or not) risk being interpreted, from this perspective, as just another form of domination and exclusion of disabled persons from social participation. Dettwyler's article clearly seems to embrace such theoretical circularity. One has just to examine the text: the author systematically opposes speculative discriminatory scenarios of archaeological inferences of inclusive caregiving behaviours towards disabled persons, *as if* inclusive caregiving attitudes would be a priori unlikely with regard to disability, and thus should be deconstructed. In the second part of her article, Dettwyler suspects any inference of care in the archaeological literature to be strongly dependent on common *prejudicial assumptions* in Western society. Such stereotypes assume that disabled people 'survive only because of the compassion of nondisabled members of the population' (Dettwyler, 1991, p. 383).

The archaeologist might then ask: how can I avoid such theoretical circularity due to contemporary political debates? What should an archaeological model of disability look like? Well, the answer I would suggest is this: ask disabled persons themselves such a question, and build a model which might be conceptually friendly with regard to *the whole content* of their corporeal experience of being impaired. If one questions only 'individuals with static impairments, which do not degenerate or cause medical complications, it is clear that it is possible to regard disability as entirely socially created' (Shakespeare, 2006b, p. 201). Of course many forms of physical or cognitive impairments exist that do not cause bodily pain nor are, in themselves, obstacles to an independent and full social life. Some disability schol-

[3] Battles (2011) and Gleeson (1999) evoke such a risk of circularity as follows: although '[there] is value for today's society in investigating disability in the more distant past' (Battles, 2011, p. 113), the historiography of disability studies 'has burdened the field with a number of [...] orthodoxies about the social context of impairment in previous societies' (Gleeson, 1999, p. 23). Such orthodoxies, which increased in anthropology in the twentieth century, present disabled people's contemporary exclusion, marginality and poverty 'by depicting them as fixed, historical conditions that have been present in most, even all, past human societies'. Accordingly, given widespread

ars have physical impairments of this kind, yet nevertheless, they often experience discrimination and environmental obstacles – which are then interpreted as social barriers. They feel disabled not because of their body, but because social norms and institutions are constructed by non-disabled persons in a way that, on many occasions, excludes them from social participation. Within this range of disabling experiences, it is as theoretically logical to be cognitively relativist and to build a dualism between the biological (impairment) and the social (disability as the varying forms of exclusionary social constructs in human societies) as it is to construct a dichotomy between gender and sexuality in feminist studies.

But apart from static impairments, which do not cause bodily pain or require intensive care, there are many others which restrict functioning, affect appearance, are degenerative or may cause premature death. If you do not deny those individuals who have a condition 'which involves pain and discomfort, it is harder to ignore the negative aspects of impairment' (Shakespeare, 2006a, 2006b, p. 201) which may sometimes require both practical healthcare and social support on daily basis. In other words, it is difficult in these cases to ignore or reject the fact that there may exist special care needs that are not social fictions but corporeal realities.

If you agree with the ethical and methodological requirements to take the whole voice of disability seriously, you will then need to rely on a third model of disability which does not reduce it to a purely socio-cognitive matter. This is precisely the up-to-date framework and definition of disability one may find in the *International Classification of Functioning, Disability and Health* of the WHO (2001), as well as in Tilley's contemporary bioarchaeological model for care analysis (Chap. 2, this volume), where the term disability is used to mean 'a state arising from body impairment, related with activity limitations and/or participation restrictions, and given specific meaning in association with the lifeways context in which the pathology is experienced'.

By relying on this definition of disability, the bioarchaeology of care assumes that, regardless of any social language or medical classifications, some impairments are cross-culturally *brute* physical facts (Vehmas & Mäkelä, 2009) *prior* their being experienced by individuals. As Tilley and Oxenham write,

> *although ways of understanding, explaining and, to some extent, experiencing health, disease and disability may be culturally determined, human biology dictates a fundamental uniformity across time and culture in physical expression of, and physiological reactions to, specific pathologies [and impairments]* (Tilley & Oxenham, 2011, p. 67).

---

assumptions of cross-cultural stigma and social exclusion of disabled people in history, 'contemporary views are based on assumptions about disability in the past such as that 'they' (people with disabilities) would not have survived under [...] harsh, 'natural' circumstances [...] (Battles, 2011, p. 113) such as those met in early prehistoric hominin communities. Given these orthodoxies, scholars may be led to think that it would be a priori unrealistic – and another non-disabled denial of a universal social condition of exclusion disabled persons experience – to interpret evidence of survival of disabled persons in prehistory as a possible indication of inclusive – or benevolent, compassionate, respectful – caregiving behaviours. To be morally and politically minimally acceptable with regard to postmodern sensibilities, care provision should be interpreted at least as just another means to deny disabled people's right to develop an autonomous and independent life. To avoid naturalization of pessimistic postmodern disability narratives, Battles (2011, p. 113) claims, at the risk of being politically incorrect: 'Anthropological investigations could refute [...] orthodoxies and contribute to denaturalizing the relationship between impairment and social disadvantage, inequality, and dependency'.

Correspondingly, inferences of caregiving behaviours from osteological and archaeological evidence can be justified, for the bioarchaeology of care approach presupposes characteristics of basic healthcare answers are also 'universal in their nature' (Tilley & Oxenham, 2011, p. 7):

> *[Where] a pathology is reliably associated with a continuum of clinical signs and symptoms there [are] certain practical requirements so fundamental to effective healthcare as to constitute 'universals' or 'constants' of care – even taking into account individual heterogeneity in response to disease. In other words, some conditions (...) generate certain requirements for care which are so essential that, if they are not met, the individual with the pathology [does not] survive – or [is] unlikely to survive for the length of time necessary to produce skeletal indicators meeting the criteria for inclusion in a bioarchaeology of care analysis* (Tilley & Oxenham, 2011, pp. 67–68).

It follows that, where there is adequate archaeological information about context, identifying biomedical effects of a specific disease or impairment allows inference of the care necessary to meet basic bodily requirements and to overcome functional limitations in situations in which the individual would probably not have survived (or at least not have flourished) without such a response.

Finally, although discerning social inclusion or exclusion in the past may be more problematic than discerning a state of physical impairment, the bioarchaeology of care approach suggests that at a case study level it is not always completely impossible. As demonstrated in bioarchaeology of care analyses (Tilley, 2015a; Tilley & Oxenham, 2011), when contextual information is available it may sometimes be possible to identify some of the likely barriers to the individual's participation in specific physical, sociocultural and economic activities and postulate that assistance would be required to overcome these (Mennear, 2013).

Bioarchaeology of care analysis is thus mid-way between cognitive universalism and cognitive relativism: though ways of explaining and experiencing health, disease and disability are still partly linguistically, socially and culturally determined and for many cases inaccessible, there exist biomedical criteria, constants of caregiving behaviours and contextual information (material, social, cultural, ecological) which sometimes open the path, at a case study level, to rationally justified bioarchaeological inferences.

Answer to Objection 3: Moral Universalism, Moral Relativism, Moral Pessimism

Before my conclusion, I have two final remarks concerning moral issues underlying bioarchaeology of care, which will have to be further developed in future works. The combining of scientific and moral questions is perhaps among the most difficult issues to be treated, but philosophical analysis is an indispensable tool for preparing the path for necessary clarifications.

First, I am inclined to think that the way Dettwyler (1991) brings her moral relativism and moral pessimism into the discussion is problematic. It is as problematic as the way a scientist like Stephen Jay Gould (1988)[4] tried to justify, a few years before Dettwyler (1991) published her article, his claim for a cross-cultural and trans-historical ethics of care by relying on one case study (Frayer et al., 1987) identifying health-related care provision in early prehistory. What is problematic in both cases is that, by justifying their moral theory on the basis of descriptive data, both sides commit what one calls a 'naturalistic fallacy' in moral philosophy, that is, the attempt to justify a normative stance on the basis of a descriptive premise (Frankena, 1939). According to philosophers who criticise the naturalistic fallacy, normative conclusions cannot be validly drawn from propositions which are non-normative.

From a moral economy specific to bioarchaeology of care, engaging in the field should require the researcher to avoid such naturalistic fallacy. This entails the need to be self-critical and honest. You may believe that a society is humane in that it takes care of those who have bodily impairments without either rejecting or marginalising them – but another scholar might think that such a criterion is morally irrelevant. Another scholar may be a moral relativist or, on the contrary, a universalist – or a mix of both. As a consequence, identification and interpretation at a case study level of health-related care provision in prehistory will be variably valued at a subjective level, depending on researcher's moral core beliefs and personal experience. The problems only come when researchers attempt to naturalise their moral beliefs by stating that these may be deduced from empirical research. Such naturalistic fallacy, whatever the moral theory it sustains, always casts a shadow on scientific practice and leads to absurdity: if sociological and ethnographic data were a direct proof in favour of a certain moral theory, then one might use any collection of empirical data as moral justification for any kind of behaviours – caregiving, murdering, torturing, and so on.

Second, I think that a unique focus on exclusion, which characterises some pessimistic postmodern disability narratives, is in some way part of the theoretical circularity I have described earlier (see answer to objection 2). A bioarchaeology of

[4] When questioning the very possibility to find empirical traces of the emergence of human moral behaviour, Stephen Jay Gould wrote: 'We have bones aplenty, but they speak to us in limited and muted ways. (…) We yearn to know how and when [this] distinctively human [trait] of […] moral decency entered our history. We wish, in short, to disinter the 'good' that lies in the bones. But goodness doesn't fossilize. (…) Since decency […] [makes] no fossils directly, the challenge for explorers of [this] most important and elusive [aspect] of human history lies in developing criteria of inference from material record. Bones tell us something. What then can we learn of compassion from a study of bones and artifacts? A remarkable discovery has just been reported from this domain of more circumstantial evidence. The November 5, 1987, issue of *Nature* […] announced the finding of an unusual skeleton from Romito, an Italian cave deposit some 11,000 years old. […] If we consider care of the handicapped (particularly at some cost of caretakers) as a key attribute of humanity, the Romito people surely practiced compassion at this level.' (Gould, 1988, pp. 16–18.). Given the antiquity of prehistoric empirical indication of caregiving behaviours, Gould states then elsewhere in his text that though progress has occurred in technology, compassionate behaviour is not a question of progress: 'We have developed a technology to aid the [disabled], but our compassion may span the age' (p. 20). When considering the traditional criteria for human worthiness, a cross-cultural and trans-historical category should then be added: 'To art and symbol, […] we should add a third category, for our usual definition of human worthiness includes kindness as well as cognition.' (p. 18).

care should remain on guard against such a risk of circularity, if it aims to contribute to a balanced and realistic vision of prehistoric human behaviours.

Of course, exclusionary behaviours and attitudes towards disability have existed throughout human history and in *all* human societies, and exclusion is a key focus in disability studies. But when we focus on exclusion, we sometimes risk endorsing a theoretical bias. We may neglect 'natural' (or 'given') inclusive practices in human groups. For example, we may come to 'take – as given – the ideological and material exclusion of people with labels of physical, sensory or cognitive impairments' (Goodley, 2010, p. xi). However, if exclusionary attitudes are considered a priori as given, 'spontaneous' inclusive behaviours among groups risk being seen a priori as improbable, if not impossible. When disability is exclusively related to social 'oppression' in the several forms of the social model of disability, it is also, of course, logical to present a pessimistic temperament, to look for empirical data which reinforce your cultural beliefs, and to be strongly sceptical about any inference of inclusive practices in past human communities: progress can only come from the future! I wonder if a substantial part of academic literature is not partly engaged in such postmodern theoretical circularity. Is it a virtuous circle? I do not believe it to be so …

As demonstrated today through empirical research in ethology (De Waal, 2009; Fashing & Nguyen, 2011; Silk, 1992), some animal societies are able to adjust to their injured members and accommodate them. Why would humans, from prehistory onwards, not partly fall within this animal continuity? At the same time, it is true that contemporary experience and empirical studies show that *Homo sapiens* welcomes in, rejects, cares for, supports, targets, excludes and includes individuals with disabilities. Given such heterogeneity, I would personally adhere to neither a pessimistic nor a romantic conception of human nature. I would adopt a non-relativistic, but intermediate, moral posture. I would argue that providing care is a complex activity of major ethical importance, given that human beings are highly dependent on the various forms of such activity to flourish, develop their capabilities and experience a fully human life.

Nevertheless, why do exclusionary behaviours exist? Why does the relationship between society and the disabled individual remain ambiguous, contradictory and unpredictable to this day? Far from leading us straight to both moral relativism and pessimism, which some researchers in the human sciences embrace when studying prehistory, I rather think that the complexity of this issue calls for a deep philosophical and ethical reflection.

Conclusion

As previous chapters of this book demonstrate, the emerging field of bioarchaeology of care research is dependent on the quality of osteological and archaeological evidence available, as well as on the advances in scientific methodology and epistemology that enable and drive its analysis. But 'objective' researchers are never purely 'neutral'. Human values, temperaments, biographies and beliefs always play a part in the shaping of 'scientific' evaluations and concepts that are used in description as well as in interpretation. Bioarchaeology of care does not escape this anthropological condition of science – there is no science without a human face.

I have suggested in this chapter that bioarchaeology of care is shaped on values, convictions and rational arguments which contrast with a field of contemporary political and moral postmodern beliefs that sometimes risk leading to theoretical circularity and excessive scepticism (if not suspicion) regarding any attempt to infer caregiving towards persons with disabilities in the past. In keeping with requirements to remain rigorously critical and cautious in their work, bioarchaeologists can now call on an applied framework that should help in building a more balanced understanding of prehistoric caregiving practices.

Given the development of this new field of research, what are the ethical considerations that inform bioarchaeology of care analysis? Though it has been impossible in a short chapter to answer this question exhaustively, I would like finally to summarise four propositions implied by the previous sections and present these for discussion:

First, respect for the moral economy of science is indubitably one of the main reasons behind growing recognition of contemporary bioarchaeology of care analysis by the scientific community. Specific virtues, values and rules required in the practice of bioarchaeology of care analysis could keep the process of inquiry explicit and fully accessible to public assessment. This seems to be one of the aims of the web-based Index of Care (Tilley & Cameron, 2014a, 2014b). From another perspective, scholars may now rely on explicit epistemological and methodological recommendations they may follow, criticise and/or improve upon, to determine evidence, inferences and build interpretations open to revision.

Second, as it is impossible to capture the way disabilities were perceived in prehistory, scholars in the field must use models of disability which are intermediate between the medical and the social, as there are past and present embodied situations which necessarily call for specific health-related care provision (within the specific corresponding bioarchaeological context) as a necessary condition for survival and continued well-being. Taking the whole experience of disabled persons seriously is precisely the path adopted by contemporary theory in bioarchaeology of care, which presents disability as a dynamic interaction between the impact of brute physical impairments and the impact of sociocultural meanings and behaviours – the latter ranging from exclusive to inclusive attitudes. Although interpretation will remain interpretation – in particular in the final dedicated methodological step of bioarchaeology of care analysis (Chap. 2, this volume) – an intermediate model of disability between the biological and the sociocultural opens the way to rational inferences of caregiving behaviours.

Third, naturalistic fallacy, that is, the attempt to *directly* infer some moral claim from empirical data (ethnographic, sociological ones, and so on), must be avoided. A moral theory requires reasons, justifications and self-critical reflection. Scholars must refrain from introducing implicit universalistic, pessimistic or relativistic moral reasoning at any stage of bioarchaeology of care analysis. Furthermore, they should make their personal moral, ideological and biographical influence explicit in analysis, since interpretation of the past is inevitably constrained by researcher's experience[5] – especially in relation to care and disability topics, which are highly sensitive to such effects. But where should one find a well-delineated approach for discussing normative issues in a bioarchaeological model for care analysis? Do we need one? Is the issue only relevant for the philosopher? Of course not, as it influences the selection of concepts used for the description and interpretation… But neither my chapter nor any of the previous chapters in this book manage this issue adequately. It is nevertheless of major importance to find a space for discussion on normative questions, as has been clearly reflected in the media and public reactions to bioarchaeology of care research over the past few years (see next chapter, this volume). This question demands discussion.

Fourth, and final, I think bioarchaeologists studying care in prehistory have the *deontological* duty to contribute to the establishment of a more balanced vision of the way our human ancestors could plausibly behave in prehistory. For many reasons, disabled persons and caregiving behaviours have not been a subject for discussion in past anthropological studies. As Groce (1985, p. 108) writes, archaeologists, anthropologists and sociologists 'have usually dismissed the disabled individuals they have encountered as liminal figures, temporary anomalies in a non-disabled population'. In the public sphere, this has led to widespread *able-bodied* histories of human evolution in which physically impaired individuals seem to have been inexistent in the past (Doat, 2014).

We only have to look at modern museums and exhibitions dedicated to prehistoric community life. I have never seen any disabled adults represented among the human figurines used in 'scientifically' reconstituted scenes of prehistoric daily life, and nor have I ever seen representations of health-related caregiving included in these diorama … Basically, what is lacking is a new narrative which, by integrating the bioarchaeology of care corpus, could give the public a more balanced perception of the presence of disabled persons, and the possible role of caregiving, in human evolution.

Acknowledgments I particularly want to thank Cécile Mathieu, Nathanaël and Camille Doat for discussions and support during the time of this work. I am also very grateful to Lorna Tilley, Alicia Shrenk and Debra Martin, who have welcomed a philosophical/critical perspective among the current chapters of this book. Finally, I thank my colleagues from the Department of Ethics and Philosophy of Lille Catholic University (France) and from the Center for the Study of Science and Philosophy of the University of Namur (Belgium), and 'Métropole Européenne Lilloise' which funding gave me the possibility to do this research.

[5] My own personal experience is strongly dependent on daily living with cognitive disabled adults who were fully included in the community where I lived for several years. Despite human vulnerabilities and complexity experienced in any common life, this is partly why I do not share a pessimistic view on relationship between disabled and non-disabled persons in human communities. Nevertheless, I am not naïve and I have also experienced exclusion, denial of autonomy and stigmatization of persons with disabilities. Such behaviours have to be fought in any society, and this is one of my strongest political and moral engagement, as I think a humane society must be fully inclusive.

References

Battles, H. (2011). Toward engagement: Exploring the prospects for an integrated anthropology of disability. *Explorations in Anthropology, 11*(1), 107–124.

Berkson, G. (2004). Intellectual and physical disabilities in prehistory and early civilization. *Mental Retardation, 42*, 195–208.

Bower, B. (2002). Care-worn fossils: Bones reopen controversy about ancient assistance. *Science News, 162*, 328–330.

Boyd, D. C. (1996). Skeletal correlates of human behaviour in the Americas. *Journal of Archaeological Method and Theory, 3*, 189–251.

Buckley, T., & Gottlieb, A. (1988). A critical appraisal of theories of menstrual symbolism. In T. Buckley & A. Gottlieb (Eds.), *Blood magic: The anthropology of menstruation* (pp. 3–50). Berkeley: University of California Press.

Daston, L. (1995). The moral economy of science. *Osiris, 10*, 2–24.

Davis, L. J. (2006). The end of identity politics and the beginning of dismodernism: On disability as an unstable category. In L. J. Davis (Ed.), *The disability studies reader* (2nd ed., pp. 231–242). New York: Routledge.

De Waal, F. (2009). *The age of empathy: nature's lessons for a kinder society*. New York: Harmony Books.

DeGusta, D. (2003). Aubesier 11 is not evidence of Neanderthal conspecific care. *Journal of Human Evolution, 45*, 91–94.

Dettwyler, K. A. (1991). Can paleopathology provide evidence for 'compassion'? *American Journal of Physical Anthropology, 84*, 375–384.

Dickel, D. N., & Doran, G. H. (1989). Severe neural tube defect syndrome from the early archaic of Florida. *American Journal of Physical Anthropology, 80*, 325–334.

DiGangi, E. A., Bethard, J. D., & Sullivan, L. P. (2009). Differential diagnosis of cartilaginous dysplasia and probable Osgood–Schlatter's disease in a Mississippian individual from East Tennessee. *International Journal of Osteoarchaeology, 20*, 424–442.

Doat, D. (2014). Evolution and human uniqueness: Prehistory, disability and the unexpected anthropology of Charles Darwin. In D. Bolt (Ed.), *Changing social attitudes toward disability: Perspective from historical, cultural, and educational studies* (pp. 15–25). New York: Routledge.

Edelman, M. (2012). E.P. Thompson and moral economies. In D. Fassin (Ed.), *A companion to moral anthropology* (pp. 49–66). Oxford: Willey-Blackwell.

Fashing, P. J., & Nguyen, N. (2011). Behavior toward the dying, diseased, or disabled among animals and its relevance to Pale pathology. *International Journal of Paleopathology, 1*, 128–129.

Fassin, D., & Lézé, S. (2013). *La question morale: Une anthologie critique*. Paris: Presses Universitaires de France.

Frankena, W. K. (1939). The naturalistic fallacy. *Mind, 48*, 464–477.

Frayer, D. W., Horton, W. A., Macchiarelli, R., & Mussi, M. (1987). Dwarfism in an adolescent from the Italian late Upper Paleolithic. *Nature, 330*, 60–62.

Gargett, R. H. (1999). Middle Palaeolithic burial is not a dead issue: the view from Qafzeh, Saint-Césaire, Kebara, Amud, and Dederiyeh. *Journal of Human Evolution, 37*, 27–90.

Gleeson, B. (1999). *Geographies of disability*. New York: Routledge.

Goodley, D. (2010). *Disability studies: An interdisciplinary introduction*. London: Sage.

Gould, S. J. (1988). Honorable men and women. *Natural History, 97*(3), 16–20.

Green, T. (2003). The archaeology of compassion. *The Humanist, 63*, 30–34.

Groce, N. (1985). *Everyone here spoke sign language: Hereditary deafness on Martha's Vineyard*. Cambridge: Harvard University Press.

Hawkes, C. (1954). Archaeological theory and method: some suggestions from the old world. *American Anthropologist, 56*, 155–168.

Hubert, J. (Ed.). (2000). *Madness, disability and social exclusion, the archaeology and anthropology of 'difference'*. London/new York: Routledge.
Hublin, J. J. (1985). Human fossils from the North African Middle Pleistocene and the origin of Homo sapiens. In E. Delson (Ed.), *Ancestors: The hard evidence* (pp. 283–288). New York: Alan R. Liss Inc.
James, W. (1984). Pragmatism. In B. Kukclick (Ed.), *William James: Writings 1902–1910* (pp. 479–624). New York: Literary Classics of the United States.
Knudson, K. J., & Stojanowski, C. M. (2008). New directions in bioarchaeology: Recent contributions to the study of human social identities. *Journal of Archaeological Research, 16*, 397–432.
Knüsel, C. J. (1999). Orthopaedic disability: Some hard evidence. *Archaeological Review from Cambridge, 15*, 31–53.
Le Pichon, X. (2009). *Ecce Homo ('Behold humanity')*. Retrieved from http://www.onbeing.org/program/fragility-and-evolution-our-humanity/feature/ecce-homo-behold-humanity/1561. Accessed 15 June 2015.
Lordkipanidze, D., Vekua, A., Ferring, R., Rightmire, G. P., Agusti, G., Kiladze, G., et al. (2005). The earliest toothless hominin skull. *Nature, 434*, 717–718.
Mallet, R., & Runswick-Cole, C. (2014). *Approaching disability: Critical issues and perspectives*. New York: Routledge.
Mennear, D. (2013). Interview with Lorna Tilley: The 'Bioarchaeology Of Care' methodology. Retrieved from https://thesebonesofmine.wordpress.com/2013/09/10/interview-with-lorna-tilley-on-the-bioarchaeology-of-care-methodology. Accessed 26 June 2015.
Merton, R. K. (1942). The normative structure of science. In N. Storer (Ed.), *The Sociology of Science: Theoretical and Empirical Investigations* (pp. 267–268). Chicago: University of Chicago Press.
Metzler, I. (1999). The paleopathology of disability in the middle ages. *Archaeological Review from Cambridge, 15*, 55–67.
Oliver, M. (1996). *Understanding disability: From theory to practice*. Macmillan: Basingstoke.
Putnam, H. (1979). *Reason, truth and history*. Cambridge: Harvard University Press.
Renfrew, J. M. (2009). Neanderthal symbolic behaviour? In C. Renfrew & I. Morley (Eds.), *Becoming human: Innovation in prehistoric material and spiritual culture* (pp. 50–60). Cambridge: Cambridge University Press.
Roberts, C. (1999). Disability in the skeletal record: Assumptions, problems and some examples. *Archaeological Review from Cambridge, 15*, 79–97.
Roca, M. G., Jiménez-Brobeil, S., Oumaoui, I. A., Tiristán, J. M., & Fernando, M. (2012). Approach to disability in a population from the Argar Culture. *Trabajos de Prehistoria, 69*(1), 162–170.
Shakespeare, T. (1999). Commentary: Observations on disability and archaeology. *Archaeological Review from Cambridge, 15*(2), 99–101.
Shakespeare, T. (2006a). *Disability rights and wrongs*. London/New York: Routledge.
Shakespeare, T. (2006b). The social model of disability. In L. J. Davis (Ed.), *The disability studies reader* (2nd ed., pp. 197–204). New York: Routledge.
Siebers, T. (2006). Disability in theory: From social constructionism to the new realism of the body. In L. J. Davis (Ed.), *The disability studies reader* (2nd ed., pp. 173–183). New York/London: Routledge.
Silk, J. B. (1992). The origins of caregiving behavior. *American Journal of Physical Anthropology, 87*(2), 227–229.
Smith, S. R. (2009). Social justice and disability: Competing interpretations of the medical and social models. In K. Kristiansen & T. Tom Shakespeare (Eds.), *Arguing about disability: Philosophical perspectives* (pp. 15–29). New York: Routledge.
Solecki, R. S. (1971). *Shanidar: The first flower people*. New York: Knopf.
Southwell-Wright, W. A. (2013a). Past perspectives: What can archaeology offer disability studies? In K. Arndt & M. Wappett (Eds.), *Emerging perspectives on disability studies* (pp. 67–97). New York: Palgrave Macmillan.

Southwell-Wright, W. A. (2013b). Past perspectives: What can archaeology offer disability studies? In K. Arndt & M. Wappett (Eds.), *Emerging perspectives on disability studies* (pp. 67–97). New York: Palgrave Macmillan.

Spikins, P. A., Rutherford, H. E., & Needham, A. P. (2010). From hominity to humanity: Compassion from the earliest archaics tomodern humans, time and mind. *The Journal of Archaeology Consciousness and Culture, 3*(3), 303–325.

Tarlow, S. (2000). Emotion in archaeology. *Current Anthropology, 41*, 713–746.

Thomas, C. (1999). *Female forms: Experiencing and understanding disability*. Buckingham: Open University Press.

Tilley, L. (2012). The bioarchaeology of care. Invited essay for 'Special forum: New directions in bioarchaeology. *The SAA Archaeological Record, 12*, 39–41.

Tilley, L. (2015a). Accommodating difference in the prehistoric past: Revisiting the case of Romito 2 from a bioarchaeology of care perspective. *International Journal of Paleopathology, 8*, 64–74.

Tilley, L. (2015b). *Theory and practice in the bioarchaeology of care*. New York: Springer.

Tilley, L., & Cameron, T. (2014a). Introducing the index of care: A web-based application supporting archaeological research into health-related care. *International Journal of Paleopathology, 6*, 5–9.

Tilley, L., & Cameron, T. (2014b). The index of care. Retrieved from http://www.indexofcare.org/. Accessed 18 June 2015.

Tilley, L., & Oxenham, M. F. (2011). Survival against the odds: Modeling the social implications of care provision to seriously disabled individuals. *International Journal of Paleopathology, 1*, 35–42.

Toyne, J. M. (2015). Tibial surgery in ancient Peru. *International Journal of Paleopathology, 8*, 29–35.

Tremain, S. (1998). Feminist approaches to naturalizing disabledbodies or, does the social model of disablement rest upon amistake?, *Paper presented at Annual Meeting of the Society for Disability Studies*. Oakland, CA.

Trinkaus, E. (1983). *The Shanidar Neandertals*. London: Academic.

Union of the Physically Impaired Against Segregation (UPIAS). (1976). *Fundamental principles of disability*. London: UPIAS.

Vehmas, S., & Mäkelä, P. (2009). The ontology of disability and impairment: A discussion of the natural and social features. In K. Kristiansen & T. Tom Shakespeare (Eds.), *Arguing about disability: Philosophical perspectives* (pp. 42–56). New York: Routledge.

Walker, A., Zimmerman, M. R., & Leakey, R. E. F. (1982). A possible case of hypervitaminosis A in Homo erectus. *Nature, 296*, 248–250.

Wittgenstein, L. J. (1969). *On certainty*. Oxford: Blackwell.

World Health Organization. (1980). *WHO International Classification of Impairments, Disabilities, andHandicaps(ICIDH)*. Retrievedfromhttp://whqlibdoc.who.int/publications/1980/9241541261_eng.pdf. Accessed 20 June 2015.

World Health Organization. (2001). *WHO International Classification of Functioning, Disability and Health (ICF)*. Retrieved from http://www.who.int/classifications/icf/en/. Accessed 20 June 2015.

Chapter 18
Highlighting the Importance of the Past: Public Engagement and Bioarchaeology of Care Research

David Joseph Mennear

Good bioarchaeological research requires the bioarchaeologist to frame questions to suit the archaeological record and with a good grasp of theoretical insights in order for the study to appeal to both anthropologists and archaeologists and the wider public …

(Christopher Knüsel, quoted in Stojanowski & Duncan, 2015, p. 51).

Introduction

The bioarchaeology of care methodology represents a fundamental shift towards understanding the concept and practicalities of caregiving in the bioarchaeological record from both the humanistic and the scientific perspective. It has helped highlight practices of caregiving in historic and prehistoric contexts, drawing on evidence from osteological remains and their archaeological contexts. Furthermore, since the publication of the Neolithic Vietnamese case study of M9 (Tilley & Oxenham, 2011), the methodology has received significant media attention, and the general public's response to this reveals a sustained interest both in understanding the implications of caregiving in archaeological contexts and in learning more about bioarchaeology as a discipline more generally.

This chapter examines the remarkable rise of public engagement and communication within archaeology by contextualising the roles of traditional and digital media in the public's understanding of archaeological practice, and it looks at the role of the bioarchaeologist, in particular, in bridging past and current populations. The role of social media, including blogging and the use of Facebook and Twitter, and the assessment of research impact in those areas, is also discussed (de Koning,

D.J. Mennear, M.Sc. (✉)
Author of web-blog These Bones of Mine, consultant bioarchaeologist, Hartlepool, United Kingdom
e-mail: thesebonesofmine@hotmail.com

© Springer International Publishing Switzerland 2017

L. Tilley, A.A. Schrenk (eds.), *New Developments in the Bioarchaeology of Care*, Bioarchaeology and Social Theory, DOI 10.1007/978-3-319-39901-0_18

2013; Meyers Emery & Killgrove, 2015; Stojanowski & Duncan, 2015). A particular area of interest that continues to define archaeological engagement with social media pertains to defining archaeological authority on the web (Perry & Beale, 2015; Perry, Shipley, & Osborne, 2015; Richardson, 2014; Stewart, 2015). Ethical guidelines and associated commentaries with regard to the use of social media are discussed as an integral feature of bioarchaeological research in general, and updated guidelines reflecting the impact of the international accessibility of the internet are also considered.

Consideration of two case studies, and their impact upon the public's understanding of the issues surrounding care in the past and the present, brings together the themes discussed in this chapter. The conclusion of the chapter raises salient points from these case studies and suggests best practice guidelines for engaging the public via traditional and digital media, and the value inherent in doing so. The bioarchaeology of care methodology represents a new beginning in recognising the evidence for caregiving activity as experienced by individuals in the archaeological record. However, it is important to examine the context in which the methodology originated to understand just *why* it is critically needed in the discipline, and owhat benefits it offers the researcher.

The Context for Research into Past Caregiving

Palaeopathology is a specialist sub-discipline of biological anthropology that focuses on the scientific study of the evolution and manifestation of disease in past populations and past individuals. While bioarchaeology (and in particular the bioarchaeology of care) draws heavily on palaeopathology, it is not synonymous with the latter, but a growing field of study that incorporates content and approaches from a wide range of disciplines in the contextualised analysis of behaviour from human remains. Recent research and new scientific applications have highlighted just how far bioarchaeology has come in the past few decades (see Hawkey, 1998; Inskip et al., 2015; Marstellar, Torres-Rouff, & Knudson, 2011 for case studies utilising interdisciplinary approaches, Martin, Harrod, & Pérez, 2014; Roberts, 2000, 2002 for bioarchaeological and palaeopathological manuals).

Any analysis of caregiving in the past must first examine the evidence for pathological changes to the skeleton (Aufderheide & Roderíquez-Martin, 1998), attempt to identify the disease responsible through a differential diagnoses (Brothwell, 2010), and then consider the possible impact(s) of the pathology on the health and functional fitness of the individual during their life, in the context of the archaeological evidence available. Dettwyler (1991), in a widely cited article, led the charge in arguing that care could not be established from the archaeological record, doubtless unintentionally understating the severity of aspects of the pathologies present in the case study examples used to support this point (see Tilley, 2015b, p. 45); she also suggested that archaeologists who claimed to identify 'care and compassion in the past' were guilty of cultural bias in their conclusions. Recent studies have challenged her conclusions, attempting an holistic life reconstruction by contextualising individuals within the archaeological record and, in this way, identifying situations in which some form of long-term care was likely needed for survival (Marstellar et al., 2011; Tilley, 2015a; Vilos, 2011).

Two important, integrative methodological approaches have significantly improved diagnoses (and our understanding of these) in palaeopathological analysis of skeletal remains in recent decades – osteobiography and biocultural analysis (see Larsen, 1997, 2002; Martin et al., 2014). Osteobiography focuses on the individual's life course, examining their remains and recorded physiological stresses and trauma within their archaeological contexts, to produce an informed narrative of what their experienced life was like (Boutin, 2012). The biocultural approach, which emphases the 'interactions between biology and culture in the disease processes', takes into account the cultural and noncultural stressors that affect a population, and is modelled appropriately within the biological and ecological context (Martin et al., 2014, p. 10). Focusing on the buffers and stressors present at any one time (as evidenced in the archaeology) allows examination of the causes of physiological stress manifested in bone.

The idea of the physically impaired, or disabled, being used as proxies for social attitudes for the vulnerable and weak in society should be used with caution, however. Significant historical studies of disability, including general studies on the changing Western conception of disability and impairment (Stiker, 1999), more culturally specific focused studies (Metzler, 2006), and the deeply personal sociological contextualisation of one's own disability (Oakley, 2007), illustrate that conceptualisations of disability differ across social and cultural contexts, and this raises implications for the consideration of care in the past. The evidence for compassion, especially in a human evolutionary context, remains difficult to quantify or qualify; however, evidence for caregiving can be confidently inferred in instances where the individual survived past a stage of severe physical impairment and where, without care, it is likely the individual would have perished (Tilley, 2015a; Tilley & Oxenham, 2011).

The topic of 'disability and care' has become a focus of interest for anthropologists, bioarchaeologists and palaeoanthropologists over the past two decades. This has, in part, been heavily influenced by the ability of researchers to use a variety of integrative approaches to investigate the physical remains of our past human and hominin populations, but also to the increased interest in the subject matter itself. One particular reason for this is more pragmatic. The World Health Organisation indicates that more than one billion people around the world today experience a disability in some form, with 200 million experiencing considerable difficulties in functioning (2011, p. xi). Disability is used as an umbrella term covering a complex phenomenon that reflects the interaction between the features of an individual's body and features of the society in which he or she lives, with the World Health Organisation defining it as a product of this interaction, rather than an attribute of the person, which hinders their full and effective participation in society (2011, p. 4). With an ageing global population, and the accompanying increased risk of both mental and physical impairment with old age, the subject of disability is of growing importance to health and social organisations (Crews, 2003). In this context, examining the various ways in which people have responded to disability in the past – including in the prehistoric past – may help to transform social beliefs and behaviours in the present. It is recognised that disability models theorised today (such as the social, medical and bio-psycho-social models) need to be carefully contextualised within their physical and cultural environment when applied to the real world (World Health Organisation, 2011). A bioarchaeological methodology that encompasses contextual variables when assessing the implications of physical impairment in the archaeological record therefore provides a bridge between the archaeological past and the present.

The Bioarchaeology of Care Methodology and the Online Index of Care Application

The bioarchaeology of care methodology, together with its non-prescriptive online Index of Care application, offers a structured case-study driven framework for identifying and analysing evidence for caregiving in the bioarchaeological record that is not limited by site, period or culture. It is an analytical and interpretive 4-stage approach (see Tilley, Chap. 2 this volume) that can be applied in any bioarchaeological context where there are human remains displaying evidence suggesting a relatively severe degree of physical impairment, likely necessitating caregiving, was present during the individual's lifetime. Perhaps most importantly, the method can be applied to either newly excavated remains *or* to remains already reported in the archaeological literature – the latter allowing for a re-examination of previous conclusions reached in determining the likelihood of caregiving (Tilley, 2015b).

Mays (2012) notes that the case study is still a dominating factor within palaeopathological studies, but the bioarchaeology of care methodology could, within reason, be used within biocultural studies of past populations to elucidate evidence of compassion and caregiving on a much larger scale. The limitations of palaeopathology should not be understated (Roberts, 2000, p. 46), but new techniques allow potential for a greater scrutiny of the lived experience of the individual as never before. The bioarchaeology of care methodology, used with the internationally accessible Index of Care application, allows for a framework that can be applied to any historic or prehistoric context and, if used with other approaches (aDNA and stable light isotope analysis), allow for a greater holistic investigation and discussion of physical impairment in a wide range of archaeological contexts (Craig & Craig, 2011; Inskip et al., 2015). Marstellar et al. (2011), for instance, have successfully integrated palaeopathological data, including biomolecular approaches, with archaeological data to understand the social context of those experiencing the effects of leishmaniasis in a Pre-Colombian Andean population. The bioarchaeology of care offers an advancement in both conceptualising physical impairment and recognising that there are different cultural approaches used in caregiving and compassion through the temporal-geographic span of humanity's history.

Vampires, Plagues Pits and Timeless Lovers: Traditional and Digital Media

Never has there been a better time to be involved with bioarchaeological research than the present for the sheer range of methodological and practical applications in examining and redefining past human populations and their behaviours (Larsen, 1997; Lewis, 2007; Martin et al., 2014). The discipline stands at an important junction, where the combined, and continual, improvements in the hard sciences (in ancient DNA analysis, 3D imaging, application and refinement of biogeochemical techniques and improved palaeopathological diagnoses) and in the social sciences (a more reflexive approach to the discipline and a new generation of researchers focused on public outreach and engagement) make it possible for bioarchaeology to be a truly interdisciplinary field. Bioarchaeology has the unique ability to help us to understand human behaviour in a deep time and cross-cultural perspective (Martin et al., 2014, p. 1), and traditional and digital media have helped develop the public's awareness of its potential. However, there is still much to do in this regard, and today's researchers need to have a long-term commitment to improving public communication if they want to improve general understanding both of bioarchaeology and of the inherent value of supporting bioarchaeological research (Killgrove, 2015).

Archaeology as a topic has always been of interest to the media, particularly where the physical remains of past populations are concerned (Larsen, 2002). This is even more the case if the individual can be identified (such as in the opening and exploration of the luxurious tomb of Tutankhamen in 1922) or if there are so-called deviant burial practices evidenced (such as plague pits and mass burials, or the so-called *Vampire burials* in Eastern Europe, which have recently been reanalysed) (Gray, 2014). These reports are often anomalies, though, and other than specialist magazines (such as British Archaeology and Current Archaeology) no traditional media outlet routinely reports on archaeological or bioarchaeological research. The physical body is one of the most emotive artefacts of the past – it humanises the past to a modern audience, who can instantly relate to the human body (Sofaer, 2006); possibly reflecting this, archaeological human remains are also a main focus of illegal trade in antiquities, although this is rarely acknowledged in the popular press (Huffer & Chappell, 2014). Action within the digital media landscape is fundamentally more social due to the ease of instant response; however, bioarchaeology had no truly international platform on established media outlets until Kristina Killgrove started blogging bioarchaeology for Forbes in May 2015 (Killgrove, 2015). It can be said, with some degree of confidence, that the online social media representation of bioarchaeology (largely through personal blogs and group blogs) is helping to change the face of traditional media reporting of bioarchaeological subjects and techniques, driven specifically by public engagement and communication (de Koning, 2013).

Public Engagement and Communication: The Rise of Social Media

Archaeologists and anthropologists have, in general, been quick to use social media sites such as Facebook and Twitter to advertise their research, companies and projects (Richardson, 2013; Stewart, 2015), and various organisations regularly use a Facebook site to update their audience on news, jobs and studies in archaeology (group titles such as BioAnthropology News has over 14,000 members, whilst Paleopathology has over 4000 members from across Europe and beyond). A new trend in archaeology in the United Kingdom has seen the rise of community archaeology units such as Elmet Archaeology or Dig Ventures, which operate on a note-for-profit basis and raise funds for projects using online public engagement sites such as Kick Starter, GoFundMe and Just Giving. These groups often make intensive use of a range of social media sites to inform project backers and the public on the results of their research and of outreach open days.

The blogging format, often defined as discrete individual posts of information using text, pictures or video, has also been widely used within the archaeology sector as a way of promoting and encouraging active engagement with the public, and as a tool to improve the communication and writing skills of the blogger themselves (Austin, 2014, p. 10). Bioarchaeology in particular has had a small, but strong, showing, with early career researchers using blogs to promote knowledge of human skeletal anatomy and bioarchaeological techniques (see Meyers Emery & Killgrove, 2015 for an in-depth discussion of the sites which regularly post content). It is worth briefly mentioning the main sites here as they are particularly effective in public engagement and communication of the importance of bioarchaeology (Table 18.1).

The sites above represent the most visited, active and recognised of the current crop of bioarchaeological blogging sites online as identified in the recent literature discussing online representation of the discipline and evidence of citation in academic journals and manuals (de Koning, 2013; Martin et al., 2014; Meyers Emery & Killgrove, 2015; Stojanowski & Duncan, 2015). A specific feature of the bioarchaeology blogs is that they are often produced by an individual acting alone rather

Table 18.1 Popular bioarchaeological blogging sites and the authors responsible for these

Powered By Osteons (poweredbyosteons.org), by Dr Kristina Killgrove, a blog focused on classical bioanthropology and public presentation of bioarchaeology, such as Bones
Bones Don't Lie (bonesdontlie.com), by doctoral candidate Katy Meyers Emery, a blog focused on mortuary and funerary archaeology which also discusses current practice and reviews academic articles
Bone Broke (bonebrokeblog.wordpress.com), by doctoral candidate Jess Beck, a blog focused on human osteology, bioarchaeology and pedagogical techniques
These Bones of Mine (thesebonesofmine.wordpress.com), by the author [David Mennear], a blog focused on human osteology, archaeology and bioarchaeology. Often highlights opportunities, such as workshops or short courses, for researchers and the public alike
Deathsplanation (deathsplaining.wordpress.com), by doctoral candidate Alison Atkin, a blog focused on issues in academia, employment and medieval bioarchaeology

than on behalf of an institution. While this is a direct reflection of their authors' dedication to extra-curricular activity, research groups and universities are now starting to recognise the importance of engaging a larger public audience online for often specialised research topics (Austin, 2014; Bertram & Katti, 2013). No satisfactory quantitative measure of blogs activity is currently recognised, with the exception of overall daily, weekly or monthly visitor statistics – but these can be impressive, as *Bones Don't Lie* by Katie Emery Meyer and *Powered By Osteons* by Kristina Killgrove, as well as my own site, *These Bones of Mine*, testify, with each receiving between 3000 and 6000 site visits per week (Meyers Emery & Killgrove, 2015). This author's blogging site, *These Bones of Mine*, has received a total of 1.5 million views since its beginning in 2011 (statistics at 17 June 2016), indicating that there is a large and sustained public interest in the fields of archaeology, bioarchaeology and heritage more generally.

The social media and digital representation of bioarchaeology, and archaeology more generally, has undergone regular review in relation to the research impact and effectiveness of this mode of public communication in the academic sphere (de Koning, 2013; Meyers Emery & Killgrove, 2015; Perry & Beale, 2015; Stojanowski & Duncan, 2015), with critical analysis of digital authority being regularly questioned and discussed (Perry et al., 2015; Richardson, 2013, 2014). Richardson, for example, raises the integral question of how researchers, or indeed students, should write about their chosen topic online when she asks 'how do we, as a discipline, converse with non-archaeologists through these Internet technologies, with relevance and academic rigour, and in a language that we can all understand?' (2013, p. 8). Although some academic researchers have been scathing of blogging, and microblogging in particular, use of current online platforms is where the most in-depth and direct form of communication with the wider public can take place within an active dialogue (Stojanowski & Duncan, 2015).

There are difficulties with assessing the content of online digital media, particularly of blog content, as no standardised methodology is currently recognised for measuring impact. Perry and Beale (2015), for instance, have highlighted the often turbulent nature of online content, both in its presentation and in its accoutrements, whilst Stewart (2015) has tried to quantitatively and qualitatively assess the impact of academic communication via Twitter. Both studies cited earlier have demonstrated the relative un-preparedness of, and the methodological difficulties faced by, research bodies and academic institutions in assessing the impact of public communication of research, in comparison to the relatively straightforward application of the standardised indices used by universities to quantify research project outcomes and the research impact of individuals (the so called *h-index*, individual indicators of research impact factors and, in the United Kingdom, the assessment of the Research Excellence Framework system) (Perry & Beale, 2015; Stewart, 2015).

Social media has also enabled the researcher to supplement and/or circumvent the traditional routes of academic publishing in journals and monographs, allowing direct uploads to 'free-to-join and use' sites such as Academia.edu, which boasts 38.5 million users who have uploaded over thirteen million academic papers, or alternatively ResearchGate.net, which boasts over 9 million users (statistics from sites' homepages at 17 June 2016). Alternatively there are also open access journals, which allow the viewing of research articles and reviews for free or for a limited time (see *Internet Archaeology* or the *AP Online Journal of Public Archaeology* for instance, both peer reviewed archaeological journals based online). Projects, such as the *Show Us Your Research*! website, set-up by the University of Coimbra and the University of Algarve in Portugal, encourage researchers to disseminate the results of anthropological projects (with a heavy focus on bioarchaeology) to the public, limiting jargon used and clearly explaining the aims, conclusions and impact of their work in short 500 word abstracts (Campanacho, Pereira, & Nunes, 2015).

What is interesting to note is that not many of the active bloggers have discussed either the impact of disability and physical impairment on individuals or long-term caregiving in the bioarchaeological record, barring Alison Atkin on her site at *Deathsplanation* (Atkin, 2015) and on my own site at *These Bones of Mine* (Mennear, 2011). This is likely a reflection of personal interest rather than a specific avoidance of the topic, however. The importance of social media, then, is recognised in its great variety and outreach – the examples cited earlier and the ongoing popularity of archaeology in traditional media formats (such as *Time Team* on television in both the UK and the US) indicate that there is an audience for archaeological and bioarchaeological outreach, one that is substantial, engaging and forward thinking. Ethics plays a fundamental part in this, especially in the context of presenting the methods and results of the discipline to the public, where situations involving human remains are complex, fluid and often confusing due to numerous legal conventions and religious beliefs across the globe (Huffer & Chappell, 2014; White & Folkens, 2005, p. 24).

Ethics in Communicating Bioarchaeology

First and foremost it is recognised here that each bioarchaeological project will be unique; and that in certain circumstances bioarchaeologists will work on projects with, or for, clients who may explicitly prohibit the publication of the research undertaken, or dictate when, how and where the information is released. This 'moral contract' between the bioarchaeologist and their first public audience, i.e. the client, may have to be renegotiated with every project undertaken. However, wherever possible, communication of research intent and findings can be used to engender greater engagement by interested parties – such as the general public, local heritage and educational groups – and should be encouraged in the initial stage of archaeology project design.

As bioarchaeologists we are in a unique position to investigate and analyse the physical remains of humans from a wide variety of prehistoric and historic contexts, but we are not the only group interested in their treatment. Nor is it correct to assume that, just because we have ethical guidelines in our professional codes of conduct, such as the Vermillion Accord on Human Remains agreed in the 1989 World Archaeology Congress (WAC), we have the final say in the analysis, curation and deposition of said remains (Huffer & Chappell, 2014). There are many legal, ethical and moral implications of working with human remains in bioarchaeological contexts and these can change dependent on situation and context of analysis. These can include, but are certainly not limited to, the claims of descendent and indigenous populations, specifications of legal permits for excavation and re-internment, research aims and reasons for examination, and/or religious or ethical considerations (Sayer, 2012). This is aptly demonstrated in the United States of America by the forging of the Native American Graves Protection and Repatriation Act (NAGPRA) in 1990 and its more recent legal amendments, which has led to greater communication between the aims of the bioarchaeologists and the consultation between, and communication with, the descendants as a priority. NAGPRA has also demonstrated its inherent value, redefining basic protocols by establishing best practice conduct and codifying the requirement to work with tribal representatives and legislative bodies (Martin et al., 2014, p. 24).

As well as the introduction of NAGPRA in the United States and the WAC Vermillion Accord, there have been a number of important professional practice guidelines containing statements of ethical behaviour as set out by various associations and institutions across the world. These include the guidelines for practitioners and the legal framework in which bioarchaeologists practice by in the United Kingdom by the British Association of Biological Anthropology and Osteoarchaeology and by the Chartered Institute of Archaeology. However, Sayer (2012, p. 137) rightly highlights the problems with the phrasing and terminology in such agreements and the fact that such best practice guidelines can be difficult to apply internationally. Further to this, Pluciennik (2005, p. 135) indicates the importance of understanding social evolutionary frameworks and ideological foundations for the understanding of the presence of bias in the researcher, the audience and the archaeological record itself. In a public engagement and communication role, it is vital that bioarchaeologists make clear their ethical and moral obligations towards the study of human remains and, if needed, their own biases. As such this author advocates the method proposed by Martin et al. (2014) – that the practitioner develops an 'ethos that encompasses how to practice an ethical bioarchaeology' (2014, p. 49). That is, an ethos in which the legitimate concerns of various groups are recognised and which leads the practitioner to engage with members of such groups as appropriate in an ethical, engaged manner, remaining flexible and adaptable as needed.

Thus, the desirable outcomes for ethical communication and engagement in bioarchaeology must include respect and sensitivity for the aims and outcomes of the project in analysing osteological material from archaeological contexts. This includes the presentation and representation of the project in traditional and digital media formats, especially so when using social media to communicate the importance and, ultimately, the aim of the research undertaken. An understanding of the target audience, including the use of terminology and explanation of the nomenclature used, should be considered, as should the appropriate use of photographic images. In the following case studies, the issues discussed earlier are grounded within their bioarchaeology of care context, indicating the interest of the public and the value of reinterpreting the evidence for care itself in bioarchaeological contexts.

Case Study Examples

Case Study 1: Introducing the Bioarchaeology of Care Methodology with the Analysis of Man Bac Burial 9, Neolithic Vietnam

This first case study describes the public's interest in research focused on physically impairment in the past, but also discusses the duties that researchers should consider in the presentation and dissemination of their work. The publication of the case study of Man Bac Burial 9 (M9), an adult male with juvenile onset quadriplegia (a complication of Klippel-Feil Syndrome type III, which left him paralysed from the waist down, with limited mobility of the upper body), discussed the functional aspects of the pathology and the daily care that this individual needed to live from childhood to his age at death (20–30 years old) (Tilley & Oxenham, 2011, p. 35, see Chap. 2, this volume). M9 needed integrated, complex, continuous and dedicated care, given in an integrated manner, to preserve his life, and the researchers speculate that this likely reflected the cultural values of his society (Tilley & Oxenham, 2011, p. 40).

The case study of M9 also signalled a sea change (following Dettwyler, 1991; Battles, 2011) in the archaeological approach to caregiving, by launching an heuristic methodology in the form of the bioarchaeology of care. This methodology allows for the construction of narratives built around the lifestyles of physically impaired individuals, based on the defensible interpretation from the bioarchaeological evidence. It was only upon Tilley's (2012) report in the Society of American Archaeology journal that the research, from Tilley and Oxenham (2011), was picked up by the public media. The *New York Times* profile of Tilley's research, which was widely circulated internationally, was particularly effective in arousing public interest (Gorman, 2012). The case study and the methodology was also discussed and debated in a number other media outlets (such as America's ABC News website and Australia's Mercatornet website) and on personal blogging sites (such as *These Bones of Mine*), where supportive comments were left by a wide range of organisations and individuals; a sample in the text box below, taken from Tilley (2015b), illustrates the content of some of these.

Text Box 18.1 A selection of comments from online sites from around the world following the article focusing on Man Bac 9, *New York Times*, December 2012 (Taken from Tilley, 2015b, pp. 295–297).

> A comment on the Atheist Universe blog, from Adriana, highlights: *I love it when science allows us a respite from ugly human behaviors such as violence and lets us focus and rejoice on wonderful facts. In this case, archaeology combined with pathological examination of… human remains, puts [forward] evidence that compassion and caring have been with our species for a very,*

(continued)

very long time, even back in the days when life was supposed to be a constant battle for survival, where survival of the fittest was supposed to be all that our species could muster. (http://atheistuniverse.net/group/thenakedape/forum/topics/compassion-and-caring-evidenced-by-archeology-and-paleopathology). Social justice advocates were quick to respond to the article on M9, with Kristina Chew's observations on the 'CARE2 (make a difference)' website representative of many views expressed: *We tend to think that we who live today are 'advanced' in regard to people in the past, especially when it comes to the treatment of the sick and those with disabilities; that, in contrast to an ancient Roman law that a 'dreadfully deformed child shall be quickly killed', we recognize the rights of individuals with disability. But disability rights activists have to routinely refute claims that they are a 'burden to society' and a 'drain' on its resources. We would do well to imitate our prehistoric forbears. I take a great deal of heart in knowing that, eons ago, people cared for those who could not care for themselves.* (http://www.care2.com/causes/ancient-bones-acts-of-kindness-eons-ago.html). Clinical groups were compared the treatment of M9 to the situation of vulnerable patients in modern healthcare systems. The Liverpool Care Pathway for the Dying Patient, a British organisation dealing with palliative care options, noted the 'gross neglect ... [evidenced in] the hundreds of deaths a year' from pressure sores in the United Kingdom; contrasting this to the care inferred for M9, it demands 'what do such examples of [modern] care, or the lack of it, say about the culture that provides it?' (http://liverpool-care-pathway-a-national-sc.blogspot.com.au/2012/12/liverpool-care-pathway-damning.html). Speaking even more directly, the Private Home Care newsletter observed: *We tend to assume that healthcare and provision for the disabled are comparatively recent concepts, reflecting a linear progression from savagery to sympathy. ... We regard the [British] National Health Service, rightly, as a mark of civilisation in contrast to systems where healthcare depends on geography, luck or money. ... Human history tends to focus on episodes of cruelty and violence, but it may be that empathy was also central to early human life. ... In prehistory, the nurse may have been just as important a figure as the fighter and hunter. As the recession forces ever more difficult choices over the funding of care for the vulnerable, it is worth recalling that we have not invented care in the community, but returned to it.* (http://www.privatehomecare.ie/news-d.asp?ART_ID=236).

It is clear that the M9 study had an emotional impact that resonated with the public – a voice was given to an individual who had survived for a decade with the assistance of his community, in an age where, without sustained and daily caregiving, he surely would have died from his condition. As Tilley (2015b) rightly states, where community-based responses to bioarchaeological research are forthcoming, these can be original and constructive, leading to new questions for, and new approaches to, the archaeological record.

Further to this it is clear that active engagement by the researcher also plays an important part in driving the research into the public and academic domain. Tilley took part in an in-depth interview with this author for *These Bones of Mine* (Mennear, 2013), which detailed the bioarchaeology of care methodology for both public and academic audiences, calling for engagement and testing of the methodology. This cannot be stressed enough. If bioarchaeologists are to have a tangible and lasting impact with their work on disability and care they need to look beyond the confines of their discipline, and engage with both the public and academics in allied fields to create a modern discourse which seeks to understand caregiving within a variety of cultural contexts. Tresgaskis (2000) and Phillips and Creighton (2010) indicate that there is a substantial interest in understanding physical impairment and disability attitudes in an archaeological context, both in the past and in the present, as the comments in the text box earlier demonstrate. If engaged with, either directly and/or through traditional and digital social media, it is evident that the public have an active interest in the representations of disability and what past experiences of this state can mean for our current understandings of physical impairment and care (Tilley, 2015b). The case of M9 has clearly demonstrated that when bioarchaeology of care research is communicated in a way that makes it accessible to all it can influence modern public discourse.

Case Study 2: Revisiting the Past: The Bioarchaeology of Care Methodology Applied to Romito 2, Upper Palaeolithic Italy

The case of M9 heralded the arrival of the bioarchaeology of care, but it is the study of Romito 2 that shows the potential of the methodology to reanalyse the existing literature and, where necessary, reassess the arguments for caregiving (Tilley, 2015a). This latter case also raises clear ethical issues in relation to both the communication of knowledge between researchers and the (physical) ownership of skeletal remains. During her research it became apparent to Tilley that Romito 2, a probable male aged 17–20 years old at death who dated from a Final Epigravettian (11,000–12,500 BP) hunter-gatherer culture, presented an academic conundrum (Tilley, 2015a, p. 64).

This individual, excavated from the rock shelter site at La Grotta del Romito in the southern Apennine mountain range in Calabria, Italy, 1963, was initially identified as a female by Messeri in 1966 (see Tilley, 2015a, p. 65), then diagnosed with chondrodystrophic dwarfism (acromesomelic dysplasia) by Frayer, Horton, Macchiarelli, and Mussi (1987), who reclassified the individual as a male (see Tilley, 2015a, and Chap. 2 this volume). As the earliest known case of dwarfism in the human skeletal record, Frayer et al. (1987, p. 60) concluded that, in the context of the hunter-gatherer economy and lifestyle in mountainous terrain, the survival of Romito 2 to his-age-at-death represented evidence for receipt of care and tolerance for a severely deformed individual. In a critical commentary, Dettwyler (1991) examined the evidence for Romito 2, along with two other prehistoric case studies and, somewhat disingenuously, assessed the likelihood of Romito 2 experiencing disability using modern ethnographic and modern western societal comparisons, without reference to Romito 2's specific lifeways context. On this basis Dettwyler (1991) concluded that his treatment in life and death likely did not represent provision of care, and also implied that Frayer et al. (1987) had overstepped the boundaries of reasonable inference. Caregiving was not the primary interest of Frayer et al.'s research, and Frayer later retracted the conclusion that Romito 2 had received care (Bower, 2002, p. 330). By this point Frayer et al.'s (1987) and Dettwyler's (1991) articles, alongside the contentious issue of who owned the skeletal remains, and access to them, had attracted attention in the media (Bower, 2002; Gould, 1988; Martin, 1988).

Tilley (2015a) explicitly challenged Dettwyler's (1991) conclusion, using the bioarchaeology of care methodology to examine the implications of Romito 2's pathology, and concluding that Romito 2's physical impairment would likely have impacted on his ability to participate in group economic activity at the level of other members of his demographic cohort, suggesting a need for provision of care in the form of 'accommodation'. For the purposes of this chapter, however, it is probably the difficulties encountered in analysing the remains of Romito 2 that are of greater relevance than the research conclusions themselves. To begin with, Frayer et al.'s (1987) analysis of Romito 2, almost 25 years after the initial excavation by Paolo Graziosi uncovered his remains, was hampered by the refusal of the Italian palaeoanthropologist Francesco Mallegni to provide access to certain skeletal elements of Romito 2 retained in his (Mallegni's) possession (Mallegni, 1988; Martin, 1988; see discussion Tilley, 2015a, p. 71). In undertaking the bioarchaeology of care reinterpretation of Romito 2, Tilley made extensive – and uniformly unsuccessful – efforts to obtain more detailed photographic and/or documentary information on the skeletal elements denied to Frayer et al. (Martin, 1988; Tilley, 2015a), with multiple requests in both English and Italian receiving little or no response (Tilley pers. comm. 2014).

Ethically, the lack of access to skeletal elements that form part of the earliest known case of dwarfism in human history does not demonstrate best practice at a professional level. It also inherently limits the opportunities for future analyses using new techniques and methodologies which can reveal new data and generate new insights into the treatment of past individuals. The Romito 2 case also demonstrates the value in revisiting and interrogating existing literature (in this case Dettwyler, 1991; Frayer et al., 1987). This is one of the strengths of the portable (accessible online) Index of Care and the bioarchaeology of care methodology.

The case study of Romito 2 demonstrates some of the practical difficulties that can face researchers in reanalysing the archaeological and osteological evidence (Tilley, 2015a, p. 71). Tilley rightly concludes that 'perhaps, as bioarchaeologist(s), it is time to review, clarify and – if necessary – refine the principles that shape the duty of care we owe our once-living subjects' (2015a, p. 72).

Lessons and Recommendations for Best Practice

It is evident that the skeletal remains of historic and prehistoric populations and individuals remain a potent symbol of a tangible link to humanity's ancestors and of mortality more generally. Caregiving, and the evidence for compassion, is a subject that is close to the heart of humanity – one only needs to realise that rarely are any individuals untouched by immediate family members needing caregiving, be it social, daily and/or medical care; it is a topic which is inherently easy to relate to. As such it is recommended that researchers integrate the archaeological and bioarchaeological evidence between the prehistoric and historical worlds to the present. No discipline is better placed, or more uniquely positioned to do this, than bioarchaeology.

The quality of reporting on archaeological research in newspapers and digital media is generally increasing. For instance, the Daily Mail newspaper (UK) has been roundly mocked, and somewhat fairly so, by some for its representations of bioarchaeological research, and it is renowned for its coverage of archaeological 'vampire' burials from Eastern Europe. However, it does sometimes interview the primary investigators on projects, and further updates readers on new theories and news regarding the archaeological discoveries it reports. In the case of the 'vampire' burials earlier, for example, cholera was subsequently named as the killer of these seventeenth- to eighteenth-century individuals, who had been identified as 'vampires' solely on the basis that they were buried in a non-normative manner (Gray, 2014). In this same article, information boxes helped to make the archaeological terminology understandable to non-specialists, performing an educational service even if the original article was written to shock.

Another example of bioarchaeology slowly becoming a staple of mainstream news is the appointment of Kristina Killgrove, a bioarchaeologist and assistant professor at the University of West Florida and prolific blogger at *Powered by Osteons*, to the Forbes online team to produce content (as often as up to four articles a week) on bioarchaeological topics, many of which have gained thousands of views within a few days of their appearance on the website. Her article on 'Industrial Revolution caused rise in cancer, obesity and arthritis, archaeologists suggest', which discusses the importance of cultural and lifestyle change on the human body and the health impacts that this can have, was published in May 2015 and as of 17 June 2016 had gained a total of 49,916 individual page views (Killgrove, 2015). Her anatomically and factually correct reporting means that the quality of the communication of bioarchaeological topics has increased awareness of bioarchaeological research and its implications for modern populations. Yet what are the suggestions for aspiring bioarchaeology bloggers, microbloggers, communicators and outreach workers with regards to best practice in public engagement and communication? How do we, as practitioners of bioarchaeological research, integrate good communication practices within the discipline?

These are challenging questions for a new and developing digital medium, one that is constantly changing and updating. Both Bertram and Katti (2013) and Meyers Emery and Killgrove (2015) indicate a number of gaps in the current social media representation of bioarchaeology, as well as suggesting a number of approaches that would develop best practices across the social media range. Some of their suggestions are particularly relevant in terms of how, and why, we should consider public engagement (using all media mediums) as a relevant, ethical and productive factor in bioarchaeological research, and these are discussed as follows.

Making Yourself, and Others, Visible

Bioarchaeologists are a tough breed to find online, due to the conflicting terminology used within bioarchaeology and related disciplines. Make your professional online presence visible by clearly defining the focus of your work and by indicating your interests in a clear and informed manner for visitors (Meyers Emery & Killgrove, 2015). It is also recommended that researchers citing digital and social media sites in academic articles, or on other social media applications, should properly reference the authors, title of post, address, and indicate the date accessed, as routine.

Exploit a Variety of Approaches

Vary the approach taken. Videos, for example, are particularly rare phenomena in bioarchaeological outreach, but have the potential to reach a vast audience – much more so than an academic article. It is well known that serialisations (such as Kristina Killgrove's Bones reviews or this author's Skeletal Series posts) keep the reader interested, whilst providing structured content. Joint posts, interviews, guest posts and video entries can also help reach different and varied audiences online and in-print (Bertram & Katti, 2013).

Provide Information on Latest Research and New Techniques

Bioarchaeology uses a range of different techniques, and new methodologies and approaches are also developed every year to investigate the archaeological record. The use of these techniques and methodologies can, and should, be discussed and contextualised in terms of, or in relation to, their use and limitations within the discipline. The majority of bioarchaeological research is published in journals in which the article itself is locked online behind a subscription block, a so-called pay wall, thus preventing interested but non-academic based readers the opportunity to learn about the detail of the latest innovations. Blogs, such as *Bones Don't Lie* by Katy Meyers Emery for example, offer the reader concise summaries of the latest published articles in a timely and free-to-access manner. Edited volumes such as this are out of the reach of the casual reader who lacks access to a specialist research or university-based library.

Try Bi, or Even Trilingual, Entries

The majority of online bioarchaeology social media content is in English. Using a second language (Spanish, Mandarin, Persian or French for example) alongside an English translation would enable readers from different areas of the globe to gain access to the content. This could be achieved through transnational projects and international academic partnerships; for example, sponsored online content or conference workshops, spanning both national and language borders, might investigate ethics 'case studies' or develop ways of promoting research best practice. Benefits would include greater exposure of research to a wider audience, achieving an increased understanding of the importance of this research, alongside the building of ethical frameworks across cultural divides. It could also lead to a more integrated approach to the physical and cultural analysis of osteological material.

Discuss Your Pedagogy and the Dangers of Digital Media

The methods by which anthropology, archaeology and bioarchaeology are taught are rarely discussed on social media sites. A pedagogical approach, such as an introduction to the elements of the human skeleton and the importance of their study, would enable the public and researchers to understand how, and why, the topics are taught in a particular manner, and the expected outcomes of this. For instance, an introduction to the terminology used in osteology designed for the lay public can help to break down the 'ivory tower' view of academia (Buckberry, Ogden, Shearman, & McCleery, 2015). Furthermore, there should be open lectures and discussion at university level alongside engagement on the pros and cons of digital and social media use, including understanding the impacts and dangers of online sexism and trolling (Armstrong & McAdams, 2010). The ethics of public communication should be considered – what are the support frameworks for the digital advocacy of bioarchaeology online?

Define Disability and Highlight Differential Diagnoses

With reference to the bioarchaeology of care methodology, discussion must be focused on the available archaeological and osteological evidence and, where the material evidence is available, the cultural context for the understanding of what a disability would entail (Battles, 2011; Doat, 2013; Spikins, Rutherford, & Needham, 2010). Due to inherent limitations in osteological evidence, a specific disease diagnosis cannot always be determined (Brothwell, 2010). Therefore in bioarchaeology of care analysis differential diagnoses must be included when examining possible disease impacts on function and the need for caregiving. Each candidate diagnosis should be considered, as these may have different effects in different cultural, geographic and economic environments.

Factor Public, Social and Digital Media Engagement into Bioarchaeological Projects

Blogging, microblogging and engaging with newspaper reporters and television producers take time and effort. Factor this into the initial research as a plan of engagement from the beginning. Identify key communication aims and develop strategies for how to achieve these aims over the course of the research project. Do not be afraid to contact bioarchaeology bloggers or other social media users with details of the project that the research team wishes to make public at a given time (this will depend on client or other stakeholder agreement and timing for release of the research via academic journals and conference presentations). Engage with users and produce content that is in line with both professional and personal ethical standards, state possible conflicts of interest if necessary, and, when discussing original research, indicate the funding bodies that have supported the work.

Meyers Emery and Killgrove (2015) indicate a number of best practice suggestions that are pertinent to repeat here. They are: to write for an educated public, to write or produce content regularly, be sensitive to your own bias and the biases of others, and to repudiate the hysteria and hype of the media in a clear, productive and informative approach. There is a responsibility on a part of all bioarchaeologists who partake in public engagement to educate and inform on the standard approaches practiced in bioarchaeology and the ethical considerations that inform this, particularly to counter sensationalism and ethical misconduct. The above are all important aspects that each bioarchaeologist should use in their approach in disseminating and discussing bioarchaeological content and approaches to public audiences.

Considerations for Future Directions

> *The bodies that we're born with, or into, are accidents: unforeseeable chance results of genes, history, time and place. We don't choose our bodies, nor much of what happens to them* (Oakley, 2007, p. 147).

This chapter has highlighted the wider themes of public engagement and communication issues that face the bioarchaeology of care methodology and the online Index of Care application; and it has also demonstrated the remarkable public interest in archaeology, specifically bioarchaeology, as evidenced by public engagement and communication across traditional and digital media platforms (Meyers Emery & Killgrove, 2015; Stojanowski & Duncan, 2015). The case studies have illustrated that such research, once released into the wild, can take on a life of their own and, as the analysis of M9 has demonstrated, can touch the feelings of many individuals from around the world. The case of Romito 2 has demonstrated the importance of re-interrogating previous research assumptions, using new theoretical frameworks and methodological approaches (Tilley, 2015a). This is a serious point to consider as the archaeological record is a finite resource, where the osteological material recovered from excavations is often of a fragile nature and subject to disintegration if not handled and stored correctly. The loss of such evidence is therefore also the loss of the individual from the record. As discussed there are the ethical and cultural concerns that must be accounted for at the onset of any research project that focuses on human skeletal material in an archaeological context. As such the author has suggested, where it is possible, a series of best practice guidelines for dissemination and communication of academic research concerning bioarchaeological projects to a wider audience.

The future of the bioarchaeology of care is rich, but it relies on researchers experimenting with and extending application of the methodology. To this end, workshops to explain and promote the use of the bioarchaeology of care approach and the Index of Care might be run for two distinct audiences: academic and public. The academic workshop would encourage bioarchaeologists to think critically about the nature of physical impairment, individual and group agency, and the importance of differential diagnoses when identifying disease processes evident on skeletal remains. The public engagement workshops could break down the 'white-coat scientist' barrier and bring a more humanistic approach to the archaeological remains of individuals (see Buckberry et al., 2015 for an integrative approach using human remains to inform on modern dietary behaviour in public and academic workshops). Demonstrations of the approach might be particularly effective at museum or education outreach open days, using and including resources already available. Interactive approaches, such as digital case studies or casts of individuals on outreach open days, could be particularly powerful in demonstrating the value of both giving and receiving care.

The author also suggests here that there are two avenues of interest for prospective bioarchaeology of care researchers. The first is the integration of quantitative analysis with the bioarchaeology of care methodology to interrogate the published literature. A case in point is the re-evaluation of the case of Romito 2 (Tilley, 2015b), which has included a perspective on the ethical quandaries surrounding the studying and the retention of human remains in bioarchaeology, and the ramifications, or lack thereof, of communication between researchers more generally.

The second suggestion is that although the bioarchaeology of care methodology is focused on the case study of the individual within their archaeological context, there is a possibility that the approach could be used to interrogate the attitudes towards disability and physical impairment at a population level. If – and only if – certain conditions of the research methodology were met (such as adequate sample size, reasonably well established archaeological context, secure dating, and osteological presentation of same, or similar, disease processes) then application of the bioarchaeology of care to studying caregiving across a cultural episode and discrete time horizon could be envisioned. This might give unprecedented access to identifying compassion in the archaeological record and potentially shed light on differential access to caregiving, for example between individuals within the same cultural group but from different economic classes.

In finishing, it is again pointed out that the public is deeply interested in bioarchaeological research, and that there is a growing audience for informed and incisive bioarchaeological content. Bioarchaeology has much to offer when it comes to a general study of the remains of past populations and individuals, both as biological and social entities (Sofaer, 2006), and the bioarchaeology of care, in particular, provides a means for questioning and informing modern attitudes and behaviours towards those with physical impairments.

Acknowledgments The author wishes to first thank the two editors of the volume, Lorna Tilley and Alecia A. Schrenk for their advice, guidance, patience and friendship in the writing of this chapter. Second, he also wishes to thank the three anonymous reviewers whose suggestions have greatly improved the body of this chapter. Finally, the author wishes to dedicate this chapter to the memory of Holly Philipa Marston, a beloved friend who saw the good in people and the value in helping to conserve the material culture of the past, for present and future generations. The laughter and love of this treasured friendship remains.

References

Armstrong, C. L., & McAdams, M. J. (2010). Believing blogs: Does a Blogger's gender influence credibility? In R. Lind (Ed.), *Race, gender and media* (pp. 30–38). Boston: Pearson.

Atkin, A. (2015). Silence in the cemetery series. *Deathsplanation*. Retrieved from https://deathsplaining.wordpress.com/?s=Silence+in+the+Cemeteryandsubmit=Search. Accessed 19 June 2015.

Aufderheide, A. C., & Roderíquez-Martin, C. (1998). *The Cambridge encyclopaedia of human palaeopathology*. Cambridge: Cambridge University Press.

Austin, M. (2014). Archaeological blogging and engagement. In D. Rocks-Macqueen & C. Webster (Eds.), *Blogging archaeology* (pp. 9–19). Landward Research: Sheffield.

Battles, H. T. (2011). Toward engagement: Exploring the prospects for an integrated anthropology of disability. *Explorations in Anthropology, 11*(1), 107–124.

Bertram, S. M., & Katti, M. (2013). The social biology professor: Effective strategies for social media engagement. *Ideas in Ecology and Evolution, 6*, 22–31.

Boutin, A. T. (2012). Crafting a bioarchaeology of personhood: Osteobiographical narratives from alalakh. In A. Baadsgaard, A. T. Boutin, & J. E. Buikstra (Eds.), *Breathing new life into the evidence of death: Contemporary approaches to bioarchaeology* (pp. 109–133). Santa Fe: School for Advanced Research Press.

Bower, B. (2002). Care-worn fossils. Bones reopen controversy about ancient assistance. *Science Newsletter, 162*, 328–330.

Brothwell, D. (2010). On problems of differential diagnosis in palaeopathology, as illustrated by a case from prehistoric Indiana. *International Journal of Osteoarchaeology, 20*, 621–622.

Buckberry, J., Ogden, A., Shearman, V., & McCleery, I. (2015). You are what you ate: Using bioarchaeology to promote healthy eating. In K. Gerdau-Radonić & K. McSweeney (Eds.), *Trends in Biological Anthropology*. Proceedings of the British Association for Biological Anthropology and Osteoarchaeology (pp. 100–111; vol. 1). Oxford: Oxbow Books.

Campanacho, V., Pereira, T., & Nunes, M. J. (2015). Show us your research! An anthropological and archaeological publication for the greater public. *Palaeopathology Newsletter, 170*, 26.

Craig, E., & Craig, G. (2011). The diagnosis and context of a facial deformity from an Anglo-Saxon Cemetery at Spofforth, North Yorkshire. *International Journal of Osteoarchaeology*.

doi:10.1002/oa.1288. Retrieved November 21, 2011, from http://onlinelibrary.wiley.com/doi/10.1002/oa.1288/full.

Crews, D. E. (2003). *Human senescence: Evolutionary and biocultural perspectives*. Cambridge: Cambridge University Press.

de Koning, M. (2013). Hello world! Challenges for blogging as anthropological outreach. *Journal of the Royal Anthropological Institute, 19*(2), 394–397. doi:10.1111/1467-9655.12040.

Dettwyler, K. A. (1991). Can palaeopathology provide evidence for 'Compassion'? *American Journal of Physical Anthropology, 84*, 375–384.

Doat, D. (2013). Evolution and human uniqueness: Prehistory, disability, and the unexpected anthropology of Charles Darwin. In D. Bolt (Ed.), *Changing social attitudes towards the disabled* (pp. 15–25). London: Routledge.

Frayer, D. W., Horton, W. A., Macchiarelli, R., & Mussi, M. (1987). Dwarfism in an adolescent from the Italian late upper palaeolithic. *Nature, 330*, 60–62.

Gorman, J. (2012). Ancient bones that tell the story of compassion. *New York Times*. Retrieved December 12, 2012, from http://www.nytimes.com/2012/12/18/science/ancient-bones-that-tell-a-story-of-compassion.html?_r=0. Accessed 1 July 2015

Gould, S. J. (1988). Honourable men and women. *Natural History, 97*(3), 16–20.

Gray, R. (2014). Polish 'Vampires' were killed by CHOLERA: Tests reveal suspected bloodsuckers were victims of epidemic. *The Daily Mail*. Retrieved from http://www.dailymail.co.uk/sciencetech/article-2850623/Polish-vampires-killed-CHOLERA-Tests-reveal-suspected-bloodsuckers-actually-early-victims-epidemic.html. Accessed 19 June 2015.

Hawkey, D. E. (1998). Disability, compassion and the skeletal record: Using musculoskeletal stress markers (MSM) to construct an osteobiography from early New Mexico. *International Journal of Osteoarchaeology, 8*, 326–340.

Huffer, D., & Chappell, D. (2014). The mainly nameless and faceless dead: An exploratory study of the illicit traffic in archaeological and ethnographic human remains. *Crime, Law and Social Change*. doi:10.1007/s10611-014-9528-4.

Inskip, S. A., Taylor, G. M., Zakrzewski, S. R., Mays, S. A., Pike, A. W. G., Llewellyn, G., et al. (2015). Osteological, biomolecular and geochemical examination of an early-saxon case of lepromatous leprosy. *PLoS One, 10*(5), e0124282. doi:10.1371/journal.pone.0124282.

Killgrove, K. (2015). Industrial revolution caused rise in cancer, obesity and arthritis, archaeologists suggest. *Forbes*. Retrieved from http://www.forbes.com/sites/kristinakillgrove/2015/05/20/industrial-revolution-caused-rise-cancer-obesity-arthritis/. Accessed 17 June 2016.

Larsen, C. (1997). *Bioarchaeology: Interpreting behaviour from the human skeleton*. Cambridge: Cambridge University Press.

Larsen, C. S. (2002). Bioarchaeology: The lives and lifestyles of past peoples. *Journal of Archaeological Research, 10*(2), 119–166.

Lewis, M. E. (2007). *The bioarchaeology of children: Perspective from biological and forensic anthropology*. Cambridge: Cambridge University Press.

Mallegni, F. (1988). Un episodio di mancanza di etica professionale? *Archivio di Antropologia Criminale, Psichiatria e Medicina Legale, XVIII*, 297–303.

Marstellar, S. J., Torres-Rouff, C., & Knudson, K. J. (2011). Pre-Columbian Andean sickness ideology and the social experience of leishmaniasis: A contextualised analysis of bioarchaeological and palaeopathological data from San Pedro de Atacama, Chile. *International Journal of Palaeopathology, 1*(1), 23–34.

Martin, R. (1988). Dwarf Star. *Explore Summer, 1988*, 12–16.

Martin, D. L., Harrod, R. P., & Pérez, V. R. (2014). *Bioarchaeology: An integrated approach to working with human remains*. London: Springer.

Mays, S. (2012). The impact of case reports relative to other types of publication in palaeopathology. *International Journal of Osteoarchaeology, 22*, 81–85.

Mennear, D. J. (2011). Fibrous dysplasia and McCune Albright syndrome. *These Bones of Mine*. Retrieved from https://thesebonesofmine.wordpress.com/2011/10/28/fibrous-dysplasia-mccune-albright-syndrome/. Accessed 19 June 2015.

Mennear, D. J. (2013). Interview with Lorna Tilley: The bioarchaeology of care methodology. *These Bones of Mine*. Retrieved from https://thesebonesofmine.wordpress.com/2013/09/10/interview-with-lorna-tilley-on-the-bioarchaeology-of-care-methodology/. Accessed 1 July 2015.

Messeri, P. (1966). *Note paleopatologiche sul materiale scheletrico umano rinvenutonella grotta del Romito a Papasidero in Calabria (Cosenza).* Atti X Riunione Sci-entifica dell'Istituto Italiano di Preistoria e Protostoria (pp. 301–307). (Cited Frayer et al. 1987, p. 562).

Metzler, I. (2006). *Disability in medieval Europe: Thinking about physical impairment during the high middle ages, c.1100–1400.* Oxon: Routledge.

Meyers Emery, K., & Killgrove, K. (2015). Bones, bodies, and blogs: Outreach and engagement in bioarchaeology. *Internet Archaeology, 39*. doi:10.11141/ia.39.5.

Oakley, A. (2007). *Fracture: Adventures of a broken body*. Bristol: The Policy Press.

Perry, S., & Beale, N. (2015). The social web and Archaeology's restructuring: Impact, exploitation, disciplinary change. *Open Archaeology, 1*(1), 153–165.

Perry, S., Shipley, L., & Osborne, J. (2015). Digital media, power and (In)Equality in archaeology and heritage. *Internet Archaeology, 38*. doi:10.11141/ia.38.4.

Phillips, T., & Creighton, J. (2010). *Employing people with disabilities: Good practice guidance for archaeologists*. IFA Professional Practice Paper No. 9. Reading: The Institute for Archaeologists.

Pluciennik, M. (2005). *Social evolution. Duckworth debates in archaeology*. London: Gerald Duckworth and Co. Ltd.

Richardson, L. (2013). A digital public archaeology? *Papers from the Institute of Archaeology, 23*(1), 1–12. doi:10.5334/pia.431.

Richardson, L. J. (2014). Understanding archaeological authority in a digital context. *Internet Archaeology, 38*. doi:10.11141/ia.38.1.

Roberts, C. A. (2000). Did they take sugar? The use of skeletal evidence in the study of disability in past populations. In J. Hubert (Ed.), *Madness, disability and social exclusion: The archaeology and anthropology of difference* (pp. 46–59). London: Routledge.

Roberts, C. A. (2002). Palaeopathology and archaeology: The current state of play. In R. Arnott (Ed.), *The archaeology of medicine* (BAR international series, Vol. 1046, pp. 1–20). Oxford: Archaeopress.

Sayer, D. (2012). *Ethics and burial archaeology. Bristol Classical Press debates in archaeology*. London: Bristol Classical Press.

Sofaer, J. R. (2006). *The body as material culture: A theoretical osteoarchaeology*. Cambridge: University of Cambridge Press.

Spikins, P. A., Rutherford, H. E., & Needham, A. P. (2010). From hominity to humanity: Compassion from the earliest archaics to modern humans. *Time and Mind, 3*(3), 303–325.

Stewart, B. (2015). Open to influence: What counts as academic influence in scholarly networked *Twitter* participation. *Learning, Media and Technology*. doi:10.1080/17439884.2015.1015547.

Stiker, H.-J. (1999). *A history of disability*. Ann Arbor: University of Michigan Press.

Stojanowski, C. M., & Duncan, W. N. (2015). Engaging bodies in the public imagination: Bioarchaeology as social science, science, and humanities. *American Journal of Human Biology*.

Tilley, L. (2012). The bioarchaeology of care. *SAA Record, 12*(3). http://onlinedigeditions.com/display_article.php?id=1078681FirefoxHTML\Shell\Open\Command. Accessed 1 July 2015.

Tilley, L. (2014). *Personal communication*. Visiting Fellow, School of Archaeology and Anthropology, Australian National University.

Tilley, L. (2015a). Accommodating difference in the prehistoric past: Revisiting the case of Romito 2 from a bioarchaeology of care perspective. *International Journal of Palaeopathology, 8*, 64–74.

Tilley, L. (2015b). *Theory and practice in the bioarchaeology of care*. New York: Springer.

Tilley, L., & Cameron, T. (2014). Introducing the index of care: A web-based application supporting archaeological research into health-related care. *International Journal of Palaeopathology, 6*, 5–9.

Tilley, L., & Oxenham, M. F. (2011). Survival against the odds: Modelling the social implications of care provision to the seriously disabled. *International Journal of Palaeopathology, 1*(1), 35–42.

Tregaskis, C. (2000). Interviewing non-disabled people about their disability-related attitudes: Seeking methodologies. *Disability and Society, 15*(2), 343–353.

Vilos, J. D. (2011). *Bioarchaeology of compassion: Exploring extreme cases of pathology in a Bronze Age Skeletal Population from Tell Abraq, U. A. E.* Master's Dissertation. Las Vegas: University of Nevada.

White, T. D., & Folkens, P. A. (2005). *The human bone manual*. London: Elsevier Academic Press.

World Health Organisation. (2011). *World report on disability*. Malta: World Health Organisation and the World Bank.

Chapter 19
Conclusion: New Developments in the Bioarchaeology of Care

Jane Buikstra

The bioarchaeology of care appears to be a subject whose time has come, indicated by several measures that will be detailed below. As noted in the introduction to this volume, this topic was first published but 5 years ago (Tilley & Oxenham, 2011) in the first issue of the *International Journal of Paleopathology* (*IJPP*), obviously meant for a professional audience. This paper was picked up quickly by a science writer for the New York Times (Gorman, 2012) and became the subject matter of an extended treatment, which stimulated public interest. The method for constructing the Index of Care, following Tilley's 4 stage schema, was subsequently made freely available on a web site (http://www.indexofcare.org/), and attention called to it once more in the *IJPP* (Tilley & Cameron, 2014). Lorna Tilley, in the meantime, completed her dissertation in 2013, and this has been revised and published (Tilley, 2015).

The bioarchaeology of care has generated enthusiasm and visibility quite rapidly. This volume and the symposium that preceded it at the 2015 annual meeting of the Society for American Archaeology are but one indication. Another is the 2015 Award for the Most Influential Article appearing in the *IJPP* over the preceding 5 years to the Tilley and Oxenham (2011) article, made jointly by the Paleopathology Association, the *IJPP*, and Elsevier. Altmetric Support, a service providing a measure of more general influence, in that social media such as blogs are considered, along with print media and Wikipedia, reports a score for the Tilley and Oxenham (2011) article in the top 5 % of all research outputs that Altmetric scores (Altmetric.com, accessed 10 February, 2016). According to Altmetric, the article has seen a global readership in the UK, US, India, and Australia. Also indicating its broad appeal is the nearly equivalent disciplinary readership distributions across the social sciences, humanities, and biological sciences.

J. Buikstra, Ph.D. (✉)
Center for Bioarchaeological Research, Arizona State University, Tempe, AZ, USA
e-mail: buikstra@asu.edu

© Springer International Publishing Switzerland 2017

L. Tilley, A.A. Schrenk (eds.), *New Developments in the Bioarchaeology of Care*, Bioarchaeology and Social Theory, DOI 10.1007/978-3-319-39901-0_19

Why then, has the bioarchaeology of care gained such traction in five brief years? A quarter century ago, Dettwyler (1991) argued strongly and apparently convincingly against any attempt to infer compassion, quality of life, or degree to which an individual was handicapped in past societies without an ethnographic record. That effectively quashed such discussions until later within the first decade of the twenty-first century when Lorna Tilley, a bioarchaeologist with a background in health care, decided to focus upon a rigorous approach to questions around health care delivery rather than on such issues as compassion, which both she and Dettwyler would agree are inaccessible through bioarchaeological analysis, no matter how detailed.

Tilley focused upon a first stage of rigorous description, both of the observed pathology and of the archaeological context, along with a rigorous differential diagnosis of the disease (Fig. 19.1.) Then the observer is asked to move on (Stage 2) to the medical literature to assess how much impact the physical limitations may have had on daily activities and if long-term accommodation and/or support would have been needed. If support and/or accommodation from others were necessary, then in Stage 3 a model of care is constructed based upon the nature of care required. Finally (Stage 4), the researcher is invited to infer individual and group responses at the social level, including identities as disabled and caregiver(s), respectively. It is important to emphasize that "care" in this context is defined in terms of behavioral support rather than care-as-compassion. Ironically, even though Tilley was quite clear with the New York Times science writer, James Gorman, about the fact that hers was not a model invoking emotional nurturance, the title of Gorman's December 17, 2012, article suggested otherwise, "Ancient Bones That Tell a Story of Compassion."

It should not be surprising to those of us who have weathered the shifting sands of processual, post-processual, postmodern, and post-structural theoretical perspectives as they have influenced anthropology to understand why bioarchaeologists in the second decade of the twenty-first century are more open to a bioarchaeology of care than those only a few decades earlier. We have read post-structuralists such as Foucault, labored to understand Bourdieu's concepts of habitus and doxa, and struggled with inferring ancient identities, such as age, gender, social status, religion, and health – not to mention their intersections.

It was not always so. Human bioarchaeology began explicitly in 1977, referencing the problem-oriented study of past peoples and their societies, population structure, heritage, diet, and health (Buikstra, 1977a). This was born of a confluence of population biology and the "New Archaeology," emphasizing community dynamics. Certainly, there is a much longer history of the study of human remains from archaeological contexts (Buikstra, 2006), but this term soon gained remarkable traction, focused by some upon the study of health and disease (Larsen, 1982, 1987, 1995). There are many bioarchaeological foci now, including the bioarchaeology of children (Lewis, 2009), bioarchaeology and identity (Knudson & Stojanowski, 2009), social bioarchaeology (Agarwal & Glencross, 2011; Tung, 2012), the bioarchaeology of violence (Martin, Harrod, & Pérez, 2012), the bioarchaeology of individuals (Stodder & Palkovich, 2012), isotopic landscapes in bioarchaeology (Grupe & McGlynn, 2015), and, of course, the bioarchaeology of care. Historical bioar-

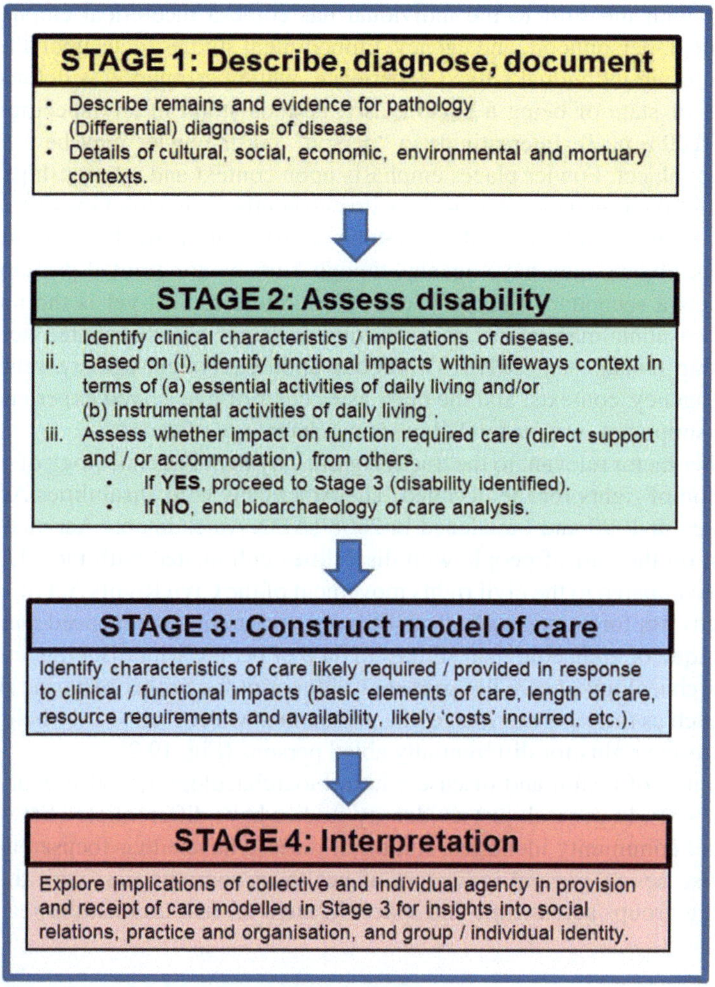

Fig. 19.1 Summary of Stages of Inference (from Tilley, 2013)

chaeology (Perry, 2012; Stojanowski, 2013) and biohistory (Stojanowski & Duncan, 2016) are also closely related.

Another parallel trend is the construction of osteobiographies, *sensu* Saul (1972; Saul & Saul, 1989). As first developed and applied by Frank Saul, the approach was very little different from bioarchaeology. It focused upon first collecting a full biological profile of individual skeletons and then combining these data to provide a picture of the ancient group. Bioarchaeology's focus more directly pertained to collecting only those data relevant to a certain research question, but the net results of study were not so very different. The term "osteobiography" has become refocused, however, to now emphasize the study of individuals, perhaps an unusual individual or context (Robb, 2002; Stodder & Palkovich, 2012).

Along with the shift to the individual has come a theoretical emphasis upon embodiment, personhood, and agency. Embodiment studies focus upon the body as the result of an individual's lived experience, while personhood is defined as "the condition or state of being a person, as it is understood in any specific context" (Fowler, 2004, p. 7). Interestingly, a "person" *sensu* Fowler may be a human or nonhuman object. Fowler places emphasis upon context and relationships between entities and their agency. "Agency" as it is currently understood may be attributed solely to humans and their volition (Robb, 2010). Alternatively, both human and nonhuman objects may have agency, though humans are granted primary agency and objects a secondary agency (Gell, 1998). More radical yet is the notion that human and nonhuman agents assume equivalent agency, distributed across their relationship (Johannsen, 2012). This focus upon equivalent agency, relationships defining agency, contexts, and the body as a center of one's lived experience are all part of a supportive milieu for Tilley's bioarchaeology of care.

Another factor relevant to the traction gained by the bioarchaeology of care is the recognition of rights for the disabled. The Americans with Disabilities Act (ADA) was passed in 1990 and broadened in 2008 (ADA Amendments Act or ADAAA). Activism on the part of people with disabilities culminated with the ADA, which has been compared to the civil rights movement of the Civil Rights Act of 1964. The 1990s activism for people with disabilities appears to have influenced Dettwyler's, 1991 critique of archaeological studies to date of people with disabling conditions. The bioarchaeology of care has provided a blueprint for further restoring rights and voice, much as the vigorous image of a person in a wheel chair is now being used to indicate usage rights for differentially abled persons (Fig. 19.2).

The study of health and disease within bioarchaeology has also evolved since the late 1970s. In general, just as identity studies have differentiated between individual and community identities, studies of disease have either focused upon individual diseases or general indicators of health in communities, with the goal of comparing groups across time and space. Matters of measurement, especially how

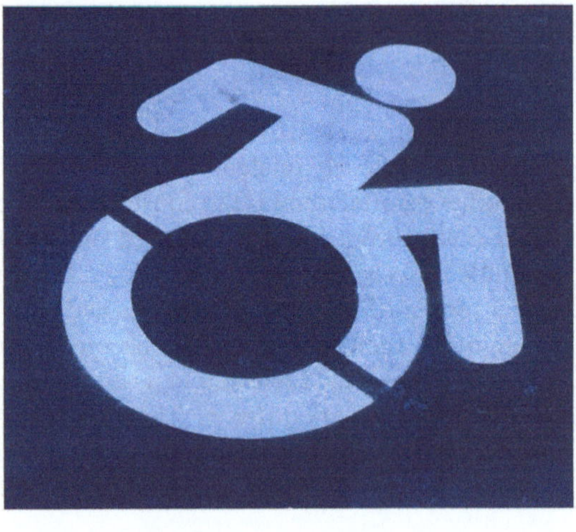

Fig. 19.2 Sign in a parking lot in Tempe, Arizona (photograph by the author)

to develop multivariate health indices (Steckel & Rose, 2002; Steckel, Larsen, Sciulli, & Walker, 2009), remain somewhat problematic.

In fact, the very definition of health itself is extremely difficult to operationalize. The World Health Organization (WHO) still relies upon the 1946 definition that was ratified in 1948 and not amended since. For the WHO (1946 [2], p. 100), "[h]ealth is a state of complete physical, mental and social well-being and not merely the absence of disease or infirmity." One cannot help but wonder if anyone, at any time, has ever been truly healthy under this definition. Is someone with a chronic disability de facto unhealthy? What about the aged? And we cannot neglect the culture-specific nature of health. For example, Australian Aboriginal people traditionally define health in terms of social, spiritual, cultural attributes. "Health does not just mean the physical well-being of the individual but refers to the social, emotional, spiritual and cultural well-being of the whole community. This is a holistic view and includes a cyclical concept of life-death-life" (NHMRC, 1996, Part 2, p. 4). Thus, while drilling down to the individual makes sense in a Western context, there are caveats imposed both for individuals and for communities far separated from us by time and space.

In my own work, I have found the concepts introduced by the bioarchaeology of care to be extremely useful. I have not formally worked through the Index of Care, being limited to the Mac (rather than PC) moiety, but even so the contemplation of the individual and the community in these instances of severe disability adds considerably to my appreciation.

I will here briefly cite three examples.

1. Juvenile Rheumatoid Arthritis, M11-2023, Moquegua Valley, Perú, 900–1050 BP (Buikstra, Poznanski, Lozada, Goldstein, & Leuschner, 1990). This individual died during late childhood or early adolescence and was buried just as were others in this cemetery. The disease had left M11-2023 with deformed, flexed joints and limbs. As s/he had no evidence of cranial modification, unlike others in the cemetery, the condition must have been evident during infancy and throughout an all-too-brief life. Today, a multidisciplinary team would have provided support, in addition to care from kin. In the best of medical worlds, this team would include a rheumatologist, an occupational therapist (OT), a physical therapist, a nurse, and social workers. But who would have been there for this Andean child, born over a millennium ago? We might infer the presence of a socially stable, cohesive kin-group and community, with individuals knowledgeable about palliative care. This care may have included manually exercising limbs and mitigating pain through medicinal plants. The individual would have endured ongoing pain and dependence upon others over the years. S/he would have watched as others in his/her peer group assumed increased independence and responsibilities during childhood and adolescence.
2. Combined Skeletal Dysplasia: Leri-Weill Dyschondrosteosis and Achondroplasia, EZ 3-7-1, Lower Illinois River valley (LIV), ~1682 BP, Middle Woodland Period (Charles, Leigh, & Buikstra, 1988; Cormier & Buikstra, Submitted; Cormier, Buikstra, & Osterholtz, Submitted). This individual was an adult female who

died during childbirth. Our recent estimation of age-at-death of between 30 and 33 years, based upon cemental annuli counts (Naji and Colard, personal communication, December 4, 2015), raises the issue of the timing of her only pregnancy and whether it developed in the context of a loving or an abusive relationship. Other examples of females thought to have died in childbirth were approximately a decade younger than EZ 3-7-1.

3. Ancient Tuberculosis (TB) in Mississippian communities in the LIV, ~1000 BP (Buikstra, 1977b; Buikstra & Cook, 1978). While there are several individuals who died with evidence of skeletal TB, the most poignant example is a female who died in her early 20s, with a severely kyphotic and ankylosed spine. One can but imagine the social and economic cost to the community in this case of chronic disability, leading to death of a young adult who would normally be prepared to take on key productive and reproductive roles.

While disease diagnosis has been central to these investigations, considering the clinical experiences of those so afflicted today extends our appreciation of their prospective social roles and the support required, sometimes over extended periods.

The Bioarchaeology of Care: This Volume

In this section, I will first briefly review the chapters that focus upon individuals, evaluating their rigor in relationship to the four-stage sequence outlined by Tilley (2013, 2015) and presented here in Fig. 19.1. I will then turn to chapters more experimental or methodological in scope.

Chapter 3 (Schrenk and Martin) is an exquisite application of the Index of Care, extended here to a situation where there are two alternative differential diagnoses: paralytic polio and cerebral palsy. The authors undertake this challenge and execute all phases of the analysis with appropriate clinical and contextual detail.

In Chap. 4, Willett and Harrod discuss the short- and long-term medical sequelae of a pelvic ring fracture. Especially significant is their consideration of traditional Pueblo healing practices and the clinical literature relevant to this example. As with Chap. 3, these authors also explicitly follow the Index of Care protocol. In Chap. 5, Worne also considers a pelvic ring fracture, in this case from an Eastern Woodlands archaeological context wherein there also exists evidence of chronic disease and recovery from scalping. Worne carefully considers possible long-term effects of the fractures seen in this middle-aged to elderly female. Ehnohistoric and archaeological data concerning aged women and status enhance this contribution.

Roberts's (Chap. 6) appropriately conservative remarks about caregiving in the past preface her study of Skeleton C148 from the cemetery of St. James and St. Mary Magdalene in Chichester, England. Following an informative, extensive description, Roberts concludes that this man had suffered from lepromatous leprosy. Following this first step, Roberts moves on to the more inferential stages of the

Index of Care, explicitly noting what can and what cannot be stated about C148's experience. Her careful approach draws appropriately upon historical and archaeological as well as clinical sources.

In Chap. 7, Matczak and Kozlowski employ an osteobiographic approach in their study of two sets of female remains from early medieval Poland. One was affected by leprosy and other by gigantism/acromegaly. The authors usefully preface their analysis with a discussion of the definitions of disability and osteobiography, also touching on theories of funerary behavior and the degree to which disability can be inferred from archaeological contexts alone. Following extensive osteobiographies, the medieval women are assessed for care needed during life and care attributed after death, the authors basing their inferences upon a wide range of clinical, historical, and archaeological evidence. While this study does not explicitly follow the stages of the Index of Care, the rich osteobiographies are enlightening and convincing.

An eighteenth century coffin burial (apparently of Mr. Samuel Lord) from the crypts of St. Bride's church was subject to extensive radiographic analysis by Conlogue et al. in Chap. 8. A temporary radiographic facility established within the crypt led to diagnosis of a severe case of kyphoscoliosis. The estimated age at death at mid-to-late 30s would seem an appropriate lower limit, with an expanded upper limit perhaps prudent. The pathological description is enhanced by radiography, including angulation of lower limb bones. The extensive discussion of Mr. Lord's ability to take care of basic activities of daily living (BADL) provides an apt evaluation, given the extent of his physical deformity. The discussion is embedded in the history of Georgian London.

Jolly and Kurin (Chap. 9) consider an Andean male from the late prehistoric highland site of Achanchi, who died as a young adult with evidence of two episodes of cranial trauma followed by trepanation. In their review, the authors consider the history of trepanation in the Andes, along with clinical literature relevant to traumatic brain injury (TBI). Following an extensive osteobiography, the probable need for short- and long-term care after TBI and surgery are considered in relationship to caregivers and the broader community.

In Chap. 10, Nystrom and Piombino-Mascali turn to the possibilities offered by extending the bioarchaeology of care to mummified remains. Noting that few examples of mummy science have explicitly addressed the subject of health care, they focus upon those wherein therapeutic treatment has been considered. These include surgical intervention, therapeutic tattooing, and the use of medicinal plants. They argue that extending the bioarchaeology of care model to mummy science would strengthen both fields.

Oxenham and Willis (Chap. 11) explicitly argue for extending the bioarchaeology of care to children, including a discussion of specific issues relevant to childhood, such as maternal health, parental nurturing, and childcare. They illustrate this focus by applying the bioarchaeology of care model to childhood markers of stress in juveniles from the 4000-year-old Vietnamese site of Man Bac. In their use of nonspecific stress indicators, which they use as a basis for inferring poor health, they have not considered the implications of the osteological paradox (Wood, Milner, Harpending, & Weiss, 1992), which must be faced in studies of this type.

As "baby-boomers" encounter increasing frailty, the issue of elder care in the past will doubtless find a ready audience. Gowland (Chap. 12) places elder care within the context of past perceptions of old age and disability. Using a life course analysis, and primarily invoking contemporary theoretical treatments, Gowland considers identity (age/gender/disabled), embodiment, and old age in studies of both contemporary and earlier people. The difficulties of identifying examples of passive and active elder abuse and neglect require careful consideration. Focus should be on the dynamic relations between an individual's identity, biography, and the disease process rather than a static vision. Gowland's arguments and her outline of issues to be faced in the study of elder care in the past suggest that this should be a productive endeavor indeed.

In Chap. 13, Wesp reminds us that the "care" given in early colonial New World hospitals may have been both bodily *and* spiritual. The interrelationship between spiritual and bodily health in Christian belief-systems is considered, with special reference to institutionalized care. The implications of this conjoined treatment in the New World is explored in context of the *Hospital Real de Indios*, located in Mexico City and redirected to the treatment of the indigenous population in 1553. Wesp's example serves as an important reminder that we must consider other than biological concepts of health and treatment when we turn to the archaeological record.

Institutions of Care are also considered by Tremblay Critcher, who emphasizes that many institutions have copious records of health care delivery. However, these records are histories written by those in power – the health care providers. The receipt of such care is apparent to us in terms of patient health, evidence of abuse, nutrition, and healing. Thus, Tremblay Critcher recommends emphasis upon the *efficacy of care* in evaluating institutional settings. She presents an example from the Oneida State Custodial Asylum in upstate New York. She notes that Stage 1–3 of the Tilley method are similar as applied to individuals within institutions, but that the final Stage 4 is entirely different. Stage 4 should assess the efficacy of care in meeting institutional goals. Another related approach would aggregate the data and assess efficacy for the total sample. Institutions could be compared; sex-specific data could be generated. This method appears promising, although a number of inherent assumptions about the nature of available samples must be considered.

Milella (Chap. 15) explores the use of data on contemporary hunter-gatherers to model the relationship of caregiving to mobility, group size, and environmental productivity. He finds that mobility is inversely correlated with juvenile mortality, which suggests to me that leaving behind polluted environments frequently enhances childhood health. Similarly, Milella interprets the lack of significant correlation between population density and mortality in terms of kin support, but what about the pathogen load anticipated in a relatively crowded community? Obviously, a much more nuanced model will become more satisfying.

The web-based support that Wilson discusses in Chap. 16 (*Digised Diseases*) will be of most use in the first stage of Index of Care development. Further extension of the database focus on clinical implications would be a desirable step in aiding the bioarchaeology of care.

Chapter 17 is by ethicist and philosopher, David Doat. Doat evaluates, from his perspective, the previous skepticism about caregiving in the past and the degree to which the bioarchaeology of care has overcome the earlier arguments. After considering three objections to inferences of caregiving (moral economy of science, cognitive relativism, and moral universalism, moral relativism, moral pessimism), Doat concludes that the bioarchaeology of care has convincingly overcome the objections previously raised by Dettwyler and others.

Ethical issues are also raised by David Mennear in Chap. 18, which focuses primarily upon the manner in which social media, such as blogs, effectively communicate bioarchaeological information. Obviously, based upon Mennear's own blog (https://thesebonesofmine.wordpress.com/), the potential for reaching the public is huge, and those promoting the bioarchaeology of care or other research topics would therefore be well advised to consider using social media for this purpose. It is our professional responsibility to communicate our research beyond the bounds of academic audiences.

In sum, this volume significantly advances the bioarchaeology of care methodology in a number of ways. Firstly, the case studies represent diverse contexts wherein the methodology works effectively in all examples. Secondly, and perhaps more tantalizing, are the possible extensions of the model to institutional settings. Finally, the assurance from the perspective of an ethicist-philosopher that our mission is on course is reassuring, as we look forward to many more applications, extensions, and enhancements of the bioarchaeology of care.

References

Agarwal, S. C., & Glencross, B. A. (Eds.). (2011). *Social bioarchaeology*. London: Wiley.

Buikstra, J. E. (1977a). Biocultural dimensions of archaeological study: A regional perspective. In R. L. Blakely (Ed.), *Biocultural adaptation in prehistoric America* (pp. 67–84). Georgia: University of Georgia Press.

Buikstra, J. E. (1977b). Differential diagnosis: An epidemiological model. *Yearbook of Physical Anthropology, 1976*, 316–328.

Buikstra, J. E. (2006). A historical introduction. In J. E. Buikstra & L. A. Beck (Eds.), *Bioarchaeology: The contextual analysis of human remains* (pp. 7–25). Amsterdam: Academic.

Buikstra, J. E., & Cook, D. C. (1978). Pre-Columbian tuberculosis: An epidemiological approach. *MCV Quarterly, 14*(1), 32–33.

Buikstra, J. E., Poznanski, A., Lozada, M. C., Goldstein, P., & Leuschner, L. (1990). A case of Juvenile rheumatoid arthritis from Pre-Columbian Peru. In J. E. Buikstra (Ed.), *A life in science: Papers in Honor of J. Lawrence Angel* (pp. 99–137). Kampsville, IL: Center for American Archeology. Scientific Papers 6.

Charles, D. K., Leigh, S. R., & Buikstra, J. E. (1988). *The Archaic and Woodland Cemeteries at the Elizabeth Site in the Lower Illinois Valley*. Published for the Illinois Dept. of Transportation by the Center for American Archeology, Kampsville Archeological Center.

Cormier, A., & Buikstra, J. E. (submitted). Impairment, disability, and identity in the Middle Woodland Period: Life at the juncture of achondroplasia, pregnancy, and infection. In J. Byrnes & J. Muller (Eds.), *Embodying impairment: Towards a bioarchaeology of disability*. New York: Springer.

Cormier, A., Buikstra, J. E., & Osterholtz, A. (submitted). Combined genetic skeletal dysplasia of a Middle Woodland Individual: A case study. *International Journal of Paleopathology.*

Dettwyler, K. A. (1991). Can paleopathology provide evidence for 'compassion'? *American Journal of Physical Anthropology, 84*, 375–384.

Fowler, C. (2004). *The archaeology of personhood: An anthropological approach.* London: Routledge.

Gell, A. (1998). *Art and agency: An anthropological theory*. Oxford: Clarendon.

Gorman, J. (2012). Ancient bones that tell a story of compassion. *New York Times* 17 December 2012. Retrieved from http://www.nytimes.com/2012/12/18/science/ancient-bones-that-tell-a--story-of-compassion.html?_r=1.

Grupe, G., & McGlynn, G. C. (Eds.). (2015). *Isotopic landscapes in bioarchaeology*. Berlin: Springer.

Johannsen, N. N. (2012) Archaeology and the inanimate agency proposition: A critique and a suggestion. In *Excavating the mind: Cross-sections through culture, cognition and materiality.* Denmark: Aarhus Universitetsforlag.

Knudson, K. J., & Stojanowski, C. M. (2009). *Bioarchaeology and identity in the Americas.* Gainesville: University Press of Florida.

Larsen, C. S. (1982). *The anthropology of St. Catherine's island 3: Prehistoric human biological adaptation.* New York: American Museum of Natural History.

Larsen, C. S. (1987). Bioarchaeological interpretations of subsistence economy and behavior from human skeletal remains. *Advances in Archaeological Method and Theory, 10*, 339–445.

Larsen, C. S. (1995). Biological changes in human populations with agriculture. *Annual Review of Anthropology, 31*, 185–213.

Lewis, M. E. (2009). *The bioarchaeology of children: Perspectives from biological and forensic anthropology.* Cambridge, UK: Cambridge Studies in Biological and Evolutionary Anthropology.

Martin, D. L., Harrod, R. P., & Pérez, V. R. (Eds.). (2012). *The bioarchaeology of violence.* Gainesville: University Press of Florida.

Naji, S., & Colard, T. (2015). Dr Stephan Naji, Department of Anthropology, New York University, USA, and Dr. Thomas Colard, Institut de Médecine Légale, Université du Droit et de la Santé Lille 2, France, personal communication.

NHMRC. (1996). *Promoting the health of indigenous Australians: A review of the infrastructure support for Aboriginal and Torres Strait Islander health advancement.* National Health and Medical Research Council, https://www.nhmrc.gov.au/_files_nhmrc/publications/attachments/hp6.pdf.

Perry, M. A. (Ed.). (2012). *Bioarchaeology and behavior: The people of the ancient near East.* Gainesville: University Press of Florida.

Robb, J. (2002). Time and biography: Osteobiography of the Italian Neolithic. In Y. Hamilakis, M. Pluciennik, & S. Tarlow (Eds.), *Thinking through the body: Archaeologies of corporeality* (pp. 153–171). London: Kluwer Academic/Plenum Publishers.

Robb, J. (2010). Beyond agency. *World Archaeology, 42*, 493–520.

Saul, F. P. (1972). *The human remains of Altar de Sacrificios: An osteobiographic analysis.* Cambridge: Peabody Museum.

Saul, F. P., & Saul, J. M. (1989). Osteobiography: A Maya example. In M. Y. İşcan & K. A. R. Kennedy (Eds.), *Reconstruction of life from the skeleton* (pp. 287–302). New York: Alan R. Liss Inc.

Steckel, R. H., Larsen, C. S., Sciulli, P. W., & Walker, P. L. (2009). The history of European Health Project: A history of health in Europe from the Late Neolithic Era to the Present. In V. Smrcka & P. L. Walker (Eds.), *Proceedings of the symposium: Social history and anthropology. Monograph 156.* Prague: Karolinum Press.

Steckel, R. H., & Rose, J. C. (Eds.). (2002). *The backbone of history: Health and nutrition in the Western Hemisphere.* Cambridge: University Press.

Stodder, A. L. W., & Palkovich, A. M. (Eds.). (2012). *The bioarchaeology of individuals.* Florida: University Press of Florida.

Stojanowski, C. M. (2013). *Mission cemeteries, mission peoples: Historical and evolutionary dimensions of intracemetery bioarchaeology in Spanish Florida*. Gainesville: University Press of Florida.

Stojanowski, C. M., & Duncan, W. N. (Eds.). (2016). *Studies in forensic biohistory: Anthropological perspectives*. Cambridge: Cambridge University Press.

Tilley, L. (2013). *Towards a bioarchaeology of care: A contextualised approach for identifying and interpreting health-related care provision in prehistory*. unpublished Ph.D. Thesis. Australian National University.

Tilley, L. (2015). *Theory and practice in the bioarchaeology of care*. New York: Springer.

Tilley, L., & Cameron, T. (2014). Introducing the index of care: A web-based application supporting archaeological research into health-related care. *International Journal of Paleopathology, 6*, 5–9.

Tilley, L., & Oxenham, M. F. (2011). Survival against the odds: Modeling the social implications of care provision to seriously disabled individuals. *International Journal of Paleopathology, 1*, 35–42.

Tung, T. A. (2012). *Violence, ritual, and the Wari empire: A social bioarchaeology of imperialism in the ancient Andes*. Gainesville: University Press of Florida.

Wood, J. W., Milner, G. R., Harpending, H. C., & Weiss, K. M. (1992). The osteological paradox: Problems of inferring prehistoric health from skeletal samples. *Current Anthropology, 33*, 343–370.

World Health Organization (WHO). (1946). Preamble to the Constitution of the World Health Organization as adopted by the International Health Conference, New York, 19–22 June, 1946.

Index

© Springer International Publishing Switzerland 2017

L. Tilley, A.A. Schrenk (eds.), *New Developments in the Bioarchaeology of Care*, Bioarchaeology and Social Theory, DOI 10.1007/978-3-319-39901-0

MIX
Papier aus verantwortungsvollen Quellen
Paper from responsible sources
FSC® C105338
FSC
www.fsc.org

If you have any concerns about our products,
you can contact us on
ProductSafety@springernature.com

In case Publisher is established outside the EU,
the EU authorized representative is:
Springer Nature Customer Service Center GmbH
Europaplatz 3, 69115 Heidelberg, Germany

Printed by Libri Plureos GmbH
in Hamburg, Germany